Oxygen Therap

Editors

WALDEMAR A. CARLO
MAXIMO VENTO

CLINICS IN PERINATOLOGY

www.perinatology.theclinics.com

Consulting Editor
LUCKY JAIN

September 2019 • Volume 46 • Number 3

ELSEVIER

1600 John F. Kennedy Boulevard • Suite 1800 • Philadelphia, Pennsylvania, 19103-2899

http://www.theclinics.com

CLINICS IN PERINATOLOGY Volume 46, Number 3
September 2019 ISSN 0095-5108, ISBN-13: 978-0-323-70876-0

Editor: Kerry Holland
Developmental Editor: Casey Potter

Clinics in Perinatology (ISSN 0095-5108) is published quarterly by Elsevier Inc., 360 Park Avenue South, New York, NY 10010-1710. Months of issue are March, June, September, and December. Business and Editorial Offices: 1600 John F. Kennedy Blvd., Ste. 1800, Philadelphia, PA 19103-2899. Customer Service Office: 3251 Riverport Lane, Maryland Heights, MO 63043. Periodicals postage paid at New York, NY and additional mailing offices. Subscription prices are $309.00 per year (US individuals), $578.00 per year (US institutions), $365.00 per year (Canadian individuals), $708.00 per year (Canadian institutions), $435.00 per year (international individuals), $708.00 per year (international institutions), $100.00 per year (US students), and $195.00 per year (Canadian and international students). International air speed delivery is included in all Clinics subscription prices. All prices are subject to change without notice. **POSTMASTER:** Send address changes to Clinics in Perinatology, Elsevier Health Sciences Division, Subscription Customer Service, 3251 Riverport Lane, Maryland Heights, MO 63043. **Customer Service: Telephone: 1-800-654-2452** (U.S. and Canada); **1-314-447-8871** (outside U.S. and Canada). **Fax: 1-314-447-8029. E-mail: journalscustomerservice-usa@elsevier.com** (for print support); **journalsonlinesupport-usa@elsevier.com** (for online support).

Reprints. For copies of 100 or more, of articles in this publication, please contact the Commercial Reprints Department, Elsevier Inc., 360 Park Avenue South, New York, NY 10010-1710. Tel. 212-633-3874; Fax: 212-633-3820; E-mail: reprints@elsevier.com.

Clinics in Perinatology is also pubilshed in Spanish by McGraw-Hill Interamericana Editores S.A., P.O. Box 5-237, 06500 Mexico D.F., Mexico.

Clinics in Perinatology is covered in MEDLINE/PubMed (Index Medicus) Current Contents, Excepta Medica, BIOSIS and ISI/BIOMED.

Contributors

CONSULTING EDITOR

LUCKY JAIN, MD, MBA
George W. Brumley Jr Professor and Chair, Emory University School of Medicine, Department of Pediatrics, Chief Academic Officer, Children's Healthcare of Atlanta, Executive Director, Emory and Children's Pediatric Institute, Atlanta, Georgia, USA

EDITORS

WALDEMAR A. CARLO, MD
Edwin M. Dixon Professor of Pediatrics, The University of Alabama at Birmingham, Division of Neonatology Director, Newborn Nurseries, Birmingham, Alabama, USA

MAXIMO VENTO, MD, PhD
Professor, Pediatrics, University of Alicante, Chief, Division of Neonatology, University & Polytechnic Hospital La Fe, Director, Neonatal Research Unit, The Health Research Institute La Fe, Valencia, Spain

AUTHORS

STEVEN H. ABMAN, MD
Professor, Pediatrics, University of Colorado, Children's Hospital Colorado, Denver, Colorado, USA

NAMASIVAYAM AMBALAVANAN, MD
Professor, Division of Neonatology, Department of Pediatrics, The University of Alabama at Birmingham, Birmingham, Alabama, USA

LISA MAREE ASKIE, PhD, MPH, BN, FHEA
NHMRC Clinical Trials Centre, University of Sydney, Camperdown, New South Wales, Australia

EDUARDO BANCALARI, MD
Professor, Pediatrics and OB/GYN, Director, Division of Neonatology, Department of Pediatrics, University of Miami Miller School of Medicine, Miami, Florida, USA

WHITTNEY BARKHUFF, MD
Assistant Professor, Department of Pediatrics, Neonatal-Perinatal Medicine, Larner College of Medicine, University of Vermont, Burlington, Vermont, USA

WALDEMAR A. CARLO, MD
Edwin M. Dixon Professor of Pediatrics, The University of Alabama at Birmingham, Division of Neonatology Director, Newborn Nurseries, Birmingham, Alabama, USA

NELSON CLAURE, MSc, PhD
Associate Professor, Pediatrics and Biomedical Engineering, Director, Neonatal Pulmonary Physiology Laboratory, Division of Neonatology, Department of Pediatrics, University of Miami Miller School of Medicine, Miami, Florida, USA

PETER G. DAVIS, MBBS, MD
Consultant Neonatologist, Neonatal Services, Director, Newborn Research Centre, The Royal Women's Hospital, Parkville, Victoria; Professor, Department of Obstetrics and Gynaecology, The University of Melbourne, Murdoch Children's Research Institute, Melbourne, Australia

JULIANN M. DI FIORE, BS
Research Engineer III, Division of Neonatology, Case Western Reserve University, Rainbow Babies & Children's Hospital, Cleveland, Ohio, USA

OSAYAME EKHAGUERE, MBBS, MPH
Department of Pediatrics, Section of Neonatal-Perinatal Medicine, Indiana University, Riley Hospital for Children at Indiana University Health, Indianapolis, Indiana, USA

SAMUEL J. GENTLE, MD
Assistant Professor, Department of Pediatrics, The University of Alabama at Birmingham, Birmingham, Alabama, USA

ROSEMARY D. HIGGINS, MD
Professor, Department of Global and Community Health, Associate Dean for Research, College of Health and Human Services, George Mason University, Fairfax, Virginia, USA

KATE A. HODGSON, MBBS (Hons), BMedSci
Neonatal Clinical/Research Fellow, Neonatal Services, Newborn Research Centre, The Royal Women's Hospital, Parkville, Victoria, Australia; PhD Candidate, Department of Obstetrics and Gynaecology, The University of Melbourne, Melbourne, Australia

ADRIENNE KIRBY, MSc
Senior Biostatistician, NHMRC Clinical Trials Centre, University of Sydney, Sydney, New South Wales, Australia

HARESH KIRPALANI, BM, MSc
Department of Pediatrics, Division of Neonatology, The Children's Hospital of Philadelphia, Philadelphia, Pennsylvania, USA

PETER M. MacFARLANE, PhD
Assistant Professor, Pediatrics, Case Western Reserve University, Rainbow Babies & Children's Hospital, Cleveland, Ohio, USA

BRETT J. MANLEY, MBBS (Hons), BMedSci, PhD
Consultant Neonatologist, Neonatal Services, Newborn Research Centre, The Royal Women's Hospital, Parkville, Victoria, Australia; Senior Lecturer, Department of Obstetrics and Gynaecology, The University of Melbourne, NHMRC Early Career Fellow, Honorary Fellow, Murdoch Children's Research Institute, Melbourne, Australia

RICHARD J. MARTIN, MD
Professor, Pediatrics, Reproductive Biology, and Physiology and Biophysics, Case Western Reserve University, Rainbow Babies & Children's Hospital, Cleveland, Ohio, USA

SHAMA PATEL, MD
Department of Pediatrics, Section of Neonatal-Perinatal Medicine, Indiana University, Riley Hospital for Children at Indiana University Health, Indianapolis, Indiana, USA

CHRISTIAN F. POETS, MD
Professor, Department of Neonatology, University Hospital, Tübingen, Germany

OLA DIDRIK SAUGSTAD, MD, PhD
Department of Pediatric Research, Oslo University Hospital, University of Oslo, Oslo, Norway; Department of Pediatrics, Robert H. Lurie Medical Research Center, Chicago, Illinois, USA; Northwestern University, Evanston, Illinois, USA

VIVEK SHUKLA, MD
Division of Neonatology, The University of Alabama at Birmingham, Birmingham, Alabama, USA

ROGER F. SOLL, MD
Wallace Professor of Pediatrics, Department of Pediatrics, Neonatal-Perinatal Medicine, Larner College of Medicine, University of Vermont, Burlington, Vermont, USA

BENJAMIN J. STENSON, MD
Professor, Neonatology, Neonatal Unit, Royal Infirmary of Edinburgh, Edinburgh, United Kingdom

WILLIAM TARNOW-MORDI, BA, MB BChir, MRCP (UK), DCH
Professor, Neonatal Medicine, Director of Neonatal and Perinatal Trials, NHMRC Clinical Trials Centre, University of Sydney, Sydney, New South Wales, Australia

TRENT E. TIPPLE, MD
Division of Neonatology, Department of Pediatrics, The University of Alabama at Birmingham, Birmingham, Alabama, USA

COLM P. TRAVERS, MD
Division of Neonatology, The University of Alabama at Birmingham, Birmingham, Alabama, USA

MAXIMO VENTO, MD, PhD
Professor, Pediatrics, University of Alicante, Chief, Division of Neonatology, University & Polytechnic Hospital La Fe, Director, Neonatal Research Unit, The Health Research Institute La Fe, Valencia, Spain

Contents

Formerly, assessing oxygenation relied on recognizing cyanosis; however, this is unreliable. Also, in neonates, a pink color, suggesting absence of severe hypoxemia, is difficult to assess. An objective and continuous assessment of oxygenation is necessary. Currently, this is best achieved noninvasively by transcutaneous partial pressure of oxygen ($PTcO_2$) monitoring or pulse oximetry. Because both $PTcO_2$ and oxygen saturation monitors (pulse oximeters) may display erroneous measurements, thorough understanding of their operating principles is required. Also, clinicians must recognize the range of values expected in healthy neonates. In this article, data on these issues are reviewed.

Fetal development occurs in a relatively hypoxemic environment, and birth represents significant oxidative stress. Premature infants are disadvantaged by a lack of maternal antioxidant transfer and impaired endogenous antioxidant responses. O_2 metabolism is essential for life and its biochemical reactions are dynamic, compartmentalized, and difficult to characterize in vivo. There is a growing appreciation for the role of reactive oxygen species in nonpathologic processes, including regulation of cell signaling and mitochondrial function. There are several gaps in the knowledge about the role of reactive oxygen species in normal development and how oxidative stress alters normal signaling and subsequent development.

Oxygen therapy is an essential part of neonatal care. Targeting oxygen saturations and preventing hypoxemia and hyperoxemia is difficult, particularly in preterm infants. The mode of oxygen delivery directly affects the stability of oxygen saturations, hypoxemia, and hyperoxemia. This stability has important clinical implications. New methods of noninvasive oxygen administration, including closed-loop automated control and servo-controlled oxygen environments, have been developed to improve oxygen saturation targeting and decrease episodes of hyperoxemia and hypoxemia.

Transition into the extrauterine world is characterized by a substantial increase in oxygen availability to tissue. Exact oxygen provision may be needed to avoid negative consequences of hypoxia or hyperoxia. For term and near-term infants, it is recommended to start with air and titrate the oxygen supplement to the saturation nomogram. However, oxygen supplementation in infants less than 32 weeks' gestation is an unsolved conundrum. At present, the inspired fraction of oxygen is set according to gestational age and blended to achieve targeted saturations and heart rates. Studies are still needed to overcome uncertainties about oxygen supplementation during preterm stabilization.

Low- and middle-income countries and resource-limited regions are major contributors to perinatal and infant mortality. Oxygen is widely used for resuscitation in high- and middle-income settings. However, oxygen supplementation is not available in resource-limited regions. Oxygen supplementation for resuscitation at birth has adverse effects in human/animal model studies. There has been a change with resultant recommendations for restrictive oxygen use in neonatal resuscitation. Neonatal resuscitation without supplemental oxygen decreases mortality and morbidities. Oxygen in resource-limited settings for neonatal resuscitation is ideal as a backup for selected resuscitations but should not be a limiting factor for implementing basic life-saving efforts.

Numerous advances in neonatal care have improved outcomes in preterm infants. Antenatal steroids, through their ability to promote lung maturation and function, have led to significant improvements in death, intraventricular hemorrhage, necrotizing enterocolitis, and respiratory distress syndrome. For years, exogenous surfactant administration has been used in conjunction with antenatal steroids to further improve outcomes for preterm infants. However, as continuous positive airway pressure has been shown to be effective in treating respiratory distress syndrome, it has become less clear how exogenous surfactant should be used. Novel approaches combining these therapies may lead to further improvement in clinical outcome.

Continuous positive airway pressure (CPAP), noninvasive intermittent positive pressure ventilation (NIPPV), and heated humidified high-flow nasal cannula (HHFNC) are modes of noninvasive respiratory support used in neonatal practice. These modes of noninvasive respiratory support may obviate mechanical ventilation, prevent extubation failure, and reduce the risk of developing bronchopulmonary dysplasia. Although the physiologic bases of CPAP and HHFNC are well delineated, and their modes and practical application consistent, those of NIPPV are unproven and varied. Available evidence suggests that NIPPV is superior to CPAP as a primary and postextubation respiratory support in preterm infants.

Kate A. Hodgson, Brett J. Manley, and Peter G. Davis

Nasal high-flow therapy (nHF) is increasingly used for neonates, with perceived benefits including reduced rates of nasal trauma and parent and nursing staff preference. Current evidence suggests that although nHF is a reasonable alternative for postextubation support of preterm infants, continuous positive airway pressure is a superior modality for primary support of respiratory distress syndrome. Minimal evidence exists for use of nHF in extremely preterm infants less than 28 weeks' gestation. Depending on clinician preference, units may still choose nHF in some settings, although careful choice of appropriate patients, and availability of rescue continuous positive airway pressure, is essential.

Juliann M. Di Fiore, Peter M. MacFarlane, and Richard J. Martin

Intermittent hypoxemia (IH) events are common during early postnatal life, particularly in preterm infants. These events have been associated with multiple morbidities, including retinopathy of prematurity, sleep disordered breathing, neurodevelopmental impairment, and mortality. The relationship between IH and poor outcomes may depend on the patterns (frequency, duration, and timing) of the IH events. Current treatment modalities used in the clinical setting have been only partially successful in reducing the incidence of apnea and accompanying IH, but the risks and benefits of more aggressive interventions should include knowledge of the relationship between IH and morbidity.

Nelson Claure and Eduardo Bancalari

Exposure to hyperoxemia from excessive oxygen supplementation and episodes of intermittent hypoxemia have been associated with damage to the eye, lung, and central nervous system in premature infants. The inherent respiratory instability of the premature infant combined with limited staffing or equipment resources often affect SpO_2 targeting and increase exposure to extreme SpO_2 levels. Multiple systems for closed loop control of inspired oxygen have been developed to improve SpO_2 targeting. This article reviews the evidence provided by clinical studies evaluating the efficacy of these systems in extreme premature infants.

Lisa Maree Askie

Participant data from approximately 5000 infants have been meta-analyzed to guide oxygen saturation policy for extremely preterm infants.

The Neonatal Oxygenation Prospective Meta-analysis showed that targeting a higher oxygen saturation range compared with a lower range resulted in decreased death and necrotizing enterocolitis and no difference in major disability but increased treated retinopathy of prematurity (ROP) and supplemental oxygen use at 36 weeks' postmenstrual age. The 91% to 95% range can be recommended for all extremely preterm infants from birth but should be accompanied by stringent surveillance for the prevention and early treatment of ROP.

Retinopathy of prematurity (ROP) is a serious disease affecting premature infants. Rates of ROP increase with decreasing gestational age. Duration of oxygen exposure is correlated with ROP. Many studies evaluating oxygen have been performed to assess impact on ROP. This article describes recent findings for oxygen saturation target studies and suggests area of future study for ROP.

Infants in the Neonatal Oxygenation Prospective Meta-analysis trials were randomized to SpO_2 targets of 85% to 89% or 91% to 95%. Group allocation was masked. Different outcomes are likely partially attributable to differences in achieved SpO_2. Infants randomized to the lower range had higher than intended readings. SpO_2 distributions of infants in the low-range group of the Benefits of Oxygen Saturation Targeting II UK trial who died or developed necrotizing enterocolitis were centered around 90% to 92%. These achieved SpO_2 distributions caution against using lower SpO_2 target ranges early or throughout the clinical course in extremely preterm infants.

The goal of oxygen therapy and oxygen saturation targeting in extremely preterm infants is to improve outcomes and balance the risks associated with both hypoxemia and hyperoxemia. Although the NeOProM trials addressed whether low or high oxygen saturation targets affect the most important outcomes of extreme prematurity including death and other co-morbidities, the trials did not evaluate infants for pulmonary hypertension. There is limited evidence for the optimal oxygen saturation targets in extremely preterm infants that can be used to prevent the development of pulmonary hypertension and manage pulmonary hypertension once developed.

This narrative review identified 23 publications in 2011 to 2019 discussing randomized trials of oxygen saturation targets of 85% to 89% versus 91%

to 95% in infants below 28 weeks' gestation. Of 18 commentaries or consensus statements, 17 recommended saturation targets above 89%. Five systematic reviews reported that the 85% to 89% target increased mortality but not the composite of death or disability. The evidence for increased mortality was assessed as of "high", "moderate," or "low," quality, reflecting substantial differences in interpreting the GRADE guidelines. Systematic reviews and guidelines without biostatisticians or epidemiologists as co-authors should be considered potentially problematic.

PROGRAM OBJECTIVE

The goal of *Clinics in Perinatology* is to keep practicing perinatologists, neonatologists, obstetricians, practicing physicians and residents up to date with current clinical practice in perinatology by providing timely articles reviewing the state of the art in patient care.

TARGET AUDIENCE

Perinatologists, neonatologists, obstetricians, practicing physicians, residents and healthcare professionals who provide patient care utilizing findings from *Clinics in Perinatology*.

LEARNING OBJECTIVES

Upon completion of this activity, participants will be able to:

1. Review the evidence for use of oxygen therapy in established pulmonary hypertension.
2. Discuss findings for oxygen saturation target studies and potential future area of study for Retinopathy of Prematurity.
3. Recognize new methods of oxygen administration being developed and implemented to improve oxygen saturation targeting in infants.

ACCREDITATION

The Elsevier Office of Continuing Medical Education (EOCME) is accredited by the Accreditation Council for Continuing Medical Education (ACCME) to provide continuing medical education for physicians.

The EOCME designates this journal-based CME activity for a maximum of 15 *AMA PRA Category 1 Credit*(s)™. Physicians should claim only the credit commensurate with the extent of their participation in the activity.

All other health care professionals requesting continuing education credit for this enduring material will be issued a certificate of participation.

DISCLOSURE OF CONFLICTS OF INTEREST

The EOCME assesses conflict of interest with its instructors, faculty, planners, and other individuals who are in a position to control the content of CME activities. All relevant conflicts of interest that are identified are thoroughly vetted by EOCME for fair balance, scientific objectivity, and patient care recommendations. EOCME is committed to providing its learners with CME activities that promote improvements or quality in healthcare and not a specific proprietary business or a commercial interest.

The planning committee, staff, authors and editors listed below have identified no financial relationships or relationships to products or devices they or their spouse/life partner have with commercial interest related to the content of this CME activity:

Steven H. Abman, MD; Namasivayam Ambalavanan, MD; Namasivayam Ambalavanan, MD; Lisa Maree Askie, PhD, MPH; Whittney Barkhuff, MD; Waldemar A. Carlo, MD; Peter G. Davis, MBBS, MD; Juliann M. Di Fiore, BSEE; Osayame Ekhaguere, MBBS, MPH; Samuel J. Gentle, MD; Rosemary D. Higgins, MD; Kate A. Hodgson, MBBS (Hons), B.Med.Sci; Kerry Holland; Lucky Jain; Alison Kemp; Adrienne Kirby, MSc; Haresh Kirpalani, BM, MSc; Peter M. MacFarlane, PhD; Brett J. Manley, MBBS (Hons), B.Med. Sci., PhD; Swaminathan Nagarajan; Richard J. Martin, MD; Shama Patel, MD; Ola Didrik Saugstad, MD, PhD; Vivek Shukla, MD; Roger F. Soll, MD; Benjamin J. Stenson, MD; William Tarnow-Mordi, BA, MB B Chir, MRCP (UK), DCH; Trent E. Tipple, MD; Colm P. Travers, MD; Maximo Vento, MD, PhD.

The planning committee, staff, authors and editors listed below have identified financial relationships or relationships to products or devices they or their spouse/life partner have with commercial interest related to the content of this CME activity:

Eduardo Bancalari, MD: receives research support and royalties and/or holds patents with Vyaire Medical, Inc.

Nelson Claure, MSc, PhD: receives research support and royalties and/or holds patents with Vyaire Medical, Inc.

Christian F. Poets, MD: participates in a speakers bureau for Masimo.

UNAPPROVED/OFF-LABEL USE DISCLOSURE

The EOCME requires CME faculty to disclose to the participants:

1. When products or procedures being discussed are off-label, unlabelled, experimental, and/or investigational (not US Food and Drug Administration [FDA] approved); and

2. Any limitations on the information presented, such as data that are preliminary or that represent ongoing research, interim analyses, and/or unsupported opinions. Faculty may discuss information about pharmaceutical agents that is outside of FDA-approved labelling. This information is intended solely for CME and is not intended to promote off-label use of these medications. If you have any questions, contact the medical affairs department of the manufacturer for the most recent prescribing information.

TO ENROLL
To enroll in the *Clinics in Perinatology* Continuing Medical Education program, call customer service at 1-800-654-2452 or sign up online at http://www.theclinics.com/home/cme. The CME program is available to subscribers for an additional annual fee of 244.40 USD.

METHOD OF PARTICIPATION
In order to claim credit, participants must complete the following:
1. Complete enrolment as indicated above.
2. Read the activity.
3. Complete the CME Test and Evaluation. Participants must achieve a score of 70% on the test. All CME Tests and Evaluations must be completed online.

CME INQUIRIES/SPECIAL NEEDS
For all CME inquiries or special needs, please contact elsevierCME@elsevier.com.

CLINICS IN PERINATOLOGY

Foreword

Oxygen and Its Checkered History in Neonatal Care

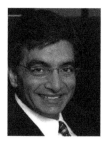

Lucky Jain, MD, MBA
Consulting Editor

If he were alive today, Dr Bill Silverman would have been anguished by how long it has taken us to bring clarity around the use of oxygen in newborns. After all, it is one of the most widely prescribed treatments in our discipline, and one that carries serious risks of harm with both overuse and underuse. Decades earlier, while referring to one of the earliest randomized clinical trials exploring the role of oxygen in causing retinopathy of prematurity,[1] Dr Silverman (**Fig. 1**) had cautioned us that "in making war with nature, there is a risk of loss in winning" (John McPhee, *The Control of Nature*).[2] The National Institutes of Health–sponsored landmark 1953 to 1954 oxygen trial provided a convincing answer to the vexing question of what was causing premature babies to go blind worldwide.[1] Prior to that, supplementation of oxygen to premature infants had become standard of care without having gone through any clinical testing. In an editorial published in 1982, Dr Silverman relented that "the euphoria after the demonstration in autumn 1954 of a firm link between prolonged exposure to high oxygen and an increased risk of retrolental fibroplasia (RLF) lasted nearly a quarter of a century,…-even though assertions concerning oxygen restriction went well beyond the narrow limits of evidence which had undergone rigorous testing."[3] The premise, of course, was that blindness due to RLF was entirely preventable if premature babies were not exposed to high concentrations of oxygen. What followed was a dictum that babies should never be exposed to oxygen concentrations greater than 40%. While a dramatic reduction in retinopathy of prematurity resulted from the curb on oxygen use, it was also secondary to the fact that the sickest babies were simply not surviving long enough to have an eye exam! Dr. Silverman concluded that, "the present uncertainties may come as a shock to those who were taught that the story of retinopathy of prematurity blindness is closed. The latest turn of events is not quite unique… nor is the current state of disbelief in the oxygen dogma particularly worrying."[3]

Clin Perinatol 46 (2019) xv–xvi
https://doi.org/10.1016/j.clp.2019.06.002
0095-5108/19/© 2019 Published by Elsevier Inc.

perinatology.theclinics.com

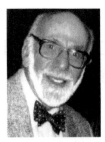

Fig. 1. William A. (Bill) Silverman MD, pictured here as winner of the 2001 William G. Bartholome Award for Ethical Excellence by the American Academy of Pediatrics. (*AAP News* October 2001, p. 166.)

Decades later, it appears that we are witnessing a remake of this 3-act play. The big difference this time is that awareness of these issues is at a very different level, as is our ability to act and adjust. Multiple networks gather and report data on a regular basis. This transparency has led to rapid changes in practice that don't have to wait a quarter of a century for data to be translated to clinically meaningful information.

A recent study[4] of 4965 infants enrolled in 5 trials (NeOProm: Neonatal Oxygen Prospective Meta-analysis) concluded that in extremely premature infants, targeting lower (85%–89%) compared with higher (91%–95%) oxygen saturations had no significant effect on the composite outcome of death or major disability or on disability alone (including blindness), but increased the average risk of death by 28 per 1000 babies treated. The authors concluded that "the tradeoffs between the benefits and harms of the different oxygen saturation target ranges may need to be assessed within local settings."[4]

These and many other important topics have been covered in this remarkable issue of the *Clinics in Perinatology* edited by Drs Carlo and Vento. As always, I am grateful to the publishing staff at Elsevier, including Kerry Holland, Lauren Boyle, and Casey Potter, for their support in covering this important topic for you.

Lucky Jain, MD, MBA
Emory University School of Medicine, and Children's Healthcare of Atlanta
1760 Haygood Drive NE
Atlanta, GA 30322, USA

E-mail address:
ljain@emory.edu

REFERENCES

1. Kinsey VE. Retrolental fibroplasia. Cooperative study of retrolental fibroplasia and the use of oxygen. AMA Arch Ophthalmol 1956;56:481–543.
2. Silverman WA. Memories of the 1953-54 oxygen trial and its aftermath. The failure of success. Control Clin Trials 1991;12:355–8.
3. Silverman WA. Retinopathy of prematurity: oxygen dogma challenged. Arch Dis Child 1982;57:731–3.
4. Askie LM, Darlow BA, Davis PG, et al. Effects of targeting lower versus higher arterial oxygen saturations on death or disability in preterm infants. Cochrane Database Syst Rev 2017;(4):CD011190. https://doi.org/10.1002/14651858.CD011190.pub2.

Preface

Oxygen Therapy for Preterm Infants

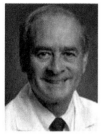 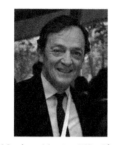

Waldemar A. Carlo, MD   Maximo Vento, MD, PhD
Editors

Randomized controlled trials and meta-analyses of higher (91%–95%) oxygen saturation targets in extremely preterm infants and room air resuscitation show improved outcomes, including increased survival. The fetal-to-neonatal transition occurs during a period of marked susceptibility to oxidative stressors due to deficits in antioxidant defenses, particularly in preterm infants. Each article in this issue is a review of the evidence that supports state-of-the-art oxygen and respiratory care practices in neonates.

Transcutaneous partial pressure of oxygen (PTco$_2$) monitoring and pulse oximetry are widely available for continuous oxygen monitoring to guide oxygen therapy in neonates. Both host advantages and shortcomings. PTco$_2$ monitoring relies heavily on skin perfusion and requires regular calibrations but is not influenced by motion. Pulse oximeters are easier to use, but abnormal hemoglobin, optical shunting, and motion may result in erroneous readings. In very unstable infants, both techniques should be used simultaneously with divergent measurements verified with direct blood-gas measurements.

Approximately 10% of all newly born infants fail to adequately adapt to extrauterine immediately after birth. Meta-analyses of randomized or quasirandomized controlled trials of air versus oxygen resuscitation in newborn infants demonstrated a 30% reduction in mortality with air resuscitation. The data on preterm infants are mixed but support targeting oxygen saturations. Resuscitation for term neonates should be started with room air. Resuscitation efforts in low-resource settings without access to supplemental oxygen should not be curtailed or limited.

Oxygen saturation targeting is important but difficult in preterm infants. Preterm infants' apnea and respiratory instability manifest with spontaneous episodes of intermittent hypoxemia. The severity and duration of these episodes can be influenced by the caregiver's response. Hyperoxemia in preterm infants receiving supplemental

Clin Perinatol 46 (2019) xvii–xviii
https://doi.org/10.1016/j.clp.2019.06.001
0095-5108/19/© 2019 Published by Elsevier Inc.

oxygen is caused by administration of excessive inspired oxygen concentrations. Maintenance of the prescribed range of Spo_2 is limited by the preterm infant's respiratory instability and staff availability. Tolerance of excessive Spo_2 is common. New methods of noninvasive oxygen administration such as closed loop Fio_2 control improve Spo_2 targeting while reducing exposure to hyperoxemia and hypoxemia.

Meta-analyses of the oxygen saturation targeting trials in extremely preterm infants show benefits of oxygen saturations targeted between 91% and 95% (vs 85% and 89%), including lower risk for mortality and necrotizing enterocolitis without long-term harms. Despite a higher rate of retinopathy of prematurity in the higher oxygen saturation group, there was no difference in the blindness rates between the groups. The trials were well designed, including allocation concealment with masking of the intervention and outcomes assessments. Furthermore, the results were homogeneous across trials (low heterogeneity based on very low I^2 statistics). Because higher oxygen saturation targets reduce mortality in extremely preterm infants, all but one of the multiple guidelines since 2011 recommend targeting oxygen saturation ranges of 91%–95% or 90%–95%, or avoiding 85%–89%. International surveys show that recommended oxygen saturation target ranges are being increasingly followed.

Noninvasive intermittent positive pressure ventilation (NIPPV) and heated humidified high-flow nasal cannula (HHFNC) are less-invasive therapies to support preterm infants, especially after extubation respiratory support in preterm infants. Available evidence suggests NIPPV is superior to continuous positive airway pressure (CPAP) for primary and postextubation respiratory support in preterm infants. Evidence indicates that CPAP is superior to HHFNC for initial noninvasive support of preterm infants with respiratory distress syndrome, but HHFNC is noninferior to CPAP for postextubation support of preterm infants greater than 28 weeks' gestation. Limited data are available for HHFNC use in extremely preterm infants or for term infants.

Thus, improvements in care focused on oxygen saturation targeting in extremely preterm infants, room air resuscitation, and noninvasive respiratory support reduce mortality and morbidities in neonates. The evidence reviewed in this issue should be used to improve current practice.

Waldemar A. Carlo, MD
Division of Neonatology Director
Newborn Nurseries
The University of Alabama at Birmingham
700 6th Avenue South
176F Suite 9380R
Birmingham, AL 35233-7335, USA

Maximo Vento, MD, PhD
University of Alicante
Division of Neonatology
University & Polytechnic Hospital La Fe
Neonatal Research Unit
The Health Research Institute La Fe
Bulevar Sur s/n
Valencia, Spain

E-mail addresses:
wcarlo@peds.uab.edu (W.A. Carlo)
Maximo.Vento@uv.es (M. Vento)

Noninvasive Monitoring and Assessment of Oxygenation in Infants

Christian F. Poets, MD

KEYWORDS

• Continuous oxygen monitoring • Pulse oximetry • PTCO$_2$ monitoring

KEY POINTS

• There are 2 techniques available for continuous oxygen monitoring: transcutaneous partial pressure of oxygen (PTcO$_2$) monitoring and pulse oximetry.
• PTcO$_2$ monitoring has the advantage that it is not influenced by motion but relies heavily on skin perfusion; it also requires regular calibrations and resiting because sensors have to be heated to 43°C to 44°C.
• Pulse oximeters are easier to use, but the presence of abnormal hemoglobins, optical shunting, and motion may result in erroneous readings. Comparability between readings from different instruments may be hampered by different averaging times and measurement algorithms.
• Particularly in very unstable infants, both techniques should ideally be used simultaneously; with divergent measurements being verified by a blood gas.

INTRODUCTION

For many years, assessing oxygenation relied on visual inspection; that is, the presence or absence of cyanosis. It has been known for almost 100 years that cyanosis becomes visible if more than 5 g/dL of deoxygenated hemoglobin are present in the peripheral blood.[1] However, this implies that a severely anemic patient will never become cyanotic, regardless how low his or her oxygen level is. Thus, cyanosis is rather unreliable as a clinical sign. Moreover, at least in neonates, a pink color, suggesting absence of severe hypoxemia, seems to be difficult to assess clinically, even by experienced neonatologists. In a video assessment study, the mean pulse oximeter saturation (SpO$_2$) at which infants were perceived to be pink by all 27 observers was 69% (ie, close to the expected value), but values ranged from 10% to 100%. The median SpO$_2$ for individual infants ranged from 42% to 93%.[2] Thus, an objective and continuous assessment of oxygenation is needed. Currently, this is

Department of Neonatology, University Hospital, Calwerstr. 7, Tübingen 72076, Germany
E-mail address: Christian-f.poets@med.uni-tuebingen.de

Clin Perinatol 46 (2019) 417–433
https://doi.org/10.1016/j.clp.2019.05.010
0095-5108/19/© 2019 Elsevier Inc. All rights reserved.

perinatology.theclinics.com

best achieved noninvasively by measuring the partial pressure of oxygen transcutaneously (transcutaneous partial pressure of oxygen [PTcO$_2$] monitoring) or measuring oxygen saturation via pulse oximetry. (See discussion of recent evidence suggesting that the optimal level of oxygenation is rather narrow, in this issue.) Thus, just relying on the absence of cyanosis by clinical examination is by no means sufficient for current neonatal care.[3] Because both PTcO$_2$ and SpO$_2$ monitors may display erroneous measurements, a thorough understanding of their operating principles is required to identify and reduce these to a minimum. Clinicians also need to know what range of values they can expect using these devices in healthy neonates. In this article, data on these issues are reviewed.

TRANSCUTANEOUS OXYGEN MONITORING
Principles of Operation

PTcO$_2$ electrodes measure the partial pressure of oxygen through the skin. PTcO$_2$ electrodes have mostly been based on the Clark electrode used in blood gas analyzers. These electrodes consist of a platinum cathode and a silver reference anode encased in an electrolyte solution and separated from the skin by a membrane permeable to oxygen. The PTcO$_2$ electrode is heated, thereby melting the crystalline structure of the stratum corneum, which otherwise would be an effective barrier to oxygen diffusion, and arterializing the blood in the capillaries underneath the electrode (**Fig. 1**). Oxygen diffuses from the capillary bed through the membrane into the electrode, where it is reduced at the cathode, generating an electric current that is converted into partial pressure measurements and displayed by the monitor.[4] The agreement between arterial and skin surface Po$_2$ depends on a fragile

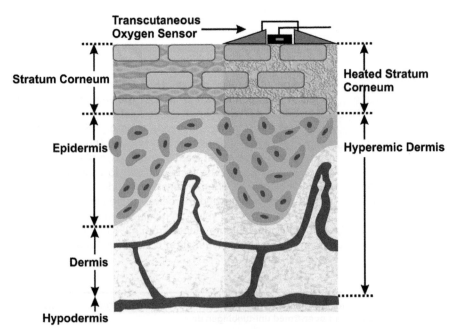

Fig. 1. A transcutaneous Po$_2$ sensor placed onto the skin. The latter is heated, thereby melting the crystalline structure of the stratum corneum, otherwise a barrier to oxygen diffusion, and arterializing the capillary bed underneath the sensor.

balance between factors that increase the P_{O_2}, namely a shift to the right of the oxygen dissociation curve and a decreased oxygen-solubility in blood, both of which are caused by the heating of the skin, as well as factors that decrease the P_{O_2}, namely the oxygen consumption in the heated skin and inside the electrode. Recently, a new optical technique for measuring PT_CO_2, called fluorescence quenching, has become commercially available that does not require calibration and was already reported to operate reliably at slightly lower electrode temperatures[5] (see later discussion).

Factors Influencing Measurements

Sensor temperature

PT_CO_2 measurements mainly depend on the temperature of the electrode. With Clark-type electrodes, arterial values are underestimated at less than 44°C, with this difference becoming larger with increasing Pa_{O_2}.[6] Therefore, to identify hyperoxemia, PT_CO_2 should not be measured at less than 44°C with these electrodes. However, at this temperature, the maximum resetting interval to prevent skin damage is only 2 to 4 hours,[7] which is unsatisfying given that there is a 10 to 15 minute interval after each resetting, during which transcutaneous values are unreliable. With the new fluorescence sensors, a recent study suggested good agreement with Pa_{O_2} already at lower temperatures, which would increase the resetting interval[5]; however, this issue requires further study.

Probe placement

The site where the PT_CO_2 sensor is placed must be chosen with care. PT_CO_2 will be falsely low if the sensor is placed over areas of thick or poorly perfused skin; for example, over a bony surface,[8] if pressure is applied to the sensor (eg, by the infant lying on it) or if too much contact gel is used. PT_CO_2 will be falsely high if there is poor contact between sensor and skin or if an insufficient amount of contact gel is used. In preterm neonates with right-to-left shunting via the ductus arteriosus, PT_CO_2 will be higher in the upper right half of the thorax and right arm than elsewhere.

Peripheral perfusion

PT_CO_2 monitors do not provide a measurement of arterial P_{O_2} but rather of the partial pressure of oxygen at the level of the arterialized cutaneous tissue. This dependence of the PT_CO_2 measurement on circulatory status has brought much unjustified discredit to the method. Yet this particular feature of PT_CO_2 monitoring, if interpreted correctly, may provide early warning of conditions such as a low cardiac output, arterial hypotension, or acidemia.[9] In neonates, the levels below which PT_CO_2 starts to significantly underread Pa_{O_2} have been defined as a systolic blood pressure of less than or equal to 33 mm Hg, a hematocrit of less than or equal to 28%, and an arterial pH of less than or equal to 7.02. Below these thresholds, PT_CO_2 may provide a reflection of cardiac output, for example, but not of Pa_{O_2}.[10]

Response times

PT_CO_2 monitors follow changes in blood oxygen levels only with some delay. This is caused by the time it takes for the oxygen to diffuse from the capillaries through the skin and from there through the membrane into the electrode. The in vitro response time (90% response to a sudden change in P_{O_2} from 19 to 0 kPa) is approximately 8 seconds.[11] The in vivo response time to spontaneous hypoxemic episodes, defined as the interval between oxygen saturation measured by pulse oximetry in the beat-to-beat mode and PT_CO_2 falling to <20 mmHg, was 16 seconds.[12]

Skin thickness

$PTcO_2$ measurements are influenced by the oxygen consumption of the skin. The latter increases with increasing skin thickness,[13] resulting in a larger difference between $PTcO_2$ and Pao_2 in older infants.[14] Studies in hemodynamically stable children and adults showed that the $PTcO_2$:Pao_2 ratio is rather constant (at around 0.8) beyond the neonatal period[14,15]; that is, Pao_2 is underestimated by about 20%.

Precision and Detection of Hypoxemia and Hyperoxemia

Under optimal measurement conditions (sensor temperature $\geq$44°C, hemodynamically stable preterm neonate, Pao_2 <13 kPa), $PTcO_2$ can be expected to be within plus or minus 1.3 to 2.0 kPa of Pao_2 95% of the time.[16] However, clinically it seems more important to know whether the $PTcO_2$ monitor will reliably detect all situations in which a patient has either too little or too much oxygen. Defining hypoxemia as a Pao_2 less than 6.7 kPa and hyperoxemia as a Pao_2 greater than 11 to 12 kPa, about 15% of both hypoxemic and hyperoxemic instances are missed by $PTcO_2$ monitors, whereas their specificity, particularly with regard to hypoxemia, is somewhat higher (**Table 1**).[16–22]

PULSE OXIMETRY
Principles of Operation

Pulse oximeters, unlike $PTcO_2$ monitors, do not measure the concentration of oxygen dissolved in plasma but the proportion of hemoglobin molecules in the arterial blood that are loaded with oxygen. Oxygenated and deoxygenated hemoglobin have different absorption spectra. Deoxygenated hemoglobin absorbs more light in the red band (600–750 nm); that is, it looks less red, whereas oxygenated hemoglobin absorbs more light in the infrared band (850–1000 nm). The oximeter probe emits light at 2 specific wavelengths (ie, 660 and 940 nm) which is transmitted through tissue (eg, a finger) and measured by a photodetector. The ratio of the light absorbances at the 2 wavelengths correlates with the proportion of oxygenated to deoxygenated hemoglobin in the tissue.

However, of all the light absorbed, only that absorbed by the pulsating parts of the tissue correlates to arterial oxygen saturation (SaO_2). Therefore, conventional pulse oximeters make use of the pulsating arterial vascular bed, which by expanding and relaxing creates changes in the light path length that modify the amount of light transmitted. The peaks and corresponding troughs of this amount are detected by measuring the transmitted light intensities several hundred times per second and then dividing them through each other, thereby obtaining a pulse-added absorbance that is independent of the absorbance characteristics of the nonpulsating parts of the tissue (**Fig. 2**). The ratio of these pulse-added light absorbances are then associated algorithmically with SaO_2 values (**Table 2**).

Current instruments use additional and/or different techniques. One such technology, for example, scans through all red-to-infrared ratios (and corresponding SpO_2 values) found in the tissue, determines the intensity of these, and chooses the rightmost peak of these intensities, which most likely corresponds to the absorbance by the arterial blood in the tissue (**Fig. 3**). It also uses frequency analysis, time domain analysis, and adaptive filtering to establish a noise reference in the detected physiologic signal, thereby improving the ability to separate between signal and noise.

Factors Influencing Measurements

Pulse oximeters are easier to use than $PTcO_2$ monitors because they do not require calibration or heating of the skin and provide immediate information about arterial

Table 1
Sensitivity and specificity of transcutaneous partial pressure of oxygen monitors in detecting hypoxemia and hyperoxemia

Reference	Electrode temperature	N patients	Age	Threshold kPa (mm Hg)	Sensitivity n	Sensitivity %	Specificity n	Specificity %
Rome et al,[60] 1984	44.0C	26	29–38 wk GA	<6.7 (50)	21/25	84	300/310	97
Martin et al,[16] 1982	44.0C	68	1–34 d	<6.7 (50)	4/4	100	64/64	100
Fanconi et al,[42] 1985	44.0C	40	1 d–19 y	<6.7 (50)	21/25	84	79/83	95
Wimberley et al,[19] 1985	44.0C	64	1–5 d	<6.7 (50)	15/22	68	397/401	99
Mok et al,[21] 1986	44.0C	19	1–61 wk	<6.7 (50)	10/12	83	15/15	100
Bossi et al,[61] 1987	44.0C	25	1–17 d	<6.7 (50)[a]	14/17	82	194/196	99
Geven et al,[18] 1987	43.5C	12	1–28 d	<6.7 (50)	40/45	89	—	—
Lafeber et al,[62] 1987	44.0C	8	5–120 d	<6.7 (50)	36/39	92	28/32	88
Southall et al,[22] 1987	44.0C	23	1–47 d	<6.7 (50)	9/11	82	43/49	88
Total or Mean	—	—	—	—	*170/200*	*85*	*1120/1150*	*97*
Duc et al,[17] 1979	44.0C	26	29–38 wk GA	>13.3 (100)	35/42	83	284/293	97
Martin et al,[16] 1982	44.0C	68	1–34 d	>10.7 (80)	33/36	92	25/32	78
Wimberley et al,[63] 1985	44.0C	64	1–5 d	>10.7 (80)	186/210	89	167/213	78
Bossi et al,[61] 1987	44.0C	25	1–17 d	>13.3 (100)[a]	23/27	85	169/186	91
Geven et al,[18] 1987	43.5C	12	1–28 d	>10.7 (80)	10/14	71	—	—
Total or Mean	—	—	—	—	*287/329*	*87*	*645/724*	*89*

Studies are sorted by year of publication. Data on hyperoxemia include only studies predominantly performed on preterm infants.
Abbreviation: GA, gestational age.
[a] Thresholds for P_{TCO_2} were 1.3 kPa (10 mm Hg) less than those for Pa_{O_2} (ie, <5.3 kPa [40 mm Hg]) and greater than 12 kPa (90 mm Hg).

Table 2
Accuracy of pulse oximeters in infants and children

Investigator, Year (Reference)	Instrument	Measurements	N patients	Range of SaO$_2$ (%)	SaO$_2$–SpO$_2$ (Bias) (%)	Precision (1 SD) (%)
Fanconi et al,[42] 1985	Nellcor N 100 (Nellcor, Medtronic, Minneapolis, MN)	108	36	58–100	–1.5	3.5
Southall rt al,[22] 1987	Nellcor N 100	92	43	70–100	–2.6	2.4
Hodgson et al,[43] 1987	Nellcor N 100	64	16	85–100	–0.8	1.8
Ramanathan et al,[44] 1987	Nellcor N 100	88	44	78–100	+0.3	2.1
	Nellcor N 100	48	24	79–100	–2.7	1.9
Jennis & Peabody,[64] 1987	Nellcor N 100	177	26	70–100	+1.7	2.2
Boxer et al,[65] 1987	Nellcor N 100	46	32	81–100	–0.6	2.3
	Nellcor N 100	62	32	40–80	–1.1	4.5
Fanconi,[66] 1988	Nellcor N 100	160	20	10–100	–4.5	7.9
Ridley,[67] 1988	Nellcor N 100	114	25	50–100	+0.7	3.1
	Ohmeda Biox 3700 (Ohmeda, GE Healthcare, Solingen, Germany)	114	25	45–100	+2.8	3.9
Barrington et al,[68] 1988	Nellcor N 100	423	—	50–100	+1.6	5.1
	Ohmeda Biox 3700	78	—	—	+3.9	5.3
	Criticare 501 (Criticare, North Kingstown, RI)	44	—	—	+4.9	2.9
Bucher et al,[57] 1989	Nellcor N 100	75	25	75–100	–2.2	2.7
	Ohmeda Biox 3700	75	25	75–100	+2.5	3.9
Russell & Helms,[69] 1990	Nellcor N 100	23	23	53–100	+0.8	3.2
	Ohmeda Biox III	24	24	53–100	+2.9	2.2
Lebecque 1991[45]	Nellcor N 100	97	47	50–100	–2.0	4.3
	Ohmeda Biox III	97	47	50–100	+0.4	4.5
Rajadurai et al,[46] 1992	Nellcor N 200	138	22	78–98	–1.3	2.3
Poets et al,[58] 1993	Kontron 7840 (Kontron, Watford, UK)	123	37	45–100	+0.6	5.2
	Nellcor N 200	123	37	45–100	+0.9	2.3
	Radiometer OXI3	123	37	45–100	+1.2	3.5

Study	Device				Bias	Precision
Thilo et al,[49] 1993	Nellcor N 100	120	30	55–100	−0.4	3.4
	Ohmeda 3700	120	30	55–100	+1.3	3.2
Schmitt et al,[50] 1993	Nellcor N 100	21	—	91–97	−0.5	2.5
	Nellcor N 100	44	—	80–90	−1.9	2.7
	Nellcor N 100	47	—	49–80	−5.8	4.8
Bell et al,[51] 1999	Ohmeda 3700band	59	18	94.3 ± 8.3	−0.5	2.2
	Ohmeda 3700clip	59	18	93.1 ± 8.8	+0.6	3.5
	Nellcor N 200band	54	18	94.5 ± 14.6	−0.2	5.1
	Nellcor N 200clip	58	18	95.8 ± 10.0	−2.0	2.5
	Novametrix 520Aband (Novametrix, Philips, Einhoven, NL)	63	18	93.3 ± 11.1	+0.2	2.7
	Novametrix 520Aclip	60	18	91.9 ± 11.4	+1.3	2.7
Bernet-Buettiker et al,[52] 2005	Radiometer Tosca/Masimo	23	23	—	−0.5	4.9
	Marquette Solar 8000 (Marquette, GE Healthcare, Sol)	23	23	—	+0.5	5.6
Sedaghat-Yazdi et al,[53] 2008	Philips M1020A (Philips, Eindhoven, NL)	48	50	66–100	−1.4	3.2[c]
	—	50	50	66–100	−2.9	3.9[d]
Rosychuk et al,[54] 2012	Masimo 4.0	122	53	65–100	−1.8	2.9
Murphy et al,[70] 2016[a]	Masimo	599	89	92 (90–99)[a]	−5.4	5.4
Griksaitis et al,[55] 2016	Masimo	270	25	75–100[a]	−2.4	12.6
	—	257	25	35–74[a]	−7.0	13.7
Harris et al,[71] 2016	Masimo SET	50	185	79 ± 6	−1.7	3.3
	Nellcor N-600	50	185	79 ± 6	−1.7	5.4
Foglia et al,[37] 2017	Masimo 7.9.1.0	21	21	60–92	−0.2	3.8
	—	14	14[b]	60–92	−1.6	4.8
	Nellcor Oximax	19	19	60–92	−3.0	5.0
	—	14	14[b]	60–92	−5.4	5.1

Studies are sorted by year of publication. Only studies reporting bias and precision based on a blood gas from an arterial line have been included. Studies are sorted by year of publication.

[a] Only children with congenital heart disease included into study.
[b] Data on infants with dark skin.
[c] Sensor placed on hand.
[d] Sensor placed on foot.

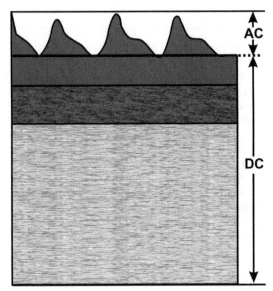

Fig. 2. Basal (DC) and pulsatile (AC) components in the light absorbances measured by the pulse oximeter. Yellow, tissue; blue, venous blood; red, arterial blood.

oxygenation. However, it is probably because of this apparent ease of use that potentially erroneous measurements on a pulse oximeter are more easily overlooked than those occurring with a $PTcO_2$ monitor. Therefore, thorough understanding of the factors potentially affecting the precision of a pulse oximeter is particularly important.

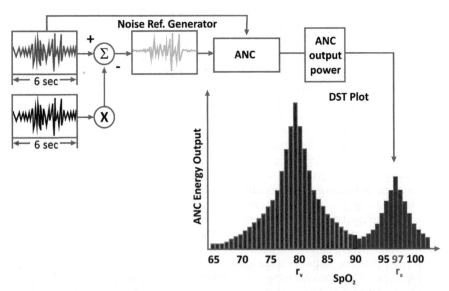

Fig. 3. Basic principle of new, more motion-resistant SpO_2 technologies. The software analyzes the red-to-infrared absorption signal and tries to describe the noisy component, thereby making it subtractable from the pulsatile (true) signal. It also scans through all absorbances found and identifies the right-most intensity peak in these absorbances. These features, among others, contribute to the relative insensitivity of this technology to motion and other artifacts. ANC, adaptive noise cancellation; DST, discrete saturation transformation; ra, arterial oxygen saturation; rv venous oxygen saturation.

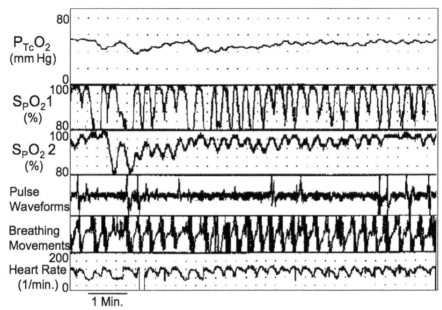

Fig. 4. Ten minute section of a simultaneous recording of SpO_2 (measured with a first-generation instrument) in the beat-to-beat mode and after averaging of the SpO_2 values over 5 to 7 seconds (default mode on this particular oximeter) during periodic breathing in a preterm infant. The beat-to-beat signal shows rapid decreases in SpO_2 to less than or equal to 80% with each apneic pause, followed by equally rapid increases to normal baseline levels of 98% to 100%. In contrast, from analysis of the averaged SpO_2 readings (and from the $PTcO_2$ signal, which is even more damped) it would appear that the patient is chronically hypoxemic but that each apneic pause has only a slight effect on oxygenation. Neither of the latter observations is correct. (*Adapted from* Poets CF, Southall DP. Noninvasive monitoring of oxygenation in infants and children: practical considerations and areas of concern. Pediatrics 1994;93:737–46; with permission.)

Probe placement

Improper probe placement may lead to the occurrence of an optical shunt; that is, the presence of light received by the photodiode without having passed through the tissue under examination. This may result from both misplacement of the sensor and exposure to ambient light. In most situations in which there is ambient light, SpO_2 will tend toward 85% (the SpO_2 value at which the ratio of red to infrared light equals 1)[23,24]; that is, SpO_2 will be falsely low, but falsely high readings (98%–100%) have also been reported[25,26] (**Fig. 5**). The light-receiving diode must be placed exactly opposite the emitting diode and both should be shielded against ambient light and not be applied with too much pressure. In addition, the sensor site should be checked every 6 to 8 hours and always if readings become implausible. It has been shown that 42% of nurses in a neonatal intermediate-care nursery exceeded a pressure on the skin of 50 mm Hg/6.7 kPa during fixation of a pulse oximeter sensor. Such high pressures may result in a reduced signal-to-noise ratio and may thus severely impair the precision of the SpO_2 measurements.[27] Highly flexible sensors provide better skin contact and thus better a signal-to-noise ratio.

Peripheral perfusion

Conventional oximeters require a pulse pressure greater than 20 mm Hg/2.7 kPa or a systolic blood pressure greater than 30 mm Hg/4 kPa to operate reliably.[28,29] Because

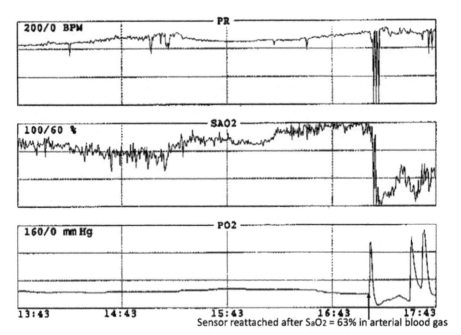

Fig. 5. Four-hour trend recording of (from top to bottom) pulse rate, SpO₂ and PTcO₂ from a 3-week old boy with severe respiratory failure resulting from diaphragmatic hernia. At 17:00, a routine arterial blood gas analysis revealed that SaO₂ was only 66%; that is, 30% lower than SpO₂. It was then found that the oximeter probe had partially come off the skin, resulting in an optical shunt. After the probe was reattached (*arrow*), the SpO₂ readings began to reflect the true severity of the hypoxemia. Analysis of the TcPO₂ signal suggests that the discrepancy between SpO₂ and SaO₂ had probably remained undetected for several hours. The spikes on the PTcO₂ signal at the end of the recording are caused by poor skin contact during bag ventilation. BPM, beats per minute; PR, pulse rate. (*From Poets CF, Southall DP. Noninvasive monitoring of oxygenation in infants and children: practical considerations and areas of concern. Pediatrics 1994;93:737–46; with permission.*)

next-generation oximeters rely less on pulse detection, they continue to operate even at lower blood pressure levels but the lowest pulse amplitude at which they still operate reliably has not been determined.

Response times
In theory, the response time of a pulse oximeter depends only on the time it takes for the blood to travel from the lung to the sensor site, which is 3 to 4 seconds in neonates.[30] However, all pulse oximeters currently available average their values over 2 to 15 seconds to level out any erroneous measurement that may occasionally occur even under optimal conditions. However, this averaging has unwanted consequences **(Fig. 4)**, including

- It delays the response to a true decrease in SpO₂ values
- It may lead to a mixing up of true with falsely low SpO₂ readings during periods of motion (eg, during feeding), which can result in the erroneous impression that the patient suffers episodes of prolonged hypoxemia
- It can lead to erroneous conclusions in situations in which a precise measurement of SpO₂ is required; for example, during sleep studies

- It hinders the definition of normal ranges for the frequency and severity of intermittent decreases in SpO_2 because such data would only be valid for the specific averaging time with which they have been obtained.

The actual influence of the averaging time on desaturation rates for 1 oximeter (Masimo Radical 7, software V4.7; Irvine, CA, USA) was studied with the help of the manufacturer who reprocessed a set of recorded raw red-to-infrared absorption data collected over a cumulative duration of 226 hours in 15 infants with apnea of prematurity using various averaging times that ranged from 3 to 15 seconds. The total number of desaturations lasting less than 20 seconds decreased from 1879 events at 3 seconds averaging to 233 events at 15 seconds averaging. For longer events, increasing the averaging time had the opposite effect: the total event number increased from 79 to 106 events when averaging time was changed from 3 to 15 seconds, probably because the latter setting resulted in several shorter desaturations being lumped together to 1 longer desaturation.[31,32] In any case, these data show the importance of knowing the averaging time used in each pulse oximeter and to standardize it for all instruments used in a neonatal unit.

Based on the linear relationship found between the logarithm of the desaturation rate and the logarithm of the averaging time, it is possible to derive a conversion formula to predict the desaturation rate (D1) obtained at 1 averaging time (T1) to that obtained with another averaging time (T2): D2 = D1 (T2/T1)c, where the exponent c depends on the desaturation threshold and the minimal desaturation duration.[32]

Motion artifact

The arterial pulsatile component contributes less than 1% to the total absorbance measured by the pulse oximeter. Hence, at least first-generation pulse oximeters were very sensitive to sudden changes in background signal; for example, due to body movements. Current instruments use various techniques to identify and read through periods with low signal-to-noise ratios as there are during motion, resulting in dramatic (>90%) decreases in false alarm rates.[33] However, some of these improvements may be achieved at the expense of not identifying true desaturation episodes,[34] which is unacceptable.

With conventional oximeters, identification of motion artifact is best done by displaying the light plethysmographic waveforms. Whenever these are distorted, SpO_2 readings become potentially unreliable. Alternatively, the pulse rate can be compared with the heart rate from an electrocardiogram monitor, which should be identical.[35] For next-generation instruments, which rely less on a clean peak-and-trough detection and thus an undisturbed pulse waveform, there is currently no independently validated method to identify periods of poor measurement conditions and thus potentially unreliable SpO_2 readings. However, Masimo's signal quality indicator, shown to reliably exclude erroneous measurements if staying at a threshold greater than 0.3,[36] may be an interesting tool in this regard. This issue is particularly important for automated oxygen controllers because their decisions to increase or reduce the Fio_2 must be based on reliable SpO_2 readings from a pulse oximeter.

Other hemoglobins and pigments

Methemoglobin (MetHb) will cause SpO_2 readings to tend toward 85% independent of SaO_2. Carboxyhemoglobin (COHb) will cause overestimation of SaO_2 by 1% for each percent COHb in the blood. Fetal hemoglobin and bilirubin do not affect pulse oximeters but may lead to a biased SaO_2 result by co-oximeters. In patients with dark skin, SpO_2 values may be falsely high, particularly during hypoxemia, and the precision of the measurement will be reduced.[37]

Algorithms

Pulse oximeters, in contrast to CO-oximeters, do not measure oxygen saturation but derive their values from a look-up table based on empirical data from healthy adults. These may vary between brands and even between different software versions from the same manufacturer. While conducting a randomized controlled trial comparing 2 different target ranges for SpO_2 (95%–89% vs 91%–95%), a British group identified a kink in the calibration curve of Masimo's oximeters. This resulted in the oximeter displaying fewer values than expected between 87% and 90% SpO_2 and to shift values greater than 87% SpO_2 upwards by 1% to 2%.[38] This caused a change in the distribution of SpO_2 values, so that correcting this calibration error resulted in a wider separation between the high and low SpO_2 group in their trial, which might explain the increased mortality in infants randomized to the low SpO_2 group seen after but not before this software upgrade. Although this hypothesis was subsequently rejected by demonstrating no change in the actual separation between SpO_2 readings in the low versus the high SpO_2 group before or after the software update,[39] it illustrates the potential relevance changes in an oximeter's calibration algorithms may have. (See discussion of further details, Maximo Vento and Ola Didrik Saugstad's article, "Targeting Oxygen in Term And Preterm Infants Starting at Birth," in this issue.)

Another influence on measurement bias and precision is that some instruments subtract a priori the typical levels of COHb, MetHb, and so forth, in healthy nonsmoking adults from their measurements and thus will display SpO_2 values that are approximately 2% to 3% lower than those displayed by other instruments. This approach; that is, to display the so-called fractional SpO_2 instead of the usual functional SpO_2 has been abandoned in recent years, probably because it resulted in an unacceptably poor ability of instruments using this approach to detect hyperoxemia.[40]

Precision and Detection of Hypoxemia and Hyperoxemia

Because the calibration curves used in pulse oximeters are from healthy adult volunteers, their calibration curves can only be attained within a range of between 70% to 80% and 100%. For this range, most manufacturers claim that 95% of their SpO_2 measurements will be within plus or minus 4% to 6% of the actual SaO_2. This is apparently also true for infants and young children. However, for saturations less than 70% to 80%, algorithms for determining SpO_2 are simply extrapolated from measurements obtained at higher SaO_2 levels. This procedure may lead to an underestimation of the true degree of hypoxemia and has led to recommendations that every patient with baseline SpO_2 values less than 75% to 80% should have her or his arterial blood oxygen saturation determined to measure the true severity of the hypoxemia.[41] However, analysis of the data plots from several validation studies, some of which included a high proportion of low SaO_2 values (**Table 3**), suggests that the pulse oximeter's sensitivity to hypoxemia (SaO_2 <80%) is not as bad as might be inferred from the previous considerations.[22,42–55] However, these data were obtained under optimal measurement conditions and may not be transferable to routine clinical conditions in which there is frequent motion artifact. Ten percent of episodes of severe hypoxemia ($PTcO_2$ <2.7 kPa) were not identified by the pulse oximeter because of motion in 1 study.[12] Thus, the true ability of pulse oximeters to detect hypoxemia in infants and children may be lower than suggested by the data summarized in **Table 3**.[48,56–58]

Pulse oximeters are also not ideally suited for detecting hyperoxemia due to the shape of the oxygen dissociation curve. Nonetheless, recent data from 5 large trials comparing these SpO_2 target ranges collectively analyzed in the neonatal oxygenation prospective meta-analysis (NeOProM) based on data from 4962 infants clearly showed that aiming for a range of 91% to 95%, instead of 86% to 89%, SpO_2 was

Table 3
Sensitivity and specificity of pulse oximeters displaying functional peripheral capillary oxygen saturation in detecting hypoxemia and hyperoxemia in infants and children

				Hypoxemia			
		N	Threshold	Sensitivity		Specificity	
Ref.	Instrument	patients	(SaO$_2$, %)	n	%	n	%
Fanconi et al,[42] 1985	Nellcor N 100	20	<80	108/121	89	37/39	95
Martin et al,[16] 1982	Nellcor N 100	8	<80	19/21	91	49/50	98
Ridley,[67] 1988	Nellcor N 100	25	<80	49/51	96	57/63	91
Lebecque et al,[45] 1981	Nellcor N100	47	<80	15/24	63	72/73	99
Gidding,[56] 1992	Nellcor	44	<80	14/18	78	47/48	98
Poets et al,[48] 1993	Nellcor N 200	37	<80	11/11	100	112/112	100
	Radiometer OXI 3	37	<80	10/11	91	111/112	99
	Kontron 7840	37	<80	9/11	82	109/112	97
Total/Mean	—	—	—	235/268	86	594/609	97

				Hyperoxemia			
			Threshold	Alarm Limit	Sensitivity		Specificity
Ref.	Instrument	N patients	(Pao$_2$, kPa)	(SpO$_2$, %)	n	%	n	%
Bucher et al,[57] 1989	N 100	25	>12	96	25/26	96	28/49	57
Poets et al,[58] 1993	N 200	50	>11	95	130/137	95	52/65	80
Bohnhorst et al,[34] 2000	Masimo	291	>11	95	179/186	96	59/105	56
	Nellcor Oxism	291	>11	95	181/186	97	44/105	42
	Agilent Viridia	280	>11	95	168/179	96	62/112	55
Total/Mean	—	—	—	95	683/714	96	245/436	58

Studies are sorted by year of publication. For hypoxemia, values are derived from the data plots shown in the individual studies; for hyperoxemia, data on sensitivity and specificity are presented for the alarm level at which the pulse oximeter would have detected at least 95% of hyperoxemic instances.

associated with a lower mortality and fewer infants with a patent ductus arteriosus or necrotizing enterocolitis requiring surgery. Yet, it also led to more retinopathy requiring treatment (but not more blindness) and more infants with bronchopulmonary dysplasia.[3] These clinical trial data show that, at least for the instrument used in the NeOProM collaboration, the question about whether the pulse oximeter detects 95% of instances in which Po$_2$ is greater than 80 mm Hg is less relevant than the question about whether the infant's oxygen levels can be maintained within a narrow range. Given the shape of the oxygen dissociation curve, this may be easier to achieve with a target range of 91% to 95% than with a target range of 86% to 89% SpO$_2$.[59]

TRANSCUTANEOUS PARTIAL PRESSURE OF OXYGEN MONITORS OR PULSE OXIMETERS?

Both devices, Pao$_2$ monitors and pulse oximeters, measure different but related variables. The relationship between Pao$_2$ and SaO$_2$ is neither linear nor constant. For example, at high SaO_2 levels, large changes in Pao_2 may occur with very small changes in SaO_2. Also, at a constant Pao_2 of, for example, 6 kPa, SaO_2 may be either 80% or 88%, depending on whether arterial pH is 7.25 to 7.40. The actual relationship between SaO_2 and Pao_2 and/or between $PTcO_2$ and SpO_2 should, therefore, be repeatedly determined, particularly in critically ill patients. In addition, both $PTcO_2$ monitors and pulse oximeters have their specific shortfalls: the $PTcO_2$ monitor is relatively difficult to use, has frequent periods when there is no reliable measurement, and reacts more slowly to sudden changes in oxygenation; whereas the pulse oximeter may fail to operate reliably whenever the patient moves, is relatively prone to erroneous measurements resulting from improper probe placement, and may be unreliable under conditions of hyperoxemia and possibly also severe hypoxemia. For these reasons, both devices should ideally be used in combination.

REFERENCES

1. Lundsgaard C, Van Slyke DD. The quantitative influences of certain factors involved in the production of cyanosis. Proc Natl Acad Sci U S A 1922;8:280–2.
2. O'Donnell CP, Kamlin CO, Davis PG, et al. Clinical assessment of infant colour at delivery. Arch Dis Child Fetal Neonatal Ed 2007;92(6):F465–7.
3. Askie LM, Darlow BA, Davis PG, et al. Effects of targeting lower versus higher arterial oxygen saturations on death or disability in preterm infants. Cochrane Database Syst Rev 2017;(4):CD011190.
4. Eberhardt P, Hammacher K, Mindt W. Perkutane Messung des Sauerstoffpartialdruckes. Methodik and Anwendungen. Stuttgart (Germany): Medizintechnik; 1972. p. 26.
5. Jakubowicz JF, Bai S, Matlock DN, et al. Effect of transcutaneous electrode temperature on accuracy and precision of carbon dioxide and oxygen measurements in the preterm infants. Respir Care 2018;63(7):900–6.
6. Rooth G, Huch A, Huch R. Transcutaneous oxygen monitors are reliable indicators of arterial oxygen tension (if used correctly). Pediatrics 1987;79(2):283–6.
7. Golden CSM. Skin craters - a complication of transcutaneous oxygen monitoring. Pediatrics 1981;67:514–6.
8. Takiwaki H, Nakanishi H, Shono Y, et al. The influence of cutaneous factors on the transcutaneous pO2 and pCO2 at various body sites. Br J Dermatol 1992;125:243–7.
9. Versmold HT, Linderkamp O, Holzmann M, et al. Transcutaneous monitoring of pO2 in newborn infants: where are the limits? Influence of blood pressure, blood volume, blood flow, viscosity and acid base state. New York: Alan R. Liss; 1979. p. 285–94.
10. Tremper KK, Waxman K, Shoemaker WC. Effects of hypoxia and shock on transcutaneous pO2 values in dogs. Crit Care Med 1979;7:526–31.
11. Okken A, Rubin IL, Martin RJ. Intermittent bag ventilation of preterm infants on continuous positive airway pressure: the effect on transcutaneous PO2. J Pediatr 1978;93:279–82.
12. Poets CF, Samuels MP, Noyes JP, et al. Home monitoring of transcutaneous oxygen tension in the early detection of hypoxaemia in infants and young children. Arch Dis Child 1991;66:676–82.
13. Falstie-Jensen J, Spaun N, Brochner-Mortensen J, et al. The influence of epidermal thickness on transcutaneous oxygen pressure measurements in normal persons. Scand J Clin Lab Invest 1988;48:519–23.

14. Vyas H, Helms P, Cheriyan G. Transcutaneous oxygen monitoring beyond the neonatal period. Crit Care Med 1988;16:844–7.
15. Tremper KK, Shoemaker WC. Transcutaneous oxygen monitoring of critically ill adults, with and without low flow shock. Crit Care Med 1981;1982:706–9.
16. Martin RJ, Robertson SS, Hopple MM. Relationship between transcutaneous and arterial oxygen tension in sick neonates during mild hyperoxemia. Crit Care Med 1982;10:670–2.
17. Duc G, Frei H, Klar H, et al. Reliability of continuous transcutaneous PO2 (Hellige) in respiratory distress syndrome of the newborn. Birth Defects Orig Artic Ser 1979;15:305–11.
18. Geven WB, Nagler E, de Boo T, et al. Combined transcutaneous oxygen, carbon dioxide tensions and end-expired CO2 levels in severely ill newborns. Adv Exp Med Biol 1987;220:115–20.
19. Wimberley PD, Frederiksen PS, Witt-Hansen J, et al. Evaluation of a transcutaneous oxygen and carbon dioxide monitor in a neonatal intensive care department. Acta Paediatr Scand 1985;74:352–9.
20. Fanconi S. Pulse oximetry and transcutaneous oxygen tension for detection of hypoxemia in critically ill infants and children. Adv Exp Med Biol 1987;220:159–64.
21. Mok J, Pintar M, Benson L, et al. Evaluation of noninvasive measurements of oxygenation in stable infants. Crit Care Med 1986;14:960–3.
22. Southall DP, Bignall S, Stebbens VA, et al. Pulse oximeter and transcutaneous arterial oxygen measurements in neonatal and paediatric intensive care. Arch Dis Child 1987;62:882–8.
23. Kelleher JF, Ruff RH. The penumbra effect: vasomotion-dependent pulse oximeter artifact due to probe malposition. Anesthesiology 1989;71:787–91.
24. Southall DP, Samuels MP. Inappropriate sensor application in pulse oximetry (letter). Lancet 1992;340:481–2.
25. Costarino AT, Davis DA, Keon TP. Falsely normal saturation reading with the pulse oximeter. Anesthesiology 1987;67:830–1.
26. Poets CF, Seidenberg J, von der Hardt H. Failure of pulse oximeter to detect sensor detachment (letter). Lancet 1993;341:244.
27. Bucher HU, Keel M, Wolf M, et al. Artifactual pulse-oximetry estimation in neonates. Lancet 1994;343:1135–6.
28. Falconer RJ, Robinson BJ. Comparison of pulse oximeters: accuracy at low arterial pressure in volunteers. Br J Anaesth 1990;65:552–7.
29. Severinghaus JW, Spellman MJ. Pulse oximeter failure thresholds in hypotension and vasoconstriction. Anesthesiology 1990;73:532–7.
30. Poets CF, Stebbens VA, Samuels MP, et al. The relationship between bradycardia, apnea, and hypoxemia in preterm infants. Pediatr Res 1993;34(2):144–7.
31. Vagedes J, Poets CF, Dietz K. Averaging time, desaturation level, duration and extent. Arch Dis Child Fetal Neonatal Ed 2013;98(3):F265–6.
32. Vagedes J, Bialkowski A, Wiechers C, et al. A conversion formula for comparing pulse oximeter desaturation rates obtained with different averaging times. PLoS One 2014;9(1):e87280.
33. Ahlborn V, Bohnhorst B, Peter CS, et al. False alarms in very low birthweight infants: comparison between three intensive care monitoring systems. Acta Paediatr 2000;89(5):571–6.
34. Bohnhorst B, Peter CS, Poets CF. Pulse oximeters' reliability in detecting hypoxemia and bradycardia: comparison between a conventional and two new generation oximeters. Crit Care Med 2000;28(5):1565–8.

35. Poets CF, Stebbens VA. Detection of movement artifact in recorded pulse oximeter saturation. Eur J Pediatr 1997;156(10):808–11.
36. Urschitz MS, Von Einem V, Seyfang A, et al. Use of pulse oximetry in automated oxygen delivery to ventilated infants. Anesth Analg 2002;94:S37–40.
37. Foglia EE, Whyte RK, Chaudhary A, et al. The effect of skin pigmentation on the accuracy of pulse oximetry in infants with hypoxemia. J Pediatr 2017;182:375–7.e2.
38. Johnston ED, Boyle B, Juszczak E, et al. Oxygen targeting in preterm infants using the Masimo SET Radical pulse oximeter. Arch Dis Child Fetal Neonatal Ed 2011. https://doi.org/10.1136/adc.2010.206011.
39. Whyte RK, Nelson H, Roberts RS, et al. Benefits of oxygen saturation targeting trials: oximeter calibration software revision and infant saturations. J Pediatr 2017;182:382–4.
40. Poets CF, Southall DP. Noninvasive monitoring of oxygenation in infants and children: practical considerations and areas of concern. Pediatrics 1994;93:737–46.
41. Baeckert P, Bucher HU, Fallenstein F, et al. Is pulse oximetry reliable in detecting hyperoxemia in the neonate? New York: Plenum Press; 1987. p. 165–9.
42. Fanconi S, Doherty P, Edmonds JF, et al. Pulse oximetry in pediatric intensive care: comparison with measured saturations and transcutaneous oxygen tension. J Pediatr 1985;107:362–6.
43. Hodgson A, Horbar J, Sharp G, et al. The accuracy of the pulse oximeter in neonates. Adv Exp Med Biol 1987;220:177–9.
44. Ramanathan R, Durand M, Larrazabal C. Pulse oximetry in very low birth weight infants with acute and chronic lung disease. Pediatrics 1987;79:612–7.
45. Lebecque P, Shango P, Stijns M, et al. Pulse oximetry versus measured arterial oxygen saturation: a comparison of the Nellcor N100 and the Biox III. Pediatr Pulmonol 1991;10:132–5.
46. Rajadurai VA, Walker AM, Yu VYH, et al. Effect of fetal haemoglobin on the accuracy of pulse oximetry in preterm infants. J Paediatr Child Health 1992;28:43–6.
47. Anderson JV. The accuracy of pulse oximetry in neonates: effects of fetal hemoglobin and bilirubin. J Perinatol 1987;7:323.
48. Poets CF, Seidenberg J, Wilken M, et al. Accuracy of measurements of Kontrol 7840, Nellcor N200 and Radiometer OX13 pulse oximeters in infants and young children. Klin Padiatr 1993;205(2):107–10 [in German].
49. Thilo EH, Andersen D, Wasserstein ML, et al. Saturation by pulse oximetry: comparison of the results obtained by instruments of different brands. J Pediatr 1993;122:620–6.
50. Schmitt HJ, Schuetz WH, Proeschel PA, et al. Accuracy of pulse oximetry in children with cyanotic congenital heart disease. J Cardiothorac Vasc Anesth 1993;7:61–5.
51. Bell C, Luther MA, Nicholson JJ, et al. Effect of probe design on accuracy and reliability of pulse oximetry in pediatric patients. J Clin Anesth 1999;11(4):323–7.
52. Bernet-Buettiker V, Ugarte MJ, Frey B, et al. Evaluation of a new combined transcutaneous measurement of PCO2/pulse oximetry oxygen saturation ear sensor in newborn patients. Pediatrics 2005;115(1):e64–8.
53. Sedaghat-Yazdi F, Torres A Jr, Fortuna R, et al. Pulse oximeter accuracy and precision affected by sensor location in cyanotic children. Pediatr Crit Care Med 2008;9(4):393–7.
54. Rosychuk RJ, Hudson-Mason A, Eklund D, et al. Discrepancies between arterial oxygen saturation and functional oxygen saturation measured with pulse oximetry in very preterm infants. Neonatology 2012;101(1):14–9.

55. Griksaitis MJ, Scrimgeour GE, Pappachan JV, et al. Accuracy of the Masimo SET(R) LNCS neo peripheral pulse oximeter in cyanotic congenital heart disease. Cardiol Young 2016;26(6):1183–6.
56. Gidding SS. Pulse oximetry in cyanotic congenital heart disease. Am J Cardiol 1992;70:391–2.
57. Bucher HU, Fanconi S, Baeckert P, et al. Hyperoxemia in newborn infants: detection by pulse oximetry. Pediatrics 1989;84:226–30.
58. Poets CF, Wilken M, Seidenberg J, et al. The reliability of a pulse oximeter in the detection of hyperoxemia. J Pediatr 1993;122:87–90.
59. Quine D, Stenson BJ. Does the monitoring method influence stability of oxygenation in preterm infants? A randomised crossover study of saturation versus transcutaneous monitoring. Arch Dis Child Fetal Neonatal Ed 2008;93(5): F347–50.
60. Rome ES, Stork EK, Carlo WA, et al. Limitations of transcutaneous pO2 and pCO2 monitoring in infants with bronchopulmonary dysplasia. Pediatrics 1984;74: 217–20.
61. Bossi E, Meister B, Pfenninger J. Comparison between transcutaneous PO2 and pulse oximetry for monitoring O2-treatment in newborns. Adv Exp Med Biol 1987; 220:171–6.
62. Lafeber HN, Fetter WPF, van der Wiel AR, et al. Pulse oximetry and transcutanous oxygen tension in hypoxemic neonates and infants with bronchopulmonary dysplasia. Adv Exp Med Biol 1987;220:181–6.
63. Wimberley PD, Pedersen KG, Olsson J, et al. Transcutaneous carbon dioxide and oxygen tension measured at different temperatures in healthy adults. Clin Chem 1985;31:1611–5.
64. Jennis MS, Peabody JL. Pulse oximetry: an alternative method for the assessment of oxygenation in newborn infants. Pediatrics 1987;79:524–8.
65. Boxer RA, Gottesfeld I, Sharanjeet S, et al. Noninvasive pulse oximetry in children with cyanotic congenital heart disease. Crit Care Med 1987;15:1062–4.
66. Fanconi S. Reliability of pulse oximetry in hypoxic infants. J Pediatr 1988;112: 424–7.
67. Ridley SA. A comparison of two pulse oximeters. Anaesthesia 1988;43:136–40.
68. Barrington KJ, Finer NN, Ryan CA. Evaluation of pulse oximetry as a continuous monitoring technique in the neonatal intensive care unit. Crit Care Med 1988;16: 1147–53.
69. Russell RIR, Helms PJ. Comparative accuracy of pulse oximetry and transcutaneous oxygen in assessing arterial saturation in pediatric intensive care. Crit Care Med 1990;18:725–7.
70. Murphy D, Pak Y, Cleary JP. Pulse oximetry overestimates oxyhemoglobin in neonates with critical congenital heart disease. Neonatology 2016;109(3):213–8.
71. Harris BU, Char DS, Feinstein JA, et al. Accuracy of pulse oximeters intended for hypoxemic pediatric patients. Pediatr Crit Care Med 2016;17(4):315–20.

Oxygen Toxicity in the Neonate

Thinking Beyond the Balance

Trent E. Tipple, MD*, Namasivayam Ambalavanan, MD

KEYWORDS

- Oxygen • Prematurity • Bronchopulmonary dysplasia • Retinopathy of prematurity
- Necrotizing enterocolitis • Glutathione • Antioxidants • Mitochondria

KEY POINTS

- Oxidative stress has traditionally been presented as an imbalance between oxidants and antioxidants but the situation is far more complex.
- Neonatal O_2 toxicity has been primarily characterized by macromolecular indices of damage that are nonspecific and are inadequate to capture dynamic biochemical processes.
- In premature infants, the fetal to neonatal transition occurs during a period of marked susceptibility to oxidative stressors caused by deficits in antioxidant defenses and impaired endogenous antioxidant response activation.
- The molecular effects of O_2 on subcellular compartments and developmental pathways are poorly understood.
- State-of-the-art oxidation-reduction biology techniques will enable more robust understanding of the global impact of O_2 toxicity in preterm neonates.

INTRODUCTION

Fetal development occurs normally in a relatively hypoxic ($\sim$20–25 Torr) environment in utero, meaning that the transition into room air at birth represents significant oxidative stress for prematurely born neonates.[1,2] However, the transition from the hypoxic environment of the womb to the relatively hyperoxic extrauterine environment occurs during a period of marked susceptibility to oxidative stressors. Preterm neonates are more susceptible to the effects of O_2 toxicity because of developmental deficits in antioxidant defenses and developmental impairments in the ability to mount rapid antioxidant responses to hyperoxia.[3–7] In general, the toxicities of O_2 during the neonatal period have been characterized by macromolecular indices of oxidative

Disclosure: Dr. Tipple received NIH grant (R01HL119280) and Dr. Ambalavanan recevied NIH grants (U01HL122626, R01HL129907, U01HL133536).
Division of Neonatology, Department of Pediatrics, The University of Alabama at Birmingham, 176 F Suite 9380, 619 19th Street South, Birmingham, AL 35249-7335, USA
* Corresponding author.
E-mail address: ttipple@peds.uab.edu

protein, lipid, and/or DNA damage. An expanding body of evidence has defined the molecular effects of hyperoxia on developmental pathways that guide organogenesis.[8,9] The sudden and dramatic increase in lung and systemic O_2 tension on preterm delivery significantly influence transcription factor activation and related downstream pathways. However, the global impact of O_2 toxicity in preterm neonates is incompletely characterized because of the lack of sensitive and specific oxidation-reduction (redox) biological techniques that adequately capture these complex biochemical reactions that undoubtedly contribute to the observed morbidity and mortality in this highly vulnerable patient population.

BASIC TENETS OF OXIDATIVE STRESS
Sources of Reactive O_2 Species

A redox reaction refers to a transfer of electrons between molecules. It is essential to remember that matter is neither created nor destroyed in chemical transformations. In the simplified scheme (**Fig. 1**), molecule A loses an electron and becomes oxidized and molecule B accepts an electron and becomes reduced. Thus, the net reaction is simply the transfer of the electron from molecule A to molecule B. In **Fig. 1**, "n" and "m" refer to the oxidation state of molecules A and B, respectively. When electrons are lost, the oxidation number increases (A^{n+1}). In contrast, when electrons are gained, the oxidation number decreases (B^{m-1}).

In order to fully comprehend the effects of O_2 tension on neonatal pathophysiology, the complexities of redox biology must be appreciated. Conceptually, this understanding must extend beyond the oxidant/antioxidant balance concept, which is that oxidative stress represents a deficiency of antioxidants in a setting of enhanced oxidant generation. This overly simplistic model suggests that oxidative stress can be overcome by exogenously administered antioxidants to restore balance. In reality, the complex biochemical reactions responsible for the reduction of O_2 are dynamic, highly compartmentalized, sensitive to clinically relevant factors such as pH and temperature, and extremely difficult to characterize in vivo with currently available techniques.[10]

Diatomic O_2 is highly reactive because of an unpaired electron in its outer orbital, and it requires 4 electrons for complete reduction (**Fig. 2**). O_2 is also the primary cellular metabolic fuel for aerobic metabolism.[10] Under normal conditions, the reactive O_2 species (ROS) generated in the process of the 4-electron reduction of O_2 to H_2O are quickly reduced (**Fig. 3**).[11] ROS generated during cellular metabolism include superoxide ($O_2^{\bullet}$) and hydrogen peroxide (H_2O_2).[10,11] Additional oxidants, including

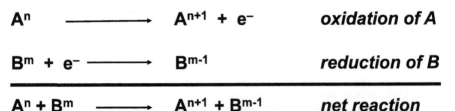

$$A^n \longrightarrow A^{n+1} + e^- \qquad \textit{oxidation of A}$$

$$B^m + e^- \longrightarrow B^{m-1} \qquad \textit{reduction of B}$$

$$A^n + B^m \longrightarrow A^{n+1} + B^{m-1} \qquad \textit{net reaction}$$

Fig. 1. Basic scheme of redox reactions. Molecule A loses an electron and becomes oxidized and molecule B accepts an electron and becomes reduced. Thus, the net reaction is simply the transfer of the electron from molecule A to molecule B. "n" and "m" refer to the oxidation state of molecules A and B, respectively. When electrons are lost, the oxidation number increases (A^{n+1}). In contrast, when electrons are gained, the oxidation number decreases (B^{m-1}).

$$e^- \quad\quad e^- \quad\quad\quad e^- \quad\quad\quad\quad\quad\quad\quad e^-$$

$$O_2 \rightarrow O_2{}^{\bullet-} \rightarrow H_2O_2 \rightarrow {}^{\bullet}OH + OH^- \rightarrow 2H_2O$$

$$2H^+ \quad\quad\quad\quad\quad\quad\quad\quad\quad\quad 2H^+$$

Fig. 2. Four-electron reduction of O_2 to H_2O with intermediate generation of reactive O_2 species including superoxide ($O2^{\bullet-}$), hydrogen peroxide (H_2O_2), and hydroxyl radical (${}^{\bullet}OH$).

peroxinitrite ($ONOO^-$), generated from the nonenzymatic reaction between $O_2{}^{\bullet-}$ and nitric oxide ($NO^{\bullet}$), and hydroxyl radical (${}^{\bullet}OH$), generated from the reaction between H_2O_2 and iron (Fe^{++}) or copper (Cu^+), are primarily formed in situations in which endogenous antioxidant systems are unable to sufficiently provide electrons for reductive processes. Although the primary focus of this article is O_2 toxicity, it is important to understand that excessive ROS generation in preterm infants comes from a variety of sources, including ischemia/reperfusion, infection, inflammation, mitochondrial respiratory chain, free iron and Fenton reaction, and hyperoxia.[12–14] The generation of ROS can lead to the disruption of normal physiologic events.[15] The extent of the effects of ROS on physiology depends on specific molecular interactions, cellular locations, and timing of exposure.[15]

The effects of ROS contribute to quantifiable cellular, tissue, and organ damage that underlies many of the morbidities of prematurity.[12] These damaging processes occur in both the placenta and the developing fetus.[13] Although premature infants that develop prematurity-related morbidities are usually exposed to only the least required amount of supplemental O_2 postnatally, they show marked evidence of oxidant stress.[6,12,14] There is evidence that excessive ROS production contributes to retinopathy of prematurity, bronchopulmonary dysplasia, intraventricular hemorrhage,

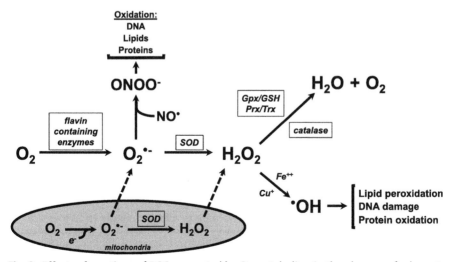

Fig. 3. Effects of reactions of ROS generated by O_2 metabolism in the absence of adequate detoxification. Nitric oxide ($NO^{\bullet}$) can react with $O2^{\bullet-}$ to form peroxinitrite ($ONOO^-$), which oxidizes DNA, lipids, and proteins. H_2O_2 can react with Fe^{++} and/or Cu^+ to cause lipid peroxidation, DNA damage, and protein oxidation. SOD, superoxide dismutase.

periventricular leukomalacia, necrotizing enterocolitis, kidney damage, and hemolysis.[13,16,17] Pathophysiologically, many diseases of prematurity likely represent a convergence between injury and ROS-induced alterations in development, probably leading to increases in susceptibility to chronic diseases in adulthood, and perhaps more rapid aging as well.[18]

The appreciation of ROS as something other than a negative entity has grown in the last 20 years. Several cellular processes are actively modulated via ROS production. ROS serve as cell signaling molecules for normal biological processes.[15] For example, nicotinamide adenine dinucleotide phosphate (NADPH) oxidases (NOXs) produce $O_2^{\bullet-}$ and/or H_2O_2 in tightly regulated and highly specific intracellular events.[19] As such, these processes are governed by transcription factors that are influenced by the redox environment of the tissue, cell, or subcellular compartment in which they are expressed. Changes in electron flux through these pathways, whether it be through reduction of O_2 or through NOX influence signaling. NOX-dependent ROS production influences developmental programming by acting on redox-sensitive transcription factors, including hypoxia-inducible factors (HIFs) and nuclear factor kappa-light-chain-enhancer of activated B cells (NF-kB). Dysregulation of HIFs and NF-kB have been linked to one another and to negative outcomes in prematurely born infants.[8,20] NOX isoforms contribute to signaling during lung development and injury and their function influences pulmonary airway and vascular cell phenotypes, including proliferation, hypertrophy, and apoptosis.[19] Oxidative stress is also associated with altered nitric oxide (NO) signaling in which ROS and reactive nitrogen species production are increased and bioavailable NO is decreased.[21]

Antioxidant Systems

Antioxidants are substances that inhibit or prevent oxidation of a substrate. Highly conserved antioxidant systems have developed to rapidly and robustly respond to alterations in cellular and subcellular redox perturbations. In the context of the previously mentioned 4-electron reduction of O_2, antioxidant systems serve as electron donors, as illustrated in **Fig. 3**.[11] Antioxidants that protect against and repair O_2-mediated injury include flavin-containing enzymes, superoxide dismutases (SODs), the glutathione (GSH) and thioredoxin (Trx) systems, heme oxygenases, and small-molecular-weight antioxidants.[1,11,22] Antioxidant capacity is lower in preterm newborns than in term infants.[14,17]

Birth represents an oxidative challenge. In the days preceding full gestation, antioxidant systems are upregulated and nonenzymatic antioxidants cross the placenta in increasing amounts.[9] These developmental changes provide for the transition from the relative hypoxia of intrauterine development to the O_2-rich extrauterine environment. Furthermore, endogenous antioxidant production is upregulated immediately before birth in term infants and is further upregulated on exposure to atmospheric O_2. Remembering that development occurs in a hypoxic environment in utero (~20–25 Torr), exposure to even room air constitutes hyperoxia for prematurely born neonates. Premature infants are at a distinct disadvantage for many reasons because they do not receive maternal antioxidants before delivery, have impaired ability to induce endogenous antioxidants before birth, and are unable to further induce endogenous antioxidant responses following delivery.[5,9] Although much has been outlined regarding associations between oxidative damage and neonatal morbidities, significant gaps in knowledge still exist regarding the role of oxidative injury in the pathogenesis of neonatal diseases.[12]

Therapeutic strategies to mitigate ROS-induced diseases in premature infants have included both enzymatic and nonenzymatic antioxidant preparations.[5]

Although logically based on the idea of antioxidant imbalance, studies in animal models and in preterm infants have yielded mixed results.[5,15] Cysteine is a precursor of GSH, the most abundant intracellular antioxidant in the body. Cysteine chloride supplementation in parenteral nutrition improved nitrogen balance in preterm infants; however, increased metabolic acidosis was also reported. N-acetylcysteine has shown promising results in preclinical models by acting as a precursor for de novo GSH synthesis. However, routine N-acetylcysteine supplementation was not found to be effective in improving respiratory outcomes in extremely low birth weight infants.[23]

One of the most promising catalytic antioxidants to undergo extensive clinical investigation in the prevention of bronchopulmonary dysplasia (BPD) was superoxide dismutase (SOD). Although the incidence of wheezing was lower in SOD-treated infants, a Cochrane meta-analysis indicated there is insufficient evidence to draw firm conclusions about the efficacy of SOD in preventing chronic lung disease of prematurity; however, it seems to be well tolerated and has no serious adverse effects.[24] Post hoc analyses of the data from infants with retinopathy of prematurity (ROP) in this trial indicated that severity greater than stage 2 was present in 42% of placebo-treated infants versus 25% of SOD-treated infants, suggesting that SOD may reduce the risk of developing ROP.[25]

O$_2$ TOXICITY–RELATED SEQUELAE OF BIRTH
Macromolecular Oxidation

In general, similar pathophysiologic mechanisms contribute to O$_2$toxicity–related morbidities in infants. As described earlier, ROS generated from metabolism, ischemia/reperfusion, infection, hyperoxia, and inflammation, when present in excess amounts, result in detectable byproducts of oxidation. These byproducts are highlighted in **Fig. 4**. Although nonspecific, the detectability of these byproducts has enabled associations between O$_2$ toxicity and neonatal disorders including BPD, intraventricular hemorrhage (IVH), ROP, necrotizing enterocolitis, and periventricular leukomalacia.[13,16]

GSH is the most abundant intracellular antioxidant in the body and cycles between thiol (GSH) and disulfide (GSSG) species. The GSH redox ratio (GSH/GSSG) is often used as a noninvasive measure of in vivo redox status. A significant negative correlation was reported between the arterioalveolar O$_2$ and blood glutathione redox ratio, with improved oxygenation inversely associated with decreased GSH/GSSG ratio.[26] Further, associations between BPD, lipid hydroperoxide (LOOH), and GSH concentrations in bronchoalveolar lavage fluid levels have suggested that early LOOH level increases in preterm infants developing BPD suggest that lung biochemical monitoring of sick infants might be possible and that BPD could be predicted early by evaluating biomarkers.[27] Extremely preterm infants have low GSH levels that impair their ability to detoxify ascorbylperoxide (AscOOH), an oxidant commonly found in parenteral nutrition. Higher first-week urinary AscOOH levels are associated with an increased incidence of BPD or death.[28]

White matter in the brains of premature infants is vulnerable to oxidative damage because of delayed expression of SOD, catalase, and GSH peroxidase enzymes.[29] Isoprostanes are a quantifiable marker of ROS-mediated tissue injury and concentrations of F$_2$-isoprostane in preterm lesions are similar to those measured in moderately severe cerebral cortical hypoxic-ischemic lesions in term infants.[29] Diffuse white matter injury involves maturation-dependent vulnerability of the oligodendrocyte lineage with selective degeneration of late oligodendrocyte progenitors triggered by oxidative

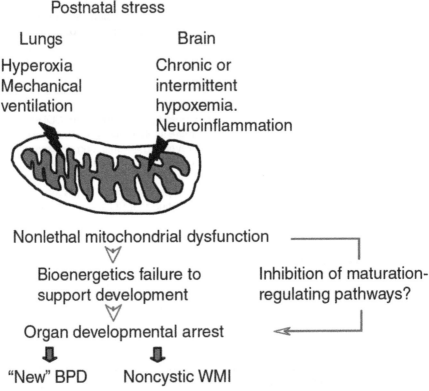

Fig. 4. Mechanisms by which perinatal mitochondrial oxidant stress contributes to white matter injury (WMI) and lung injury in preterm infants. (*From* Ten VS. Mitochondrial dysfunction in alveolar and white matter developmental failure in premature infants. *Pediatr Res.* 2017;81(2):286-292; with permission.)

stress and other insults.[29] Oxidative damage triggers cell death in preterm human white matter and the magnitude of oxidative damage is comparable with that sustained in the cerebral cortex after severe perinatal asphyxia.[29]

Redox-Dependent Alterations in Cell Signaling

As presented earlier, there has been increasing recognition of O_2 toxicity as an alteration in redox-dependent cellular and subcellular function. When viewed from this perspective, even subtle changes in redox balance can have persistent effects on organogenesis, tissue repair, and cellular function. As an example, multiple growth factors and signaling cascades play important roles in normal lung vascular development.[30,31] One of the most extensively studied endothelial growth factors is vascular endothelial growth factor (VEGF). VEGF, a potent endothelial cell mitogen produced by type 2 alveolar epithelial cells, is significantly involved in alveolar development and its expression is regulated by HIFs.[32–34] Numerous studies in newborn animal models have shown the importance of normal VEGF signaling to lung alveolar development.[35–41] Premature delivery has deleterious effects on the O_2-dependent biological processes that mediate lung development; in particular, the HIF/VEGF pathways.[8]

NF-kB regulates angiogenesis by acting upstream of HIF/VEGF.[20] Direct effects of ROS on signaling pathways include redox-sensitive transcription factors (eg, HIF; nuclear factor, erythroid derived 2, like 2 [Nrf2]; and NF-kB) as well as indirect effects through inactivation of NO-based signaling.[15] For example, NF-kB is a direct regulator of VEGF receptor-2 (VEGFR2), in the neonatal pulmonary vasculature.[42] Similar to BPD, altered HIF/VEGF signaling also mechanistically contributes to ROP. O_2 toxicity can directly damage pulmonary parenchyma and vessels.[43] Treatment with iNO can enhance additional ROS formation in the form of $ONOO^-$ leading to NO depletion and enhanced arterial pulmonary vascular constriction.[43]

O_2-mediated activation of NOX enzymes modulates angiogenesis or apoptotic pathways in the retina and contributes to the pathophysiology of ROP. The magnitude of NOX activation from O_2 fluctuations is associated with the degree of ROP.[44] VEGF-induced VEGFR2 alters the interaction between NOX and phosphorylated VEGFR2, suggesting that NOX4 may be a target to alter ROS generation to modulate VEGFR2 signaling and reduce ROP.[45] Patients with BPD frequently show alterations in pulmonary vascular remodeling and tone that manifest as pulmonary hypertension (PH).[46] ROS and NO signaling pathways are disrupted in PH, as shown by increased NOX expression, uncoupling of endothelial NO synthase, and reduced mitochondrial number and function.[21]

Redox Effects in the Mitochondria

More than 90% of ATP in mammalian cells is produced by oxidative phosphorylation through the action of mitochondrial ATP synthase.[47] Mitochondrial bioenergetic dysfunction has been proposed as a cause of altered organ development in premature infants (see **Fig. 4**).[48] Mitochondria are now thought of as among the cell's most sophisticated and dynamic responsive sensing systems.[49] Specific signatures of mitochondrial dysfunction that are associated with disease pathogenesis and/or progression are increasingly recognized as being important.[49] Although the specific pathways that regulate alveolar and white matter development are different in premature infants, both postnatal pulmonary and white matter development depend on proper mitochondrial function.[48,50] At birth, both the lungs and brains of premature infants are structurally and functionally immature, and growth also requires substantial energy.[48] Mitochondrial dysfunction is increasingly appreciated as a key pathologic feature in the development of lung disease.[49,50]

Mitochondria govern the response to altered O_2 tension and mitochondrial quality control.[51] Premature neonates show lower mitochondrial functional capacity, likely because of maturational delays in critical mitochondrial complexes and increased degradation of mitochondrial proteins.[47] Although the role of mitochondrial processes in diseases of prematurity is complex, recent evidence suggests that mitochondria offer the potential for novel diagnostics and therapeutics in lung diseases.[49] Vascular endothelial mitochondrial function at birth was recently shown to be a potential biomarker for BPD susceptibility in preterm infants.[50] Mitochondrial dysfunction in human-derived vascular endothelial cells isolated from umbilical cords at the time of birth strongly predicted the risk of poor pulmonary outcomes.[50] In vitro, hyperoxia causes reduced O_2 consumption, increased uncoupling, and altered insulin secretion in human beta cells. Using ultradeep sequencing, Kleeberger and colleagues[52] identified mitochondrial DNA (mtDNA) sequence variation and differences in heteroplasmy between inbred mouse strains that associate with pulmonary phenotypes on hyperoxic exposure in neonatal mice. The effects of these differences on mitochondrial function is an area of active investigation for the Kleeberger group. Ballinger and colleagues[53] recently showed that differences in mitochondrial bioenergetics and mtDNA damage associated with maternal ancestry may contribute to endothelial dysfunction and vascular disease. Collectively, these data highlight the need for a greater understanding of the impacts of mitochondrial dynamics, mitochondrial metabolism, mtDNA sequence variability, and mitochondrial protein expression in the context of neonatal diseases.[49]

GAPS IN KNOWLEDGE
Effects of Genetics on Redox Biology in the Neonate

O_2 toxicity alters developmental pathways through a variety of mechanisms.[54] Similarly, differential responses to O_2 toxicity are also influenced by genetics in individual patients, including ROS production, antioxidant responses, and genetics of underlying developmental pathways. VEGF and endothelial nitric oxide synthase (eNOS) haplotypes are associated with differential effects of O_2 on the development of RDS, BPD, IVH, and ROP in a population of 342 neonates less than 29 weeks old.[55] Collectively, the data indicated that haplotypes of VEGF and eNOS genes may also independently affect birth weight and gestational age, and act as protecting or risk markers for prematurity complications.[55]

With respect to antioxidants, genetic polymorphisms of SOD and catalase were recently shown to influence the incidence of morbidities in premature infants.[43] Genetic variations in antioxidant enzymes may contribute to the pathogenesis of redox-mediated prematurity complications. In an investigation of a cohort of 451 infants less than 30 weeks old, a single-nucleotide polymorphism related to the Nox family altered the susceptibility to oxidative stress–related complications of prematurity, including RDS, BPD, and ROP.[56] Furthermore, it has been estimated that the effects of gestational age and the duration of supplemental O_2 administration may account for up to 70% of the variance in ROP susceptibility.[57]

In general, SNPs of antioxidant enzymes have been poorly studied.[43,58] With respect to GSH metabolism during the neonatal period, levels of oxidative stress markers in boys are greater compared with girls. This discrepancy is likely caused by alterations in estrogen metabolism, which promotes the activation of glutathione metabolism.[59] Thus, it is possible that considerations regarding sex must be factored into nutritionally focused antioxidant therapies that target GSH metabolism.[59] After adjustment for epidemiologic confounders, sequence variants of NAD(P)H quinone oxidoreductase-1 and Nrf2 SNPs were associated with BPD and severe BPD, respectively.[60] Additional study of genetic polymorphisms could help identify high-risk populations that would benefit from targeted antioxidant strategies.[43]

Enhancing Endogenous Antioxidant Responses

Nrf2 is a transcription factor that coordinates the basal expression and inducible activation of antioxidant and xenobiotic genes. For a comprehensive overview of Nrf2 and associated processes, the reader is directed to the excellent review by Tonelli and colleagues[61] (**Fig. 5**). Briefly, Nrf2 regulates de novo GSH synthesis, NADPH production, as well as autophagy, stem cell activation, and the unfolded protein response.[61] O_2 is a potent Nrf2 stimulus and, based on the availability of binding partners, competition or cooperation with other activators and repressors, and crosstalk with other signaling pathways, Nrf2 epigenetically alters target gene promoters.[61] Nrf2 is currently being

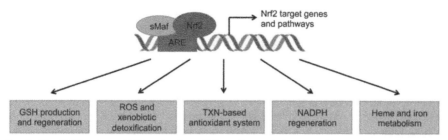

Fig. 5. The Nrf2 system. Nrf2 activation elicits enhanced de novo GSH synthesis, detoxification of ROS and xenobiotics, enhancement of the thioredoxin (TXN) antioxidant system, regeneration of NADPH, and heme metabolism. ARE, Antioxidant Response Element; sMaf, small musculoaponeurotic fibrosasoma. (*Adapted from* Tonelli C, Chio IIC, Tuveson DA. Transcriptional Regulation by Nrf2. Antioxid Redox Signal. 2018;29(17):1727-1745; with permission.)

investigated as a potential therapeutic target to enhance endogenous antioxidant responses to attenuate the impacts of O_2 toxicity on the premature infant.

Trace elements, including copper, zinc, iron, and selenium (Se), are essential for normal antioxidant enzyme function. Preterm infants have well-documented perinatal deficiencies in Se, as recently reviewed by our group.[62] Data indicate that trace mineral supplementation could optimize total antioxidant capacity.[63] Although Se supplementation was associated with a reduction in sepsis in preterm infants, it did not improve survival, reduce BPD, or reduce ROP incidence.[64] Using BPD models, the Kleeberger group has used bioinformatics to identify novel Nrf2-dependently modulated genes that regulate downstream targets in order to screen for chemicals or drugs that modulate expression. These types of approaches could help lead to the identification of new Nrf2 modulating therapies to prevent morbidities of prematurity.[65] There is much interest in understanding the intersection between trace mineral status on the efficacy of Nrf2 modulating therapies in diseases of prematurity.[66]

Methodologically, analyses of oxidative stress biomarkers have not translated into routine clinical practice because of lack of automation and cost.[67] In addition, the lack of specificity, especially as it relates to redox-regulated developmental processes, creates significant technical challenges, and economic difficulties constitute a challenge for the immediate future because accurate evaluation of oxidative stress would contribute to improve the quality of care of our neonatal patients.[67] New techniques such as surface-enhanced Raman spectroscopy may improve the ability to measure oxidative stress biomarkers using low sample volumes and in real time.[67,68]

O_2 TOXICITY: BEYOND THE BALANCE

It is clear that ROS have important regulatory and signaling roles in the newborn. Thus, antioxidant manipulation is likely to have implications for redox-sensitive developmental pathways that guide proper organogenesis.[16] Given the evolving understanding of oxidative stress in the neonate, future research must include evaluations of the prognostic and therapeutic value of oxidative stress biomarkers and antioxidants in premature infants.[12] The lack of enhanced induction of antioxidants by O_2 in preterm infants highlights the need to better understand the mechanisms responsible for differential responses and burden of disease in this highly vulnerable population.[9] Clinicians are also currently unable to determine which infants are likely to achieve maximal benefit from therapies that replace antioxidants or enhance endogenous antioxidant responses.[16]

NF-kB has a major role in lung and brain development, suggesting that therapeutic strategies to selectively block or enhance discrete components of this pathway may hold promise in preventing or treating diseases of prematurity.[20,42] It is also possible that preservation of mitochondrial function or prevention of mitochondrial dysfunction may be a novel strategy to prevent morbidities in prematurely born infants.[48] Enhancement of NO signaling and prevention of eNOS uncoupling by NOX inhibition could help prevent mitochondrial dysfunction and/or restore mitochondrial function.[21] In addition, use of high-throughput evaluation of mitochondrial biology of human umbilical vein endothelial cells or peripheral blood mononuclear cells may help modify therapeutic strategies to decrease risk for adverse outcomes in susceptible infants.[50]

REFERENCES

1. Asikainen TM, White CW. Pulmonary antioxidant defenses in the preterm newborn with respiratory distress and bronchopulmonary dysplasia in evolution: implications for antioxidant therapy. Antioxid Redox Signal 2004;6(1):155–67.
2. Welty SE. Is there a role for antioxidant therapy in bronchopulmonary dysplasia? J Nutr 2001;131(3):947S–50S.
3. Stenmark KR, Abman SH. Lung vascular development: implications for the pathogenesis of bronchopulmonary dysplasia. Annu Rev Physiol 2005;67:623–61.
4. Baydas G, Karatas F, Gursu MF, et al. Antioxidant vitamin levels in term and preterm infants and their relation to maternal vitamin status. Arch Med Res 2002; 33(3):276–80.
5. Lee JW, Davis JM. Future applications of antioxidants in premature infants. Curr Opin Pediatr 2011;23(2):161–6.
6. Smith CV, Hansen TN, Martin NE, et al. Oxidant stress responses in premature infants during exposure to hyperoxia. Pediatr Res 1993;34(3):360–5.
7. Jain A, Mehta T, Auld PA, et al. Glutathione metabolism in newborns: evidence for glutathione deficiency in plasma, bronchoalveolar lavage fluid, and lymphocytes in prematures. Pediatr Pulmonol 1995;20(3):160–6.
8. Thebaud B, Abman SH. Bronchopulmonary dysplasia: where have all the vessels gone? Roles of angiogenic growth factors in chronic lung disease. Am J Respir Crit Care Med 2007;175(10):978–85.
9. Davis JM, Auten RL. Maturation of the antioxidant system and the effects on preterm birth. Semin Fetal Neonatal Med 2010;15(4):191–5.
10. Davies KJ. Oxidative stress, antioxidant defenses, and damage removal, repair, and replacement systems. IUBMB Life 2000;50(4–5):279–89.
11. Nordberg J, Arner ES. Reactive oxygen species, antioxidants, and the mammalian thioredoxin system. Free Radic Biol Med 2001;31(11):1287–312.
12. Ozsurekci Y, Aykac K. Oxidative stress related diseases in newborns. Oxid Med Cell Longev 2016;2016:2768365.
13. Perrone S, Santacroce A, Longini M, et al. The free radical diseases of prematurity: from cellular mechanisms to bedside. Oxid Med Cell Longev 2018;2018: 7483062.
14. Perrone S, Bracciali C, Di Virgilio N, et al. Oxygen use in neonatal care: a two-edged sword. Front Pediatr 2016;4:143.
15. Auten RL, Davis JM. Oxygen toxicity and reactive oxygen species: the devil is in the details. Pediatr Res 2009;66(2):121–7.
16. Jankov RP, Negus A, Tanswell AK. Antioxidants as therapy in the newborn: some words of caution. Pediatr Res 2001;50(6):681–7.

17. Aceti A, Beghetti I, Martini S, et al. Oxidative stress and necrotizing enterocolitis: pathogenetic mechanisms, opportunities for intervention, and role of human milk. Oxid Med Cell Longev 2018;2018:7397659.
18. Meiners S, Hilgendorff A. Early injury of the neonatal lung contributes to premature lung aging: a hypothesis. Mol Cell Pediatr 2016;3(1):24.
19. Harijith A, Natarajan V, Fu P. The role of nicotinamide adenine dinucleotide phosphate oxidases in lung architecture remodeling. Antioxidants (Basel) 2017;6(4) [pii:E104].
20. Alvira CM. Nuclear factor-kappa-B signaling in lung development and disease: one pathway, numerous functions. Birth Defects Res A Clin Mol Teratol 2014; 100(3):202–16.
21. Tabima DM, Frizzell S, Gladwin MT. Reactive oxygen and nitrogen species in pulmonary hypertension. Free Radic Biol Med 2012;52(9):1970–86.
22. Asikainen TM, White CW. Antioxidant defenses in the preterm lung: role for hypoxia-inducible factors in BPD? Toxicol Appl Pharmacol 2005;203(2):177–88.
23. Soghier LM, Brion LP. Cysteine, cystine or N-acetylcysteine supplementation in parenterally fed neonates. Cochrane Database Syst Rev 2006;(4):CD004869.
24. Suresh GK, Davis JM, Soll RF. Superoxide dismutase for preventing chronic lung disease in mechanically ventilated preterm infants. Cochrane Database Syst Rev 2001;(1):CD001968.
25. Parad RB, Allred EN, Rosenfeld WN, et al. Reduction of retinopathy of prematurity in extremely low gestational age newborns treated with recombinant human Cu/Zn superoxide dismutase. Neonatology 2012;102(2):139–44.
26. Nemeth I, Boda D. Blood glutathione redox ratio as a parameter of oxidative stress in premature infants with IRDS. Free Radic Biol Med 1994;16(3):347–53.
27. Fabiano A, Gavilanes AW, Zimmermann LJ, et al. The development of lung biochemical monitoring can play a key role in the early prediction of bronchopulmonary dysplasia. Acta Paediatr 2016;105(5):535–41.
28. Mohamed I, Elremaly W, Rouleau T, et al. Ascorbylperoxide contaminating parenteral nutrition is associated with bronchopulmonary dysplasia or death in extremely preterm infants. JPEN J Parenter Enteral Nutr 2017;41(6):1023–9.
29. Back SA. White matter injury in the preterm infant: pathology and mechanisms. Acta Neuropathol 2017;134(3):331–49.
30. Kumar VH, Ryan RM. Growth factors in the fetal and neonatal lung. Front Biosci 2004;9:464–80.
31. D'Angio CT, Maniscalco WM. The role of vascular growth factors in hyperoxia-induced injury to the developing lung. Front Biosci 2002;7:d1609–23.
32. van Tuyl M, Liu J, Wang J, et al. Role of oxygen and vascular development in epithelial branching morphogenesis of the developing mouse lung. Am J Physiol Lung Cell Mol Physiol 2005;288(1):L167–78.
33. Choi KS, Bae MK, Jeong JW, et al. Hypoxia-induced angiogenesis during carcinogenesis. J Biochem Mol Biol 2003;36(1):120–7.
34. Shweiki D, Itin A, Soffer D, et al. Vascular endothelial growth factor induced by hypoxia may mediate hypoxia-initiated angiogenesis. Nature 1992;359(6398):843–5.
35. Kunig AM, Balasubramaniam V, Markham NE, et al. Recombinant human VEGF treatment transiently increases lung edema but enhances lung structure after neonatal hyperoxia. Am J Physiol Lung Cell Mol Physiol 2006;291(5):L1068–78.
36. Jakkula M, Le Cras TD, Gebb S, et al. Inhibition of angiogenesis decreases alveolarization in the developing rat lung. Am J Physiol Lung Cell Mol Physiol 2000; 279(3):L600–7.

37. Galambos C, Ng YS, Ali A, et al. Defective pulmonary development in the absence of heparin-binding vascular endothelial growth factor isoforms. Am J Respir Cell Mol Biol 2002;27(2):194–203.

38. Gerber HP, Hillan KJ, Ryan AM, et al. VEGF is required for growth and survival in neonatal mice. Development 1999;126(6):1149–59.

39. Thebaud B, Ladha F, Michelakis ED, et al. Vascular endothelial growth factor gene therapy increases survival, promotes lung angiogenesis, and prevents alveolar damage in hyperoxia-induced lung injury: evidence that angiogenesis participates in alveolarization. Circulation 2005;112(16):2477–86.

40. Kunig AM, Balasubramaniam V, Markham NE, et al. Recombinant human VEGF treatment enhances alveolarization after hyperoxic lung injury in neonatal rats. Am J Physiol Lung Cell Mol Physiol 2005;289(4):L529–35.

41. Maniscalco WM, Watkins RH, D'Angio CT, et al. Hyperoxic injury decreases alveolar epithelial cell expression of vascular endothelial growth factor (VEGF) in neonatal rabbit lung. Am J Respir Cell Mol Biol 1997;16(5):557–67.

42. Iosef C, Alastalo TP, Hou Y, et al. Inhibiting NF-kappaB in the developing lung disrupts angiogenesis and alveolarization. Am J Physiol Lung Cell Mol Physiol 2012;302(10):L1023–36.

43. Dani C, Poggi C. The role of genetic polymorphisms in antioxidant enzymes and potential antioxidant therapies in neonatal lung disease. Antioxid Redox Signal 2014;21(13):1863–80.

44. Saito Y, Uppal A, Byfield G, et al. Activated NAD(P)H oxidase from supplemental oxygen induces neovascularization independent of VEGF in retinopathy of prematurity model. Invest Ophthalmol Vis Sci 2008;49(4):1591–8.

45. Wang H, Yang Z, Jiang Y, et al. Endothelial NADPH oxidase 4 mediates vascular endothelial growth factor receptor 2-induced intravitreal neovascularization in a rat model of retinopathy of prematurity. Mol Vis 2014;20:231–41.

46. Alvira CM. Aberrant pulmonary vascular growth and remodeling in bronchopulmonary dysplasia. Front Med (Lausanne) 2016;3:21.

47. Honzik T, Wenchich L, Bohm M, et al. Activities of respiratory chain complexes and pyruvate dehydrogenase in isolated muscle mitochondria in premature neonates. Early Hum Dev 2008;84(4):269–76.

48. Ten VS. Mitochondrial dysfunction in alveolar and white matter developmental failure in premature infants. Pediatr Res 2017;81(2):286–92.

49. Cloonan SM, Choi AM. Mitochondria in lung disease. J Clin Invest 2016;126(3):809–20.

50. Kandasamy J, Olave N, Ballinger SW, et al. Vascular endothelial mitochondrial function predicts death or pulmonary outcomes in preterm infants. Am J Respir Crit Care Med 2017;196(8):1040–9.

51. Schumacker PT, Gillespie MN, Nakahira K, et al. Mitochondria in lung biology and pathology: more than just a powerhouse. Am J Physiol Lung Cell Mol Physiol 2014;306(11):L962–74.

52. Nichols JL, Gladwell W, Verhein KC, et al. Genome-wide association mapping of acute lung injury in neonatal inbred mice. FASEB J 2014;28(6):2538–50.

53. Krzywanski DM, Moellering DR, Westbrook DG, et al. Endothelial cell bioenergetics and mitochondrial DNA damage differ in humans having African or West Eurasian maternal ancestry. Circ Cardiovasc Genet 2016;9(1):26–36.

54. Saugstad OD, Sejersted Y, Solberg R, et al. Oxygenation of the newborn: a molecular approach. Neonatology 2012;101(4):315–25.

55. Poggi C, Giusti B, Gozzini E, et al. Genetic contributions to the development of complications in preterm newborns. PLoS One 2015;10(7):e0131741.

56. Huizing MJ, Cavallaro G, Moonen RM, et al. Is the C242T polymorphism of the CYBA gene linked with oxidative stress-associated complications of prematurity? Antioxid Redox Signal 2017;27(17):1432–8.

57. van Wijngaarden P, Brereton HM, Coster DJ, et al. Hereditary influences in oxygen-induced retinopathy in the rat. Doc Ophthalmol 2010;120(1):87–97.

58. Cuna A, George L, Sampath V. Genetic predisposition to necrotizing enterocolitis in premature infants: current knowledge, challenges, and future directions. Semin Fetal Neonatal Med 2018;23(6):387–93.

59. Lavoie JC, Tremblay A. Sex-specificity of oxidative stress in newborns leading to a personalized antioxidant nutritive strategy. Antioxidants (Basel) 2018;7(4) [pii:E49].

60. Silva DM, Nardiello C, Pozarska A, et al. Recent advances in the mechanisms of lung alveolarization and the pathogenesis of bronchopulmonary dysplasia. Am J Physiol Lung Cell Mol Physiol 2015;309(11):L1239–72.

61. Tonelli C, Chio IIC, Tuveson DA. Transcriptional regulation by Nrf2. Antioxid Redox Signal 2018;29(17):1727–45.

62. Tindell R, Tipple T. Selenium: implications for outcomes in extremely preterm infants. J Perinatol 2018;38(3):197–202.

63. Perrone S, Tataranno ML, Buonocore G. Oxidative stress and bronchopulmonary dysplasia. J Clin Neonatol 2012;1(3):109–14.

64. Darlow BA, Austin NC. Selenium supplementation to prevent short-term morbidity in preterm neonates. Cochrane Database Syst Rev 2003;(4):CD003312.

65. Cho HY, Wang X, Li J, et al. Potential therapeutic targets in Nrf2-dependent protection against neonatal respiratory distress disease predicted by cDNA microarray analysis and bioinformatics tools. Curr Opin Toxicol 2016;1:125–33.

66. Tindell R, Wall SB, Li Q, et al. Selenium supplementation of lung epithelial cells enhances nuclear factor E2-related factor 2 (Nrf2) activation following thioredoxin reductase inhibition. Redox Biol 2018;19:331–8.

67. Torres-Cuevas I, Parra-Llorca A, Sanchez-Illana A, et al. Oxygen and oxidative stress in the perinatal period. Redox Biol 2017;12:674–81.

68. Panikkanvalappil SR, James M, Hira SM, et al. Hyperoxia induces intracellular acidification in neonatal mouse lung fibroblasts: real-time investigation using plasmonically enhanced Raman spectroscopy. J Am Chem Soc 2016;138(11): 3779–88.

New Methods for Noninvasive Oxygen Administration

Colm P. Travers, MD, Waldemar A. Carlo, MD*

KEYWORDS

- Oxygen • Hypoxemia • Hyperoxemia • Targeting • Intermittent hypoxemia
- Nasal cannula • Environment • Noninvasive

KEY POINTS

- Oxygen saturation targeting is important but difficult in preterm infants.
- New methods of noninvasive oxygen administration improve oxygen saturation targeting and reduce intermittent hypoxemia.
- Closed-loop automated control and servo-controlled oxygen environment systems have not yet been shown to improve important clinical outcomes.

INTRODUCTION

Oxygen is one of the most commonly used drugs in neonatology.[1] There are risks and benefits of various modes of supplemental oxygen administration in different clinical settings.[2] The aim of supplemental oxygen therapy is to maximize the amount of time spent in the appropriate target oxygen saturation range while minimizing hypoxemia and hyperoxemia[3] as well as lung injury. However, preterm infants have respiratory instability,[4] which makes targeting oxygen saturations challenging and labor intensive for the bedside nurse and clinician. Owing to a combination of immature control of breathing and lung disease, preterm infants may spend a considerable proportion of time outside their intended oxygen saturation ranges.[5–7] Novel methods of oxygen administration are being developed and implemented to improve oxygen saturation targeting in infants.

HISTORICAL PERSPECTIVE

The first use of supplemental oxygen in neonates to treat cyanosis was described as early as 1780, not long after its rediscovery by Joseph Priestley. However, widespread

Disclosures: W.A. Carlo is on the Board of Mednax.
Division of Neonatology, The University of Alabama at Birmingham, Suite 9380 WIC, 1700 6th Avenue South, Birmingham, AL 35249, USA
* Corresponding author.
E-mail address: wcarlo@peds.uab.edu

Clin Perinatol 46 (2019) 449–458
https://doi.org/10.1016/j.clp.2019.05.012
0095-5108/19/© 2019 Elsevier Inc. All rights reserved.

adoption of supplemental noninvasive oxygen therapy to treat neonates did not occur until the 1940s.[8] Oxygen therapy at that time was typically provided via incubator flooding to create a high ambient "oxygen environment" for the spontaneously breathing infant. At that time, preterm infants with signs of respiratory distress were frequently nursed in incubators with a fraction of inspired oxygen (Fio_2) ranging from 0.4 to 0.8. This practice changed in the United States starting in 1955 after a randomized controlled trial demonstrated that preterm infants nursed in lower Fio_2 environments had a decreased incidence of retinopathy of prematurity with no difference in mortality compared with infants nursed in higher Fio_2 environments.[9] With new technology allowing continuous measurements of Pao_2 and oxygen saturations, the practice shifted toward targeting narrower ranges of oxygen saturations culminating in a series of large randomized controlled trials defining the optimal range of oxygen saturations.[10–13] Practice has now shifted toward optimizing the amount of time spent in these target ranges and the clinical meaningfulness of time spent above and below these target ranges.

NONINVASIVE OXYGEN ADMINISTRATION METHOD AND TARGETING

Recent meta-analyses have shown that targeting oxygen saturations from 91% to 95% in preterm infants is associated with a lower rate of mortality and severe necrotizing enterocolitis, with the tradeoff of higher rates of severe retinopathy of prematurity requiring treatment but not a higher rate of blindness.[13] This difference in important clinical outcomes occurred despite the expected overlap in achieved oxygen saturations between the higher and lower target groups.[10,12] The maintenance of oxygen saturations in this tight range remains especially challenging among infants at the lowest gestations[7] on both invasive and noninvasive oxygen therapy[14] and in particular among infants with bronchopulmonary dysplasia.[3] Preterm infants have frequent episodes of transient hypoventilation, which results in frequent episodes of intermittent hypoxemia. Episodes of intermittent hypoxemia have been defined as episodes of oxygen saturations at 85% or less for 10 or more seconds, and episodes of severe intermittent hypoxemia, which have been defined as episodes of oxygen saturation 80% or less for 10 or more seconds.[14] One recent study reported a median of 117 to 130 episodes of intermittent hypoxemia per day and a median of 39 to 47 episodes of severe intermittent hypoxemia per day in a cohort of 25 very low birth weight infants.[14]

Severe episodes of intermittent hypoxemia have been associated with a greater risk for neurodevelopmental impairment and retinopathy of prematurity in preterm infants, although these data are observational and may be prone to bias, because sicker infants are likely to have longer hospitalizations, remain in these studies for longer, and have more episodes of intermittent hypoxemia.[15–17] Although avoiding hypoxemia is important, prolonged hyperoxemia can lead to oxidative stress and injury, particularly to vascular beds in the eyes. Hyperoxemia is known to cause retinopathy of prematurity. Hyperoxemia can occur when additional supplemental oxygen is given either to avoid episodes of hypoxemia or to treat episodes of hypoxemia.[3] Such rapid fluctuations in oxygen saturation have been associated with changes in vascular tone and injury to vascular beds in the brain and eyes in animal models.[18,19]

Efforts to limit exposure to oxygen saturations above target range may increase episodes of hypoxemia, whereas efforts to limit hypoxemia may lead to exposure to oxygen saturations above the target range.[3] In the SUPPORT and COT trials both the lower and higher oxygen saturation groups achieved higher saturations than the targets.[10,11] In the BOOST II trials, infants in the lower target saturation group also achieved higher oxygen saturations than the target.[12] In a multicenter prospective cohort study from the era before the oxygen saturation target trials, 84 extremely preterm infants had high-resolution pulse oximetry data recorded for 72 hours each week for the first 4 weeks after birth.[6] Infants on oxygen or respiratory support spent 36% of the time above individual center target ranges compared with 16% below the target range, and the amount of time spent outside the target range was higher in centers with narrower target ranges.

Targeting lower oxygen saturations is likely to lead to more episodes of intermitted hypoxemia. One hundred fifteen extremely preterm infants participating in the SUPPORT trial had additional high-resolution pulse oximetry continuously recorded until 36 weeks postmenstrual age or they were off respiratory support.[16] Infants in this subcohort who were randomized to the lower oxygen saturation target range had more episodes of intermittent hypoxemia.

Oxygen delivery modes may affect oxygen saturation targeting. A prospective study followed 71 infants weighing less than 1500 g receiving oxygen supplementation until they reached 31 weeks' postmenstrual age[20] and noted that infants on nasal cannulae spent a greater proportion of time above the target range compared with infants on noninvasive positive pressure ventilation/continuous positive airway pressure (mean $\pm$ standard deviation, 60 $\pm$ 14% vs 41 $\pm$ 17%; $P<.002$), although presumably the infants requiring noninvasive positive pressure ventilation/continuous positive airway pressure were sicker. New methods of oxygen administration have been developed to mitigate this difficulty with oxygen stability and targeting given the potentially important clinical implications.

CLOSED-LOOP AUTOMATED CONTROL SYSTEMS

Closed-loop systems were developed to decrease the proportion of time infants spend outside target oxygen saturation ranges by decreasing overshoot and undershoot responses to hypoxemia and hyperoxemia, respectively.[3] A recent metaanalysis identified 10 randomized controlled trials comparing automated Fio_2 control with manual Fio_2 control in preterm infants on positive pressure respiratory support.[21] Automated control using closed-loop systems were more effective at maintaining oxygen saturation targets compared with manual control, increasing the proportion of time spent within the targeted saturation range (**Fig. 1**) and decreasing the time spent above the target range with hyperoxia and with severe hypoxemia ($SpO_2 < 80\%$). The proportion of time with an oxygen saturation below the target range was not

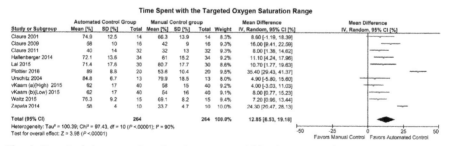

Time Spent with the Targeted Oxygen Saturation Range

Study or Subgroup	Automated Control Group Mean [%]	SD [%]	Total	Manual Control group Mean [%]	SD [%]	Total	Weight	Mean Difference IV, Random, 95% CI [%]
Claure 2001	74.9	12.5	14	66.3	13.9	14	8.3%	8.60 [-1.19, 18.39]
Claure 2009	68	10	16	42	9	16	9.3%	16.00 [9.41, 22.59]
Claure 2011	40	14	32	32	13	32	9.3%	8.00 [1.38, 14.62]
Hallenberger 2014	72.1	13.6	34	61	15.2	34	9.2%	11.10 [4.24, 17.96]
Lal 2015	71.4	17.8	30	60.7	17.7	30	8.6%	10.70 [1.77, 19.63]
Plottier 2016	89	8.8	20	53.6	10.4	20	9.6%	35.40 [29.43, 41.37]
Urschitz 2004	84.8	6.7	13	79.9	18.5	13	8.0%	4.90 [-5.80, 15.60]
vKaam (a)(High) 2015	62	17	40	58	15	40	9.2%	4.00 [-3.03, 11.03]
vKaam (b)(Low) 2015	62	17	40	54	16	40	9.1%	8.00 [0.77, 15.23]
Waltz 2015	76.3	9.2	15	69.1	8.2	15	9.4%	7.20 [0.96, 13.44]
Zapata 2014	58	4	10	33.7	4.7	10	10.0%	24.30 [20.47, 28.13]
Total (95% CI)			**264**			**264**	**100.0%**	**12.85 [6.53, 19.18]**

Heterogeneity: Tau^2 = 100.39; Chi^2 = 97.43, df = 10 ($P<.00001$); I^2 = 90%
Test for overall effect: Z = 3.98 ($P<.00001$)

Favors Manual Control   Favors Automated Control

Fig. 1. Forest plots comparing the time spent within the targeted saturation range in a metaanalysis of automated versus manual control of inspired oxygen to target oxygen saturation in preterm infants. Automated control of inspired oxygen increased the proportion of time spent within the targeted saturation range. (*From* Mitra S, Singh B, El-Naggar W, et al. Automated versus manual control of inspired oxygen to target oxygen saturation in preterm infants: a systematic review and meta-analysis. J Perinatol 2018;38(4):351–360; with permission.)

decreased. Recently this technology has been applied in a prospective cohort study of 20 very preterm infants on nasal continuous positive airway pressure or high-flow nasal cannula using a closed-loop oxygen blender. During a 4-hour testing period the automated system had a greater proportion of time in the target range owing to a combination of less time above and below the target range, as well as a lower proportion of time at less than 80%. Although closed-loop systems offer much promise, clinical trials to date have not focused on mortality or major morbidities. Closed-loop systems have not yet been studied in preterm infants who are not receiving positive pressure support.

SERVO-CONTROLLED OXYGEN ENVIRONMENT SYSTEMS

Servo-controlled systems for environmental oxygen have been studied recently in preterm infants off positive pressure support. In a randomized crossover study of 25 preterm infants with gestational age of 27 ± 2 weeks (mean ± standard deviation) and a birth weight of 933 ± 328 g on noninvasive supplemental oxygen, an oxygen environment maintained by a digitally set servo-controlled incubator system was compared with low-flow nasal cannula (defined as flows of ≤1.0 L/kg/min).[14] Infants had a decreased number of episodes of intermittent hypoxemia per 24 hours while on oxygen environment (117 ± 77 episodes; median, 98; range, 4–335) compared with nasal cannula (130 ± 63 episodes; median, 136; range, 16–252; $P = .002$) (**Table 1**). Infants

Table 1
Outcomes by mode of supplemental oxygen therapy

	Oxygen Environment	Nasal Cannula	P Value
No. of episodes of IH per 24 h	117 ± 77 (98, 4–335)	130 ± 63 (136, 16–252)	.002
Proportion of time SpO_2 of <85%	0.05 ± 0.03 (0.04, 0.00–0.14)	0.06 ± 0.03 (0.06, 0.01–0.13)	<.001
Proportion of time SpO_2 of <91%	0.28 ± 0.09 (0.28, 0.12–0.44)	0.29 ± 0.09 (0.27, 0.11–0.49)	.27
Proportion of time SpO_2 from 91% to 95%	0.50 ± 0.09 (0.51, 0.24–0.69)	0.49 ± 0.10 (0.48, 0.21–0.67)	.13
Proportion of time SpO_2 of >95%	0.22 ± 0.14 (0.18, 2–55)	0.22 ± 0.12 (0.20, 0.04–0.61)	.52
No. of episodes of severe IH per 24 h	47 ± 47 (28, 0–175)	48 ± 36 (39, 3–145)	.005
No. of episodes of bradycardia per 24 h	6 ± 5 (5, 1–9)	6 ± 7 (3, 2–10)	.90
Coefficient of variation of SpO_2	0.05 ± 0.02 (0.04, 0.02–0.09)	0.05 ± 0.01 (0.05, 0.03–0.09)	.02
Effective FiO_2 during study	0.25 ± 0.04 (0.24, 0.21–0.38)	0.26 ± 0.04 (0.25, 0.21–0.43)	.11
No. of FiO_2 adjustments per 24 h	5 ± 3 (5, 0–11)	6 ± 3 (7, 0–11)	.002
No. of recorded interventions per 24 h	5 ± 3 (3, 0–22)	5 ± 3 (3, 0–33)	.24

Values are mean ± SD (median, range).
Abbreviation: IH, intermittent hypoxemia.
From Travers CP, Carlo WA, Nakhmani A, Bhatia S, Gentle SJ, Amperayani VA, et al. Environmental or Nasal Cannula Supplemental Oxygen for Preterm Infants: A Randomized Cross-Over Trial. J Pediatr 2018;200:98–103.

on oxygen environment also had decreased episodes of severe intermittent hypoxemia per 24 hours (47 ± 47 episodes; median, 28; range, 0–175) in the oxygen environment group compared with (48 ± 36 episodes; median, 39; range, 3–145) infants in the nasal cannula group ($P = .005$). Infants on oxygen environment had a lower proportion of time with oxygen saturations of less than 85% (0.05 ± 0.03 vs 0.06 ± 0.03; $P<.001$; **Fig. 2**) and a lower coefficient of variation of oxygen saturation ($P = .02$), indicating improved stability of oxygen saturations. In addition, infants had a decreased number of adjustments in Fio_2 while on oxygen environment compared with nasal cannula (5 ± 3 per 24 hours on oxygen environment vs 6 ± 3 per 24 hours on nasal cannula; $P = .002$). This study showed that, for preterm infants receiving supplemental oxygen, servo-controlled oxygen environment decreases hypoxemia compared with nasal cannula. Improvements in oxygen stability and targeting with oxygen environment can be attributed to more stable effective hypopharyngeal Fio_2 concentration, which does not fluctuate with changes in infant breathing patterns and mouth breathing. However, the clinical significance of these findings on important infant outcomes has not been studied.

DEVICES FOR NONINVASIVE OXYGEN ADMINISTRATION

Nasal cannula, nasal catheter, and nasopharyngeal catheter oxygen administration provide oxygen flow from a source (which may be blended or unblended) via narrow plastic tubing to the infant nares. Nasal catheters are thin, flexible tubes placed into the nasal passage with the tip of the catheter sitting in the posterior nasal passages. The correct length can be estimated as the distance from the outside of the nostril to the inner margin of the eyebrow.[2] Nasopharyngeal catheters are similar thin flexible tubes placed deeper than the nasal catheter, passing beyond the nasal passages so that the tip is positioned in the posterior pharynx. The correct length can be estimated as the distance from the outside of the nostril to the tragus of the ear. When correctly positioned the tip of the catheter can be seen in the posterior pharynx just below the soft palate.[2] An advantage of both catheter types is that they are easily secured. A disadvantage is that both these catheter types are at risk of becoming

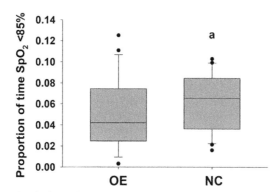

Fig. 2. Box plot with whiskers showing the proportion of time with oxygen saturations of less than 85% on oxygen environment (OE) versus nasal cannula (NC). Infants on oxygen environment had oxygen saturations of less than 85% for a lower proportion of time compared with infants on nasal cannula oxygen therapy. [a] Indicates significant difference with a *P* value of <.05. (*From* Travers CP, Carlo WA, Nakhmani A, Bhatia S, Gentle SJ, Amperayani VA, et al. Environmental or Nasal Cannula Supplemental Oxygen for Preterm Infants: A Randomized Cross-Over Trial. J Pediatr 2018;200:98–103; with permission.)

blocked with mucus, particularly if nonhumidified gases are used. Nasopharyngeal catheters may require frequent replacement or humidification to prevent obstruction from occurring. One study reported complete nasal obstruction in 44% of infants and children from 2 weeks to 5 years of age when heated and humidified gas was not used.[22] A nasogastric or orogastric tube should be in place when a nasopharyngeal catheter is used to allow gastric decompression in case of inadvertent advancement of the catheter into the esophagus.

There are relatively few data comparing these different interfaces in the neonatal population. Nasal cannula and nasopharyngeal catheters were compared in a crossover study of 11 infants on supplemental oxygen with no difference observed in effective hypopharyngeal Fio_2, respiratory rates, or pulmonary mechanics between these interfaces.[23] Nasal and nasopharyngeal catheters have been compared in a nonrandomized crossover study of 12 children less than 2 years old with lower respiratory tract infections.[24] This study showed a lower transcutaneous oxygen tension when the catheter tip was withdrawn from the pharyngeal position to the nasal position (mean difference of 56 mm Hg; 95% confidence interval, 34–78 mm Hg) indicating more entrainment of air with a nasal catheter compared with a nasopharyngeal catheter. Therefore, nasal catheters would be expected to require either a higher Fio_2 or higher flow rates to maintain similar oxygenation compared with nasopharyngeal catheters. This study also compared nasopharyngeal catheters with head box oxygen administration. This study showed that a flow of oxygen ($Fio_2 = 1.0$) at 0.15 L/kg/min through an 8F cannula provided transcutaneous oxygen tensions similar to those of head box oxygen at Fio_2 of 0.5.[24] In a randomized crossover study comparing oxygen modes of delivery in 60 children with respiratory tract infections, those on nasal cannula required an average of 26% higher flow rates ($P = .003$) compared with nasopharyngeal oxygen to achieve similar oxygen saturations.[22] This was likely due to the generation of inadvertent positive end-expiratory pressure with the use of these interfaces at higher flow rates. Nasopharyngeal oxygen has been shown to generate positive end-expiratory pressure even at flows as low as 0.5 L/min in spontaneously breathing newborn infants.[25] Neither nasal catheters nor nasopharyngeal catheters are typically used in neonatal care now, having been largely superseded in practice by nasal cannulae; however, there are pros and cons with each interface.

Nasal cannulae, which are now the most common interface for noninvasive oxygen administration, end in short (0.5–1.0 cm in length) binasal prongs with a 1- to 3-mm internal diameter and sit just inside the nostrils. Low-flow nasal cannula oxygen delivery, arbitrarily defined as flows of less than or equal to 1 to 2 L per min, are used in neonatal intensive care units globally and are the preferred method for home oxygen delivery; however, they have not been well-studied.[26] Nasal cannulae may be complicated by nasal obstruction with complete obstruction, which was observed in 13% of infants and children treated with nasal cannula oxygen in 1 randomized controlled trial.[22] Low-flow nasal cannulae, when correctly positioned, allow entrainment of air with infant breaths[27] so that the effective oxygen concentration will be affected by nasal versus mouth breathing as well as breathing rate, volume, and inspiratory time, which are likely to fluctuate in spontaneously breathing infants.[28,29]

The approximate effective hypopharyngeal Fio_2 can be calculated using formulae incorporating the Fio_2, cannula flow, and minute ventilation.[29–31] Standardized charts based on infant weight, set Fio_2, and cannula flow have been validated to allow for a relatively accurate estimation of the effective Fio_2,[32] but these estimations do not consider the wide fluctuations in inspiratory flow that occur, especially in patients with respiratory disease. In centers in the Neonatal Research Network, some infants on nasal cannula are managed with effective Fio_2 concentrations of 0.21.[26] Of 187 infants who underwent an oxygen challenge test, 87 (46.5%) passed the 30-minute room air challenge.[32] Fifty-two infants were prescribed an effective oxygen concentration of less than 0.23 whereas 16 infants were being managed with effective Fio_2 concentrations of 0.21. Seventy-two percent of the infants prescribed an effective oxygen concentration of less than 0.23 passed the oxygen challenge test. As expected, infants receiving an effective Fio_2 of 0.23 or less had a lower rate of oxygen challenge test failure ($P<.001$).

Head-box (hood) oxygen and oxygen environment avoids the difficulty of needing to calculate effective oxygen concentrations and decisions about whether to wean Fio_2 versus flow, because the set oxygen concentration is equal to the hypopharyngeal oxygen concentration. These modes of noninvasive oxygen administration deliver a stable, effective Fio_2 despite mouth breathing or irregular breathing patterns among neonates. Although servo-controlled oxygen environments rapidly adjust the oxygen concentration so that the set oxygen environment is generally maintained during infant care, other systems do not self-adjust and may lead to decreased oxygen concentration during infant care. Both head-box oxygen and oxygen environment allow a precise determination of inspired oxygen with an oxygen analyzer and titration of the Fio_2 with the use of oxygen blenders. Some modern incubators are fitted with a servo-controlled oxygen environment system for inspired oxygen administration to maintain a digitally set oxygen environment from 21% to 65% inside the incubator, which has been demonstrated to decrease hypoxemia and improve oxygen stability in spontaneously breathing preterm infants.[14]

OXYGEN OR FLOW

There has been debate about how best to wean infants from nasal cannula oxygen. Infants on nasal cannula receive flow, which could provide pressure to maintain upper airway patency and thus decrease episodes of desaturation.[33,34] In a randomized crossover study of 25 preterm infants comparing low-flow nasal cannula (typically set at 0.5 L/kg/min) with oxygen environment, there was no difference in the number of episodes of bradycardia between oxygen environment and nasal cannula at flows of 1 L/kg/min or less,[14] suggesting that low-flow nasal cannula do not stimulate or support breathing. In a randomized crossover trial of 14 infants less than 33 weeks gestation comparing low-flow oxygen or low-flow air at a rate of 0.1 L/min through nasal cannulae, as expected, oxygen was more effective in decreasing episodes of hypoxemia in preterm infants compared with low-flow air or sham treatment.[35] This study found that low-flow oxygen decreased treatment failure (defined as 6 episodes of hypoxemia, 4 episodes of hypoxemia requiring stimulation, 2 episodes of hypoxemia requiring free flow oxygen, or an SpO_2 of <80% for >3 minutes) compared with low-flow air or sham treatment (14% vs 50%). In addition, there was no difference in efficacy between low-flow air and sham treatment, suggesting that low-flow air does not support breathing.

In contrast, flows of more than 1 L/min or 1 L/kg/min generate positive pressure, which can support infant oxygenation and breathing.[36] However, it is not clear whether high-flow nasal cannula improve outcomes compared with other noninvasive methods of oxygen administration[36] or when it is appropriate to switch from high-flow nasal cannula to noninvasive oxygen administration.[37] Few studies have evaluated the optimal method of weaning off nasal cannula. A quality improvement initiative followed 90 infants receiving oxygen therapy with nasal cannulae as part of a protocol to standardize the use of nasal cannulae.[28] Infants were managed with 1 of 2 algorithms for the use of nasal cannulae, but could be switched to the other group as per physician preference. One group was managed with stable Fio_2 and weaned by adjusting the flow (n = 12). The other group was maintained on a stable flow and weaned by adjusting the Fio_2 (n = 53). There were also infants who used more than 1 algorithm in the switched group (n = 25). The small number of infants in the stable flow only group who were managed on flows of 0.5 to 1.0 L required fewer oxygen days compared with infants in the stable Fio_2 only group (9.4 ± 14 days vs 36.7 ± 45 days; P = .008). This study suggested a potential benefit for weaning the Fio_2 rather than flow to decrease the number of oxygen days, but the results were biased by a lack of randomization and allowing physicians to switch infants between groups without intention to treat.

SUMMARY

Targeting oxygen saturation is difficult in preterm infants. Newer modalities of oxygen delivery including servo-controlled oxygen environment and closed-loop automated control systems decrease the number of episodes of intermittent hypoxemia and improve oxygen saturation targeting. Data from large oxygen saturation targeting trials suggest that lower rates of episodes of intermittent hypoxemia and a few percent right shift in oxygen saturation histograms improve major clinical outcomes. However, there are not major studies to determine whether newer oxygen delivery modalities improve important clinical outcomes.

REFERENCES

1. Saugstad OD, Aune D. Optimal oxygenation of extremely low birth weight infants: a meta-analysis and systematic review of the oxygen saturation target studies. Neonatology 2014;105:55–63.
2. Frey B, Shann F. Oxygen administration in infants. Arch Dis Child Fetal Neonatal Ed 2003;88(2):F84–8.
3. Claure N, Bancalari E. Closed-loop control of inspired oxygen in premature infants. Semin Fetal Neonatal Med 2015;20:198–204.
4. Martin RJ, Wang K, Köroğlu O, et al. Intermittent hypoxic episodes in preterm infants: do they matter? Neonatology 2011;100:303–10.
5. Claure N, Bancalari E, D'Ugard C, et al. Multicenter crossover study of automated control of inspired oxygen in ventilated preterm infants. Pediatrics 2011;127(1): 76–83.
6. Hagadorn JI, Furey AM, Nghiem TH, et al, for the AVIOx Study Group. Achieved versus intended pulse oximeter saturation in infants born less than 28 weeks' gestation: the AVIOx study. Pediatrics 2006;118:1574–82.
7. Hallenberger A, Poets CF, Horn W, et al, CLAC Study Group. Closed-loop automatic oxygen control (CLAC) in preterm infants: a randomized controlled trial. Pediatrics 2014;133:379–85.
8. Cummings JJ, Polin RA, COMMITTEE ON FETUS AND NEWBORN. Oxygen targeting in extremely low birth weight infants. Pediatrics 2016;138(2):e20161576.
9. Kinsey VE. Retrolental fibroplasia; cooperative study of retrolental fibroplasia and the use of oxygen. AMA Arch Ophthalmol 1956;56(4):481–543.
10. Carlo WA, Finer NN, Walsh MC, et al, for the SUPPORT Study Group of the Eunice Kennedy Shriver NICHD Neonatal Research Network. Target ranges of oxygen saturation in extremely preterm infants. N Engl J Med 2010;362(21):1959–69.
11. Schmidt B, Whyte RK, Asztalos EV, et al, for the Canadian Oxygen Trial (COT) Group. Effects of targeting higher vs lower arterial oxygen saturations on death

or disability in extremely preterm infants: a randomized clinical trial. JAMA 2013; 309(20):2111–20.

12. Tarnow-Mordi W, Stenson B, Kirby A, et al, for the BOOST-II Australia and United Kingdom Collaborative Groups. Outcomes of two trials of oxygen-saturation targets in preterm infants. N Engl J Med 2016;374(8):749–60.

13. Askie LM, Darlow BA, Finer N, et al, for the Neonatal Oxygenation Prospective Meta-Analysis (NeOProM) Collaboration. Association between oxygen saturation targeting and death or disability in extremely preterm infants in the neonatal oxygenation prospective meta-analysis collaboration. JAMA 2018;319(21): 2190–201.

14. Travers CP, Carlo WA, Nakhmani A, et al. Environmental or nasal cannula supplemental oxygen for preterm infants: a randomized cross-over trial. J Pediatr 2018; 200:98–103.

15. Poets CF, Roberts RS, Schmidt B, et al, for the Canadian Oxygen Trial Investigators. Association between intermittent hypoxemia or bradycardia and late death or disability in extremely preterm infants. JAMA 2015;314:595–603.

16. Di Fiore JM, Walsh M, Wrage L, et al, for the SUPPORT Study Group of Eunice Kennedy Shriver National Institute of Child Health and Human Development Neonatal Research Network. Low oxygen saturation target range is associated with increased incidence of intermittent hypoxemia. J Pediatr 2012;161:1047–52.

17. Di Fiore JM, Bloom JN, Orge F, et al. A higher incidence of intermittent hypoxemic episodes is associated with severe retinopathy of prematurity. J Pediatr 2010; 157:69–73.

18. Ratner V, Kishkurno SV, Slinko SK, et al. The contribution of intermittent hypoxemia to late neurological handicap in mice with hyperoxia-induced lung injury. Neonatology 2007;92:50–8.

19. Winners-Mendizabal OG, Orge FH, Martin RJ, et al. Hypoxia-hyperoxia paradigms in the development of oxygen-induced retinopathy in a rat pup model. J Neonatal Perinatal Med 2014;7:113–7.

20. Arawiran J, Curry J, Welde L, et al. Sojourn in excessively high oxygen saturation ranges in individual, very low-birthweight neonates. Acta Paediatr 2015; 104:51–6.

21. Mitra S, Singh B, El-Naggar W, et al. Automated versus manual control of inspired oxygen to target oxygen saturation in preterm infants: a systematic review and meta-analysis. J Perinatol 2018;38(4):351–60.

22. Weber MW, Palmer A, Oparaugo A, et al. Comparison of nasal prongs and nasopharyngeal catheter for the delivery of oxygen in children with hypoxemia because of a lower respiratory tract infection. J Pediatr 1995;127(3):378–83.

23. Wilson J, Arnold C, Connor R, et al. Evaluation of oxygen delivery with the use of nasopharyngeal catheters and nasal cannulas. Neonatal Netw 1996;15(4):15–22.

24. Shann F, Gatchalian S, Hutchinson R. Nasopharyngeal oxygen in children. Lancet 1988;2(8622):1238–40.

25. Frey B, McQuillan PJ, Shann F, et al. Nasopharyngeal oxygen therapy produces positive end-expiratory pressure in infants. Eur J Pediatr 2001;160(9):556–60.

26. Walsh M, Engle W, Laptook A, et al, for the National Institute of Child Health and Human Development Neonatal Research Network. Oxygen delivery through nasal cannulae to preterm infants: can practice be improved? Pediatrics 2005; 116:857–61.

27. St Clair N, Touch SM, Greenspan JS. Supplemental oxygen delivery to the nonventilated neonate. Neonatal Netw 2001;20(6):39–46.

28. Jackson JK, Ford SP, Meinert KA, et al. Standardizing nasal cannula oxygen administration in the neonatal intensive care unit. Pediatrics 2006;118(2):187–96.

29. Vain NE, Prudent LM, Stevens DP, et al. Regulation of oxygen concentration delivered to infants via nasal cannulas. Am J Dis Child 1989;143:1458–60.

30. Benaron DA, Benitz WE. Maximizing the stability of oxygen delivered via nasal cannula. Arch Pediatr Adolesc Med 1994;148(3):294–300.

31. Finer NN, Bates R, Tomat P. Low flow oxygen delivery via nasal cannula to neonates. Pediatr Pulmonol 1996;21:48–51.

32. Walsh MC, Wilson-Costello D, Zadell A, et al. Safety, reliability, and validity of a physiologic definition of bronchopulmonary dysplasia. J Perinatol 2003;23(6):451–6.

33. Locke RG, Wolfson MR, Shaffer TH, et al. Inadvertent administration of positive end-distending pressure during nasal cannula flow. Pediatrics 1993;91(1):135–8.

34. Sreenan C, Lemke RP, Hudson-Mason A, et al. High-flow nasal cannulae in the management of apnea of prematurity: a comparison with conventional nasal continuous positive airway pressure. Pediatrics 2001;107(5):1081–3.

35. Hensey CC, Hayden E, O'Donnell CP. A randomised crossover study of low-flow air or oxygen via nasal cannulae to prevent desaturation in preterm infants. Arch Dis Child Fetal Neonatal Ed 2013;98:388–91.

36. Wilkinson D, Andersen C, O'Donnell CP, et al. High flow nasal cannula for respiratory support in preterm infants. Cochrane Database Syst Rev 2016;(2):CD006405.

37. Farley RC, Hough JL, Jardine LA. Strategies for the discontinuation of humidified high flow nasal cannula (HHFNC) in preterm infants. Cochrane Database Syst Rev 2015;(6):CD011079.

Targeting Oxygen in Term and Preterm Infants Starting at Birth

Maximo Vento, MD, PhD[a],*, Ola Didrik Saugstad, MD, PhD[b,c,d]

KEYWORDS

- Oxygen • Resuscitation • Newborn infant • Preterm • Oxygen saturation
- Pulse oximetry

KEY POINTS

- Approximately 10% of all newly born infants fail to adequately adapt immediately after birth; moreover, the number of very preterm infants needing intervention to achieve postnatal stabilization is significantly higher. Positive pressure ventilation with an adjusted inspired fraction of oxygen (Fio_2) is the mainstay of newborn stabilization.
- Term babies are initially ventilated with air and oxygen is titrated to keep oxygen saturation (Spo_2) within the published nomogram.
- In preterm infants, optimal oxygen supplementation to avoid injury caused by hyperoxia and/or hypoxia is still under debate. Only a few studies with different designs including aa small number of preterm infants are available for analysis. Recent studies have shown that extremely low birthweight (ELBW) infants not achieving Spo_2 greater than or equal to 80% and/or heart rates greater than 100 beats/min at 5 minutes are at a greater risk for morbidities and mortality. Moreover, ELBW infants receiving an initial Fio_2 less than 0.4 are at a greater risk of not achieving desired Spo_2 or heart rates at 5 minutes.
- Adequately designed and powered studies are being launched aiming to solve the uncertainties relative to the oxygen management in the delivery room in preterm infants.

INTRODUCTION

Evidence is still lacking regarding the optimum amount of oxygen required in the first minutes of life for newborn infants, especially for those who are premature or asphyxiated, who may need supplemental oxygen but at the same time are poorly equipped

Disclosure: The authors disclose no commercial or financial conflicts of interest in relation to this article. M. Vento acknowledges PI17/0313 grant from the Instituto de Salud Carlos III (Ministry of Science, Innovation and Universities, Kingdom of Spain).
[a] Division of Neonatology, University and Polytechnic Hospital La Fe, Avenida Fernando Abril Martorell 106, Valencia 46026, Spain; [b] Department of Pediatric Research, Oslo University Hospital, University of Oslo, Postboks 4950 Nydalen, Oslo 0424, Norway; [c] Department of Pediatrics, Robert H Lurie Medical Research Center, Chicago, IL, USA; [d] Northwestern University, Evanston, IL, USA
* Corresponding author.
E-mail address: maximo.vento@uv.es

Clin Perinatol 46 (2019) 459–473
https://doi.org/10.1016/j.clp.2019.05.013
perinatology.theclinics.com

to deal with oxidative stress. At birth, placental gas exchange is abruptly substituted by air breathing. The initial breaths increase arterial partial pressure of oxygen (Pao_2) within the first minutes of life from 25 to 30 mm Hg (3.3 kPa) in the fetus to 75 to 85 mm Hg (10.5 kPa) in the newborn (**Fig. 1**). This abrupt and dramatic 3-fold increase in oxygenation requires a seamless cardiovascular and pulmonary transition.[1] In addition, such a tremendous increase in oxygenation, and therefore oxidative stress, requires well-developed antioxidant defense mechanisms. However, preterm infants do not have sufficient antioxidant defense, either de novo or passively acquired from the mother, until the third trimester, which increases susceptibility to oxidative stress with potentially long-term effects imposed on the infant (see **Fig. 1**).[2]

In term infants experiencing intrapartum events/birth asphyxia, the oxidative load following oxygen supplementation might also be toxic in spite of a more developed antioxidative defense than in the premature infant.[3] In preterm infants, especially in the very preterm, positive pressure ventilation with supplemental oxygen is frequently needed and this adds to the risk of oxidant injury.[4] Oxidant injury can have acute consequences, such as an increased mortality or morbidity, can have a higher risk of intracranial hemorrhage, can favor conditions such as bronchopulmonary dysplasia (BPD) or retinopathy of prematurity,[3,4] or can induce epigenetic changes in the methylome with unknown long-term consequences (**Fig. 2**).[5] The optimal way to oxygenate newborn infants with a suboptimal transition is therefore still not known. Even if the normal development of oxygenation after birth were known, the optimal development of oxygenation in preterm and in term asphyxiated newborn infants is not. Although this field has moved fast in recent years, there are still several unanswered questions.

This article provides readers with an updated insight into the conundrum of how to supplement oxygen to term and preterm infants during postnatal stabilization under different circumstances, underscoring a lack of evidence that prompts the need for further studies.

PHYSIOLOGIC CHANGES IN THE FETAL TO NEONATAL TRANSITION
Cardiocirculatory and Antioxidant Characteristics of Fetal Life

Fetal life is characterized by a lower partial arterial pressure of oxygen (Pao_2) in circulating blood compared with the newborn infant, intracardiac (foramen ovale) and

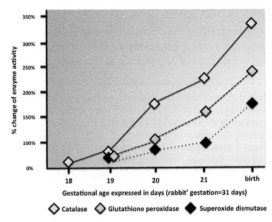

Fig. 1. Maturation of the antioxidant defense system during gestation in a rabbit model. (*Modified from* Frank L, Groseclose EE. Preparation for birth into an O2-rich environment: the antioxidant enzymes in the developing rabbit lung. Pediatr Res 1984;18:240-4.)

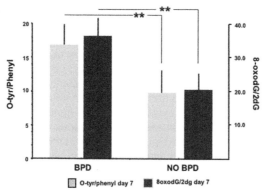

Fig. 2. The use of higher oxygen ($Fio_2 = 0.9$) in preterm infants less than or equal to 28 week's gestation caused a significant increase in biomarkers of oxidative damage to proteins as measured by the urinary elimination of Ortotyrosine/phenylalanine ratio (O-tyr/Phenyl) and DNA as measured by 8-oxodihydroguanosine/2-deoxiguanosine ratio (8-oxodG/2dG ratio). The concentration of both biomarkers in urine correlated with the development of bronchopulmonary dysplasia (BPD) **p<0.01. (*Modified from* Vento M, Moro M, Escrig R, et al. Preterm resuscitation with low oxygen causes less oxidative stress, inflammation, and chronic lung disease. Pediatrics 2009;124:e439–49.)

extracardiac (ductus arteriosus) shunting of the lung circulation, and an immature anti-oxidant defense system. The presence of contracted pulmonary arteries with an augmented wall thickness in the fetus causes an increased pulmonary arterial pressure (PAP) and concomitantly a high pulmonary vascular resistance (PVR). As a consequence, a substantial proportion of the cardiac afterload is diverted from the pulmonary circulation to the low-resistance placental territory where gas exchange will take place. The high PVR during the fetal period is caused by a combination of mechanical factors, various vasoconstrictor mediators such as endothelin and thromboxane, and a relative hypoxemia.[6,7] Oxygenation of the fetus directly depends on the oxygen partial pressure gradient between the maternal side of the intervillous space and fetal blood oxygen content. During embryogenesis in the first 8 to 10 weeks' gestation, fetal partial pressure of oxygen is approximately 20 mm Hg, reaching a plateau around 40 to 50 mm Hg with placental maturation.[8]

The activity of the antioxidant enzyme defenses only matures late in gestation paralleling the maturation of pulmonary surfactant, which contains significant amounts of superoxide dismutases (SODs), catalase (CAT), and glutathione peroxidases (GPx) to prevent surfactant inactivation by free radicals (see **Fig. 1**).[2] However, during gestation the fetal redox balance is regulated by the antioxidant activity of the placenta.[2] When born prematurely, despite the administration of antenatal steroids, extremely low birthweight infants do not reach the antioxidant capacity of term babies and are prone to oxidative stress and damage.[9]

Circulatory and Metabolic Changes in the Fetal to Neonatal Transition

Following birth, the decrease in the PVR and PAP is the consequence of the initiation of breathing. The initial respiratory movements enhance oxygenation, cause pulmonary vessel vasodilatation, decrease PVR, and increase pulmonary blood flow. In addition, there is rapid involution of the medial smooth muscle and thinning of the small pulmonary arteries, which greatly contribute to decreasing PVR and PAP. In addition, changes in the balance between vasoconstrictor factors, such as endothelin-1 and thromboxane, and vasodilator mediators, such as prostacyclin and endothelium-derived nitric oxide, on the pulmonary artery smooth muscles cells contribute to pulmonary vessel vasodilatation and redirection of the afterload to the lung circulation.[6,7] As a consequence, there is an abrupt increase in Pao_2 and closure of the intracardiac and extracardiac shunts.[10] Inspiratory efforts cause lung expansion and extrusion of pulmonary fluid to the interstitial tissue, contributing to lung aeration. In addition, expiratory breaking maneuvers and surfactant alignment on the alveolar surface prevent expiratory collapse and help establish a functional residual capacity that will facilitate an adequate gas exchange just with gentle contractions of the diaphragm.[11–13] Under these circumstances, failure to vasodilate the pulmonary vascular bed secondary to asphyxia, infection, pulmonary artery smooth muscle cell hypertrophy, lung hypoplasia, malformations, and so forth inevitably causes a hypoxemic respiratory failure in the newborn infant immediately after birth.[14] In preterm infants, additional circumstances, such as the immaturity of the thoracic cage and weakness of respiratory muscles, hinder lung fluid extrusion to the interstitium and subsequently lung aeration.[13] Moreover, lack of surfactant, increased elastic recoil, and absence of effective breaking maneuvers cause expiratory lung collapse. Thus, preterm infants are already predisposed to respiratory insufficiency in the first minutes after birth and frequently need respiratory support and oxygen in the delivery room.[15]

OXIDATIVE STRESS IN THE FETAL TO NEONATAL TRANSITION

Classic experimental studies in rabbits showed that the expression and activity of relevant antioxidant enzymes, including SOD, CATs, and GPx, only mature at the end of gestation (see **Fig. 1**).[16] Moreover, additional experimental studies also showed the inability of preterm rabbits to respond to hyperoxia by increasing antioxidant gene expression.[17,18] In preterm infants the activity of antioxidant enzymes SOD, CAT, and GPx were significantly lower than in term newborn infants and, despite the use of antenatal steroids, activities of antioxidant enzymes never reached term infants' values.[9] In addition, the capability to synthesize glutathione, the most relevant nonenzymatic intracellular antioxidant, is also substantially reduced because expression of the limiting enzyme γ-cystathionase is reduced in very preterm neonates.[19,20] Further, availability of other relevant antioxidant defenses, such as thioredoxin (TRx), hemoxygenases, vitamin C, vitamin E, beta carotene, and transition metal chelators, is not achieved until the end of gestation.[21] In experimental studies, the reduced to oxidized glutathione ratio (GSH/GSSG) in isolated hepatocytes of rat fetuses was significantly reduced in the fetal to neonatal transition[22] and the administration of N-acetyl-cysteine an L-cysteine donor that favors GSH synthesis to pregnant rats significantly reduced oxidative stress in offspring.[23] Healthy newborn infants show a reduction of GSH/GSSG ratio and increased antioxidant enzyme activities in whole blood immediately after birth.[24] Oxidative stress under physiologic conditions in the fetal to neonatal transition contributes to the activation of adaptive metabolic pathways such as the transsulfuration pathway relevant to the synthesis of L-cysteine and DNA methylation.[20]

Under certain circumstances, such as prematurity, hypoxic respiratory distress, or birth asphyxia, neonatologists apply positive pressure ventilation with an admixture that contains a high inspired fraction of oxygen ($Fio_2 > 0.21$).

Oxygen in excess causes a burst of reactive oxygen species (ROS), some of which are highly aggressive free radicals that may overcome the antioxidant defense system of the newborn infant and cause oxidative stress (**Fig. 3**). Free radicals are atomic or molecular species capable of independent existence that contain 1 or more unpaired electrons in their molecular orbitals. Oxygen free radicals react with vital cell constituents, such as membrane lipids, structural or functional proteins, DNA, and RNA,

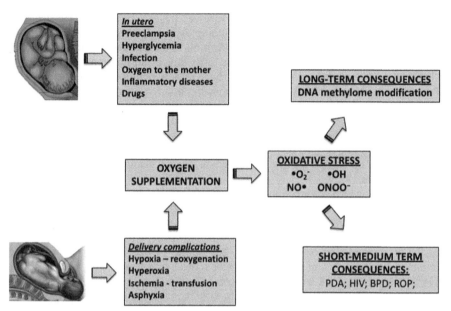

Fig. 3. In utero conditions that affect the fetus and complications in the fetal to neonatal transition often predispose the newly born infant to hypoxemia or respiratory distress. The use of high oxygen concentration causes a burst of ROS that may cause acute or long-term damage to the baby. HIV, human immunodeficiency virus; PDA, patent ductus arteriosus; ROP, retinopathy of prematurity. (*From* Torres-Cuevas I, Parra-Llorca A, Sánchez-Illana A, et al. Oxygen and oxidative stress in the perinatal period. Redox Biol 2017;12:674–681; with permission.)

altering their chemical composition and structure and leading to dysfunction. Because most ROS are generated within the mitochondria, oxidative stress leads to mitochondrial dysfunction, energy exhaustion, and activation of proinflammatory and proapoptotic pathways.[25] Free radicals are generated when oxygen is not completely reduced. One electron reduction of oxygen leads to the formation of anion superoxide $(O_2^{\bullet}-)$. Dismutation of anion superoxide with 1 additional electron forms hydrogen peroxide (H_2O_2), which is not a free radical but a signaling molecule. In addition, the addition of 1 electron to hydrogen peroxide through Fenton chemistry in the presence of a transition metal, especially iron, leads to the formation of the extremely reactive hydroxyl radical $(OH\bullet)$. In the presence of nitric oxide $(\bullet NO)$, oxygen-derived free radicals react, forming reactive nitrogen species (RNS) such as peroxynitrite $(ONOO-)$. ROS and RNS are potent oxidizing and reducing agents that subtract electrons from any nearby standing molecules, altering their structure and function, and begetting them into free radicals.[26] Aerobic cells generate ROS through enzymatic and nonenzymatic reactions that occur in subcellular organelles such as mitochondria, endoplasmic reticulum, nuclear membranes, peroxisomes, plasma membranes, and the cytoplasm. All these structures have enzymatic systems allowing the transfer of electrons from the Krebs cycle using the specific transporters nicotinamide adenine dinucleotide (NADH) or phosphorylated nicotinamide adenine dinucleotide (NADPH) to molecular oxygen in the mitochondria where the bulk of ROS is generated.[27] Concomitantly, other potential enzymatic sources of ROS include arachidonic acid metabolism by cyclooxygenase/lipoxygenase, NO synthase, cytochrome P450, the NADPH-oxidase (Nox) family of proteins, and xanthine oxidoreductase.[28] Hyperoxia, intermittent hypoxia, or prolonged hypoxia followed by reoxygenation, especially with high Fio_2, activates the Nox family enzyme complex[29] and/or the xanthine reductase-oxidase pathway[30] to generate ROS in great amounts and cause oxidative damage to cell structures. Hypoxia leads to increase of Krebs cycle intermediates, such as α-ketoglutarate, succinate, and fumarate. These intermediates decrease more slowly after resuscitation with 100% oxygen, suggesting that hyperoxia leads to mitochondrial dysfunction.[31] Succinate is a gatekeeper that regulates the electron flow across the electron respiratory chain. After intense hypoxia during reoxygenation with increased concentrations of oxygen, it also creates the so-called reverse electron transport from complex II to complex I, which generates a many-fold increased production of ROS compared with the conventional forward electron transport from complex I to complex II.[32]

Reoxygenation with higher oxygen concentrations induces inflammation not only in the lungs but also in the brain and probably in other organs as well, as has been extensively shown in different experimental animal models (for a review see Ref.[33]). Clinical studies have shown that asphyxia and resuscitation of term babies with high Fio_2 causes an exacerbated oxidative stress, damage to myocardium and kidneys, and increased mortality,[3,34] or in preterm babies BPD or intraventricular hemorrhage (IVH)[35–37] (see **Fig. 3**). Even a brief (minutes) hyperoxic exposure immediately after birth has been epidemiologically linked to conditions associated with inflammation and DNA damage, such as childhood malignancies.[38,39]

OXYGEN SATURATION AT BIRTH AND GUIDELINES' RECOMMENDATIONS

With the initiation of breathing, Pao_2 increases form 3.3 kPa (25–30 mm Hg) to 10.5 kPa (75–85 mm Hg) in the first minutes after birth. The increase in Pao_2 both in term and preterm infants is gradual in the first minutes after birth. This time is needed to expand and aerate the lungs, extrude lung fluid from the respiratory airways, and establish a functional residual capacity.[40] The incorporation of pulse oximetry in the delivery room allowed investigators to monitor preductal and-postductal pulse oximetry in term and preterm infants born by vaginal delivery or cesarean section from birth until stabilization. Studies showed that healthy term or near-term newborn infants needed several minutes for arterial oxygen saturation (Spo_2) to plateau ≈90%. Moreover, time for stabilization showed a great interindividual variability, especially in extremely preterm infants, who often needed 5 minutes or more to achieve Spo_2 greater than 85%.[3,41]

In a prospective observational study, Dawson and colleagues[42] monitored and registered preductal pulse oximetry in 308 term and 160 preterm healthy newborn infants with normal deliveries for 10 minutes after birth. Spo_2 interquartile ranges at 3, 5, and 10 minutes were 81% (71%–90%), 92% (83%–96%), and 97% (94%–98%) respectively for term infants and 76% (67%–83%), 86% (80%–92%), and 94% (91%–97%) respectively for preterm infants. Of note, preterm infants only represented 34% of all babies participating in the study and preterm less than 32 weeks' gestation only 8% of the total. Hence, the ranges obtained for preterm infants were representative of late (33–36 weeks) but not of very preterm (<32 weeks) babies.[42] The recent guidelines of the American Heart Association recommended Spo_2 targets at 3, 5, and 10 minutes of 70% to 75%, 80% to 85% and 85% to 95% respectively.[43]

To date, no target ranges for oxygen saturation for very preterm infants are yet available. In a recent international search in public databases to determine current recommendations guiding oxygen management for stabilization of preterm infants in the delivery room, only 80% of the guidelines provided specific recommendations according to gestational age. The most frequently recommended initial Fio_2 ($iFio_2$) was 0.21 to 0.3.[44] Although most guidelines suggested titrating oxygen to meet Spo_2 targets recommended by expert committees, specific 5-minute targets substantially differed between countries (from 70% to 90%), underpinning the lack of evidence behind these recommendations.[44]

OXYGEN IN THE DELIVERY ROOM
In Term Infants

Birth asphyxia is one of the 3 most important causes of early neonatal death globally. In 2013, neonatal mortality reached 2.62 million newborn infants, representing 41.6% of deaths in children less than 5 years old.[45] Of note, although these deaths had a significant 64% reduction since 1970, neonatal deaths accounted for 41.6% compared with 37.4% in 1990.[46] Moreover, early neonatal death (ENN), defined as newborn death before 7 days after birth, still represents the bulk of neonatal deaths in low-income countries.[47] Among the causes of ENN, birth asphyxia (BA) has consistently accounted for about 25% of ENN in low-income and middle-income countries over the past decade,[48] and in high-income countries BA accounts for 7.1% of mortality, taking into consideration all gestational ages.[48] Despite the benefits derived from the introduction of therapeutic hypothermia in high-income countries, the picture is different in low-income and middle-income countries. The low quality of recent hypothermia trials, including the lack of comprehensive follow-up, provides evidence of neither safety nor efficacy of hypothermia as neuroprotection for sequelae of neonatal hypoxic-ischemic encephalopathy such as cerebral palsy, hearing and/or vision impairment, epilepsy, and mental retardation.[49]

In the 20 years up to the 1990 it was accepted that newborns should be resuscitated with pure oxygen. This idea began to be challenged from the late 1970s and in the 1990s animal studies showed that newborn resuscitation can be performed with air.[31] This possibility was supported by 2 clinical studies showing a tendency to lower mortality when air substituted oxygen. In addition, time to first breath occurred 30 seconds earlier.[50,51] The practice of giving pure oxygen at birth therefore had suppressed newborn spontaneous ventilation the last 200 years.[52]

Further clinical studies found that a brief exposure to pure oxygen during resuscitation at birth triggered long-term increases in oxidative stress and levels of inflammatory markers for at least 3 weeks, and damage to specific organs such as heart and kidney.[24,53,54] Thus a few minutes of oxygen exposure in the delivery room triggered long-term effects, perhaps for the rest of the life, in the babies given pure oxygen.

Subsequent meta-analyses including more than 2000 infants randomized or quasirandomized to air or oxygen resuscitation eventually showed a significant 30% reduction in mortality if air substituted 100% oxygen during resuscitation.[55] The last meta-analysis showed, in low-income countries, a decrease in mortality from 18.1% in infants traditionally resuscitated with pure oxygen compared with 13.3% (odds ratio [OR], 0.74; 95% confidence interval [CI], 0.57–0.95) in infants resuscitated with air. Data from European countries in the study, Spain and Romania, were analyzed separately. Mortalities were lower, but the relative reduction in mortality was even more dramatic than in low-income areas; from 3.9% to 1.1% (OR, 0.32; 95% CI, 0.12–0.84).[34]

This dramatic finding indicated that as many as 250,000 lives could be saved globally each year by air resuscitation. In addition, another 300,000 so-called fresh stillbirths could be rescued; these infants often had not be resuscitated previously because of lack of oxygen.[56] Mortality caused by BA has decreased by approximately 300,000 in the last 25 years.[57]

In Preterm Infants

The $iFiO_2$ for preterm infants in the delivery room still represents a relevant conundrum for neonatologists. The risk of hyperoxia with the subsequent oxidative stress and damage to lung, kidneys, or eyes should be balanced with the risks of hypoxia and the consequences for the central nervous system. Preliminary studies in 1995 performed by Lundstrøm and colleagues[58] showed that the use of higher FiO_2 of 0.8 compared with 0.21 caused a significant reduction in cerebral blood flow. The first feasibility studies performed in very preterm infants comparing air versus 100% oxygen showed that babies in the air group had difficulties overcoming bradycardia and hypoxemia in the first minutes and therefore needed supplemental oxygen.[59] Rabi and colleagues[60] also showed that preterm infants stabilized with air significantly failed to achieve preestablished targeted saturations compared with infants initially resuscitated with an FiO_2 of 1.0 and titrated according to response. Escrig and colleagues,[61] in a feasibility study, randomized very preterm infants less than 28 weeks' gestation with an initial FiO_2 of 0.3 or 0.9. No differences between the groups were found in evolving SpO_2 and heart rate during the first minutes after birth and/or in the achievement of targeted saturations. Furthermore, in a following study with a similar design, the use of lower initial FiO_2 (0.3) compared with higher FiO_2 (0.9–1.0) significantly decreased oxidant stress and proinflammatory biomarkers and the incidence of BPD (see **Fig. 2**).[35] In a subsequent study, Kapadia and colleagues[37] showed that higher oxygen loads in the delivery room in preterm infants led to an increase in incidence of BPD, oxygen needs, days of mechanical ventilation, and length of hospital stay. Apparently, the use of an $iFiO_2$ of 0.3 was sufficient to avoid profound bradycardia and hypoxemia in the first minutes after birth, thus avoiding the need for higher supplemental oxygen and the ensuing negative consequences, especially for extremely preterm infants.

In this scenario, the largest study examining effects of high (60%–100%) versus low (21%–30%) initial FiO_2 in the delivery room for premature infants is the Targeted Oxygen in the Resuscitation of Preterm Infants (Torpido) trial.[62] This trial was a randomized, unmasked study designed to determine major disability and death at 2 years in infants less than 32 weeks' gestation after delivery room resuscitation was initiated with either air or 100% oxygen, and pulse oximetry was adjusted to target 65% to 95% at 5 minutes and 85% to 95% until neonatal intensive care unit (NICU) admission.[62] Out of 6291 eligible infants, only 292 were enrolled and 290 randomized; 145 were allocated to each group. In the air group, 1 newborn infant was excluded because of lung hypoplasia, and in the 100% oxygen group 2 infants were excluded because of hypertrophic cardiomyopathy and 1 with congenital diaphragmatic hernia. Mean gestation was 28.9 weeks. Recruitment ceased in June 2014, per the recommendations of the Data and Safety Monitoring Committee owing to loss of equipoise for the use of 100% oxygen. There was no difference in death for the whole data set; thus, 10% died in the air group and 4% in the oxygen group. OR 2.3 (95% CI, 0.9–5.7). However, in a post hoc nonprespecified analysis, infants less than 28 weeks who received air resuscitation had higher mortality during hospital stay (air, 22% versus 100% oxygen, 6%; risk ratio [RR], 3.9; 95% CI, 1.1–13.4; $P = .01$). Although these results should be considered cautiously, the investigators warned about the use of air in extremely low gestational age infants, although it was underscored that the study was underpowered to render this post hoc analysis reliable.[62]

A recent meta-analysis,[63] which included the Torpido trial[62] and other studies that compared outcomes when using higher vs lower $iFiO_2$ in preterm infants in the delivery room, showed no differences in the major outcomes, such as hospital deaths (RR,

0.99; 95% CI, 0.52–1,91), BPD (RR, 0.88; 95% CI, 0.68–11.4), IVH grade greater than or equal to 3 (RR, 0.81; 95% CI, 0.52–1.27), retinopathy of prematurity (ROP) greater than or equal to grade 3 (RR, 0.82; 95% CI, 0.46–1.46), necrotizing enterocolitis Bell stage greater than or equal to 2 (RR, 1.61; 95% CI, 0.77–3.36), or patent ductus arteriosus (PDA) (RR, 0.95; 95% CI, 0.80–1.14). However, babies with lower initial Fio_2 needed more time to achieve the preestablished Spo_2 (**Fig. 4**).

Randomized blinded studies in babies less than or equal to 32 weeks' gestation showed a lower risk of death in the low-Fio_2 groups in which researchers were not involved in Fio_2 manipulation (0.46 [0.23–0.92]; $P = .03$); in contrast, in unmasked studies in which clinicians controlled the Fio_2 in response to Spo_2, the low-oxygen group showed higher mortality (1.94 [1.02–3.68]; $P = .04$).[64] Lui and colleagues[64] published a Cochrane Database Systematic Review to determine the influence on relevant outcomes of lower (Fio_2 >0.4) or higher (Fio_2<0.4) initial inspired oxygen when titrated according to oxygen saturation targets during the stabilization of preterm infants. A total of 10 randomized and nonrandomized eligible trials including 914 infants were identified. Meta-analysis showed no difference in mortality to discharge between lower and higher initial Fio_2 targeted to oxygen saturation (RR, 1.05; 95% CI, 0.68, 1.63). In addition, no differences were found for other outcomes, such as use of intermittent positive pressure ventilation or intubation in the delivery room, ROP, IVH, periventricular leukomalacia, necrotizing enterocolitis, PDA, chronic lung disease, or mortality to

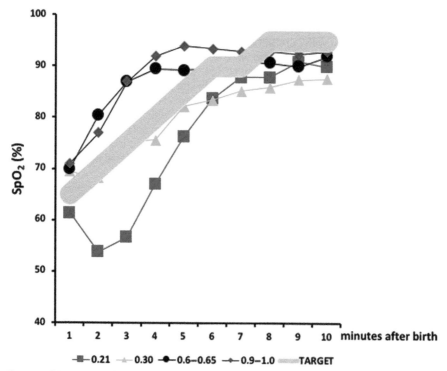

Fig. 4. Achievement of targeted saturations of 80% to 85% at 5 minutes after birth in preterm infants receiving different inspiratory fractions of oxygen in the delivery room. (*From* Oei JL, Vento M, Rabi Y, et al. Higher or lower oxygen for delivery room resuscitation of preterm infants below 28 completed weeks gestation: a meta-analysis. Arch Dis Child Fetal Neonatal Ed 2017;102:F24–F30.)

follow-up. However, the reviewers underscored that the quality of the evidence was very low.[64]

FOLLOW-UP IN PRETERM BABIES STABILIZED WITH HIGHER OR LOWER INITIAL FRACTION OF INSPIRED OXYGEN

Few studies have approached the correlation between the initial Fio_2 used during delivery room stabilization and long-term clinical outcomes of preterm babies (a summary is given in **Table 1**). Boronat and colleagues[65] followed preterm infants less than 32 weeks' gestation enrolled in 2 randomized controlled double-blinded trials and compared outcomes at 24 months postnatal age. A total of 206 (81.4%) babies completed the follow-up. No differences in mortality at hospital discharge or when follow-up was completed were found. The Bayley III scale scores including motor, cognitive, and language composites and neurosensorial handicaps, cerebral palsy, or language skills did not significantly differ.[65] In a retrospective study, Soraisham and colleagues[66] analyzed the database of level III NICUs pertaining to the Canadian Neonatal Network for a 2-year period (2010–2011) and compared the neurodevelopmental outcomes at 18 to 21 months of corrected age of infants born at less than 29 weeks' gestation. During this study period there was no national guideline and each NICU followed local protocols. The investigators compared neurodevelopmental outcomes between infants that received an $iFio_2$ during delivery room stabilization of 0.21, 1.0, or intermediate. The members of the follow-up clinic were unaware of the $iFio_2$ received by the patients. The assessment included Bayley III scales, and the Gross Motor Function Classification System was used to classify the functional impairment in children with cerebral palsy. Visual and hearing impairment were also assessed.[66] The outcomes measured were composite of death or neurodevelopmental impairment (NDI) and death or severe NDI at 18 to 21 months of corrected age. Out of 1509 infants, 445 received room air, 483 received intermediate oxygen concentrations, and 581 received 100% oxygen. Results showed no significant difference in the primary composite outcomes of death or NDI and death or severe NDI at 18 to 21 months. However, the use of pure oxygen was associated with increased odds of severe NDI among survivors compared with room air, and increased incidence of BPD, IVH, or neurologic injury.[66] In a retrospective observational study by Kapadia

Table 1
Follow-up of preterm infants resuscitated with higher or lower inspired fraction of oxygen

Author, Reference	Population	Fio_2	Study Design	Evaluation	Results Between Groups
Boronat et al[65]	≤32 wk GA	0.3 vs 0.6–0.65	RCT, blinded	Bayley III Visual Hearing	No difference
Lui et al[64]	≤29 wk GA	0.21, intermediate, 1.0	Retrospective observational cohort	Bayley III Visual Hearing	No difference
Soraisham et al[66]	≤28 wk GA	0.21 vs 1.0	Retrospective observational cohort	Bayley III Visual Hearing	No difference
Kapadia et al[67]	≤32 wk GA	0.21 vs 1.0	RCT, unblinded	Bayley III Visual Hearing	No difference

Abbreviations: GA, gestational age; RCT, randomized controlled trial.

and colleagues,[67] low-oxygen versus high-oxygen strategy in babies less than or equal to 28 weeks' gestation was compared. Low-oxygen and high-oxygen strategies were defined as initiating the stabilization with an Fio_2 of 0.21 or 1.0 respectively. Oxygen was titrated thereafter according to evolving Spo_2 and heart rate to meet Neonatal Resuscitation Program–recommended transitional target saturations. No difference in mortality was found, but neonates in the low-oxygen group had higher motor composite scores on Bayley III scale (91[85,97] vs 88 [76, 94]; $P<.01$).[67] However, in the Torpido trial,[65] infants less than 28 weeks' gestation randomized to an $iFio_2$ of 0.21 had a higher mortality before hospital discharge (22%) compared with infants given 100% oxygen (6%) (RR, 3.9; 95% CI, 1.1–13.4; $P = .01$). Similarly, the Canadian Neonatal Network in a retrospective cohort study compared severe neurologic injury in infants less than or equal to 27 weeks' gestation in 2 different periods. Before 2006, preterm babies were initially resuscitated with 100% oxygen. Thereafter, the policy changed and babies received less than 100% oxygen that was blended according to $Spo2$.[68] Adjusted OR for the primary outcome of severe neurologic injury or death was significantly higher in the low-oxygen group or room air than in the 100% oxygen group.[68] In addition, NDI at 2 to 3 years of age using Bayley Scales of Development (III) or the Ages and Stages Questionnaire by intention to treat were assessed in 240 children born at less than 32 weeks that had been randomized to room air or 100% oxygen at birth. No differences in death or NDI could be established.[69]

These conflicting results in NICUs with high standards of care represent a conundrum that has not yet been resolved. Hence, although the European studies are more recent, were blinded, and were designed for specifically targeted saturations, the Torpido and the Canadian studies included centers with different oxygenation protocols and no Spo_2 reference ranges. It is plausible that during this transition period, without clear Spo_2 targets, Fio_2 adjustments began to evolve with progressively more clinician experience.[70]

EXPERTS' PROPOSAL FOR INITIAL INSPIRED FRACTION OF OXYGEN AT BIRTH ACCORDING TO GESTATIONAL AGE

Based on these data a recent suggestion by experts (**Table 2**) recommends the use of an initial Fio_2 of 0.3 for preterm infants less than or equal to 28 weeks' gestation, 0.21 to 0.3 Fio_2 and Spo_2 for preterm infants less than or equal to 32 weeks' gestation, and 0.21 for preterm infants from 33 to 36 weeks' gestation and term newborn infants, with the corresponding saturation ranges.[71] Fio_2 should be titrated to achieve a target Spo_2 of 80% to 85% at 5 minutes after complete expulsion of the fetus.

Table 2
Experts' suggestions for the use of oxygen in the delivery room

Gestational Age (wk)	Initial Fio_2	Saturation Target at 5 min[a] (%)	Fio_2 Change
≥37 (term)	0.21	85–90	0.1 × 30 s
≥32; <37	0.21	85	0.1 × 30 s
≥28–31	0.21–0.3	80–85	0.1 × 30 s
<28	0.3	80	0.1 × 30 s
<26	0.3–0.4	80	0.1 × 30 s

[a] Time is considered after the entire fetal body is expelled from the mother.
Data from Thamrin V, Saugstad OD, Tarnow-Mordi W, et al. Preterm infant outcomes after randomization to initial resuscitation with Fio_2 0.21 or 1.0. J Pediatr 2018;201:55–61; with permission.

REFERENCES

1. Vento M, Escobar J, Cernada M, et al. The use and misuse of oxygen during the neonatal period. Clin Perinatol 2012;39:165–76.
2. Davis JM, Auten RL. Maturation of the antioxidant system and the effects on preterm birth. Semin Fetal Neonatal Med 2010;15:191–5.
3. Vento M. Oxygen supplementation in the neonatal period: changing the paradigm. Neonatology 2014;105:323–31.
4. Kapadia VS, Rabi Y, Oei JL. The goldilocks principle. Oxygen in the delivery room: when is it too little, too much, and just right? Semin Fetal Neonatal Med 2018;23(5):347–54.
5. Lorente-Pozo S, Parra-Llorca A, Núñez-Ramiro A, et al. The oxygen load supplied during delivery room stabilization of preterm infants modifies the DNA methylation profile. J Pediatr 2018;202:70–6.e2.
6. Gao Y, Raj JU. Regulation of the pulmonary circulation in the fetus and newborn. Physiol Rev 2010;90:1291–335.
7. Vali P, Lakshminrusimha S. The fetus can teach us: oxygen and the pulmonary vasculature. Children 2017;4:67–78.
8. Schneider H. Oxygenation of the placental-fetal unit in humans. Respir Physiol Neurobiol 2011;178:51–8.
9. Vento M, Aguar M, Escobar J, et al. Antenatal steroids and antioxidant enzyme activity in preterm infants: influence of gender and timing. Antioxid Redox Signal 2009;11:2945–55.
10. Vali P, Mathew B, Lakshminrusimha S. Neonatal resuscitation: evolving strategies. Matern Health Neonatol Perinatol 2015;1:4.
11. Vyas H, Field D, Milner AD, et al. Determinants of the first inspiratory volume and functional residual capacity at birth. Pediatr Pulmonol 1986;2:189–93.
12. Siew ML, Wallace MJ, Kitchen MJ, et al. Inspiration regulates the rate and temporal pattern of lung liquid clearance and lung aeration at birth. J Appl Physiol 2009; 106:1888–95.
13. Hooper SB, Te Pas AB, Kitchen MJ. Respiratory transition in the newborn: a three-phase process. Arch Dis Child Fetal Neonatal Ed 2016;101:F266–71.
14. Storme L, Aubry E, Rakza T, et al, French Congenital Diaphragmatic Hernia Study Group. Pathophysiology of persistent pulmonary hypertension of the newborn: impact of the perinatal environment. Arch Cardiovasc Dis 2013;106:169–77.
15. Sweet D, Carnielli V, Greisen G, et al. European consensus guidelines on the management of respiratory distress syndrome – 2016 update. Neonatology 2017;111:107–25.
16. Frank L, Groseclose EE. Preparation for birth into an O_2-rich environment: the antioxidant enzymes in the developing rabbit lung. Pediatr Res 1984;18:240–4.
17. Frank L, Sosenko IR. Failure of premature rabbits to increase antioxidant enzymes during hyperoxic exposure: increased susceptibility to pulmonary oxygen toxicity compared with term rabbits. Pediatr Res 1991;29:292–6.
18. Sosenko IR, Chen Y, Price LT, et al. Failure of premature rabbits to increase antioxidant enzyme activities after hyperoxic exposure: antioxidant enzyme gene expression and pharmacologic intervention with endotoxin and dexamethasone. Pediatr Res 1995;37:469–75.
19. Viña J, Vento M, García-Sala F, et al. L-cysteine and glutathione metabolism are impaired in premature infants due to cystathionase deficiency. Am J Clin Nutr 1995;61:1067–9.

20. Martín JA, Pereda J, Martínez-López I, et al. Oxidative stress as a signal to up-regulate gamma-cystathionase in the fetal-to-neonatal transition in rats. Cell Mol Biol (Noisy-le-grand) 2007;53(Suppl):OL1010–7.
21. Escobar J, Cubells E, Enomoto M, et al. Prolonging in utero-like oxygenation after birth diminishes oxidative stress in the lung and brain of mice pups. Redox Biol 2013;1:297–303.
22. Pallardo FV, Sastre J, Asensi M, et al. Physiological changes in glutathione metabolism in foetal and newborn rat liver. Biochem J 1991;274:891–3.
23. Sastre J, Asensi M, Rodrigo F, et al. Antioxidant administration to the mother prevents oxidative stress associated with birth in the neonatal rat. Life Sci 1994;54:2055–9.
24. Vento M, Asensi M, Sastre J, et al. Resuscitation with room air instead of 100% oxygen prevents oxidative stress in moderately asphyxiated term neonates. Pediatrics 2001;107:642–7.
25. Vento M, Hummler H, Dawson JA, et al. Use of oxygen in the resuscitation of neonates. In: Dennery PA, Buonocore G, Saugstad OD, editors. Perinatal and prenatal disorders. 1st edition. New York: Springer Science+Business Media; 2014. p. 213–44.
26. Torres-Cuevas I, Parra-Llorca A, Sánchez-Illana A, et al. Oxygen and oxidative stress in the perinatal period. Redox Biol 2017;12:674–81.
27. Cave AC, Brewer AC, Narayanapanicker A, et al. NADPH oxidases in cardiovascular health and disease. Antioxid Redox Signal 2006;8:691–728.
28. Pendyala S, Natarajan V. Redox regulation of Nox proteins. Respir Physiol Neurobiol 2010;175:265–71.
29. Sies H, Berndt C, Jones DP. Oxidative stress. Annu Rev Biochem 2017;86:715–48.
30. Saugstad OD. Resuscitation of newborn infants: from oxygen to room air. Lancet 2010;376:1970–1.
31. Solberg R, Enot D, Deigner HP, et al. Metabolomic analyses of plasma reveals new insights into asphyxia and resuscitation in pigs. PLoS One 2010;5(3):e9606.
32. Chouchani ET, Pell VR, Gaude E, et al. Ischaemic accumulation of succinate controls reperfusion injury through mitochondrial ROS. Nature 2014;515:431–5.
33. Saugstad OD, Sejersted Y, Solberg R, et al. Oxygenation of the newborn: a molecular approach. Neonatology 2012;101:315–25.
34. Saugstad OD, Ramji S, Soll RF, et al. Resuscitation of newborn infants with 21% or 100% oxygen: an updated systematic review and meta-analysis. Neonatology 2008;94(3):176–82.
35. Vento M, Moro M, Escrig R, et al. Preterm resuscitation with low oxygen causes less oxidative stress, inflammation, and chronic lung disease. Pediatrics 2009;124:e439–49.
36. Tataranno ML, Oei JL, Perrone S, et al. Resuscitating preterm infants with 100% oxygen is associated with higher oxidative stress than room air. Acta Paediatr 2015;104:759–65.
37. Kapadia VS, Chalak LF, Sparks JE, et al. Resuscitation of preterm neonates with limited versus high oxygen strategy. Pediatrics 2013;132:e1488–96.
38. Naumburg E, Bellocco R, Cnattingius S, et al. Supplementary oxygen and risk of childhood lymphatic leukaemia. Acta Paediatr 2002;91:1328–33.
39. Spector LG, Klebanoff MA, Feusner JH, et al. Childhood cancer following neonatal oxygen supplementation. J Pediatr 2005;147(1):27–31.
40. Vento M, Saugstad OD. Role of management in the delivery room and beyond the evolution of bronchopulmonary dysplasia. In: Abman SH, editor.

Bronchopulmonary dysplasia. 1st edition. New York: Informa Healthcare USA Inc; 2010. p. 292–313.

41. Dawson JA, Morley CJ. Monitoring oxygen saturation and heart rate in the early neonatal period. Semin Fetal Neonatal Med 2010;15:203–7.

42. Dawson JA, Kamlin CO, Vento M, et al. Defining the reference range for oxygen saturation for infants after birth. Pediatrics 2010;125:e1340–7.

43. Wyckoff MH, Aziz K, Escobedo MB, et al. Part 13: neonatal resuscitation: 2015 American Heart Association guidelines update for cardiopulmonary resuscitation and emergency cardiovascular care. Circulation 2015;132(18 Suppl 2):S543–60.

44. Wilson A, Vento M, Shah PS, et al. A review of international clinical practice guidelines for the use of oxygen in the delivery room resuscitation of preterm infants. Acta Paediatr 2018;107:20–7.

45. Wang H, Liddell CA, Coates MM, et al. Global, regional, and national levels of neonatal, infant, and under-5 mortality during 1990-2013: a systematic analysis for the Global Burden of Disease Study 2013. Lancet 2014;384(9947):957–79.

46. Lehtonen L, Gimeno A, Parra-Llorca A, et al. Early neonatal death: a challenge worldwide. Semin Fetal Neonatal Med 2017;22:153–60.

47. Lawn JE, Blencowe H, Oza S, et al. Every newborn: progress, priorities, and potential beyond survival. Lancet 2014;384(9938):189–205.

48. Office of National Statistics for England and Wales. Gestation specific infant mortality 2013. Office of National Statistics; 2015. Available at: http://www.ons.gov.uk/peoplepopulationandcommunity/healthandsocialcare/causesofdeath/bulletins/pregnancyandethnicfactorsinfluencingbirthsandinfantmortality/. Accessed 14 October, 2015.

49. Shankaran D. Outcomes of hypoxic-ischemic encephalopathy in neonates treated with hypothermia. Clin Perinatol 2014;41:149–59.

50. Ramji S, Ahuja S, Thirupuram S, et al. Resuscitation of asphyxic newborn infants with room air or 100% oxygen. Pediatr Res 1993;34:809–12.

51. Saugstad OD, Rootwelt T, Aalen O. Resuscitation of asphyxiated newborn infants with room air or oxygen: an international controlled trial: the Resair 2 study. Pediatrics 1998;102:e1.

52. Obladen M. History of neonatal resuscitation. Part 2: oxygen and other drugs. Neonatology 2009;95:91–6.

53. Vento M, Asensi M, Sastre J, et al. Oxidative stress in asphyxiated term infants resuscitated with 100% oxygen. J Pediatr 2003;142:240–6.

54. Vento M, Sastre J, Asensi MA, et al. Room-air resuscitation causes less damage to heart and kidney than 100% oxygen. Am J Respir Crit Care Med 2005;172:1393–8.

55. Saugstad OD, Ramji S, Vento M. Resuscitation of depressed newborn infants with ambient air or pure oxygen: a meta-analysis. Biol Neonate 2005;87(1):27–34.

56. Carlo WA, Goudar SS, Jehan I, et al. Newborn-care training and perinatal mortality in developing countries. N Engl J Med 2010;362:614–23.

57. Ariff S, Lee AC, Lawn J, et al. Global burden, epidemiologic trends, and prevention of intrapartum-related deaths in low-resource settings. Clin Perinatol 2016;43:593–608.

58. Lundstrøm KE, Pryds O, Greisen G. Oxygen at birth and prolonged cerebral vasoconstriction in preterm infants. Arch Dis Child 1995;73:F81–6.

59. Wang CL, Anderson C, Leone TA, et al. Resuscitation of preterm neonates by using room air or 100% oxygen. Pediatrics 2008;121:1083–9.

60. Rabi Y, Singhal N, Nettel-Aguirre A. Room-air versus oxygen administration for resuscitation of preterm infants: the ROAR study. Pediatrics 2011;128:e374–81.

61. Escrig R, Arruza L, Izquierdo I, et al. Achievement of targeted saturation values in extremely low gestational age neonates resuscitated with low or high oxygen concentrations: a prospective, randomized trial. Pediatrics 2008;121:875–81.

62. Oei JL, Saugstad OD, Lui K, et al. Targeted oxygen in the resuscitation of preterm infants, a randomized clinical trial. Pediatrics 2017;139:e20161452.

63. Oei JL, Vento M, Rabi Y, et al. Higher or lower oxygen for delivery room resuscitation of preterm infants below 28 completed weeks gestation: a meta-analysis. Arch Dis Child Fetal Neonatal Ed 2017;102:F24–30.

64. Lui K, Jones LJ, Foster JP, et al. Lower versus higher oxygen concentrations titrated to target oxygen saturations during resuscitation of preterm infants at birth. Cochrane Database Syst Rev 2018;(5):CD010239.

65. Boronat N, Aguar M, Rook D, et al. Survival and neurodevelopmental outcomes of preterms resuscitated with different oxygen fractions. Pediatrics 2016;138: e20161405.

66. Soraisham AS, Rabi Y, Shah PS, et al. Neurodevelopmental outcomes of preterm infants resuscitated with different oxygen concentrations at birth. J Perinatol 2017;37:1141–7.

67. Kapadia VS, Lal CV, Kakkilaya V, et al. Impact of the neonatal resuscitation program-recommended low oxygen strategy on outcomes of infants born preterm. J Pediatr 2017;191:35–41.

68. Rabi Y, Lodha A, Soraisham A, et al. Outcomes of preterm infants following the introduction of room air resuscitation. Resuscitation 2015;96:252–9.

69. Thamrin V, Saugstad OD, Tarnow-Mordi W, et al. Preterm infant outcomes after randomization to initial resuscitation with FiO_2 0.21 or 1.0. J Pediatr 2018;201: 55–61.

70. Vento M, Schmoelzer G, Cheung PY, et al. What initial oxygen is best for preterm infants in the delivery room? A response to the 2015 neonatal resuscitation guidelines. Resuscitation 2016;101:e7–8.

71. Saugstad OD, Oei JL, Lakshminrusimha S, et al. Oxygen therapy of the newborn from molecular understanding to clinical practice. Pediatr Res 2019;85(1):20–9.

Newborn Resuscitation in Settings Without Access to Supplemental Oxygen

Vivek Shukla, MD[a], Waldemar A. Carlo, MD[a],*,
Maximo Vento, MD, PhD[b]

KEYWORDS

- Oxygen • Resuscitation • Developing countries • Asphyxia neonatorum
- Adverse effects of oxygen • Oxygen, supply and distribution

KEY POINTS

- Oxygen has been overused in neonatal resuscitation for many years.
- Resuscitation for term neonates should be started with room air and resuscitation for preterm neonates should be started with restrictive oxygen concentration in settings with supplemental oxygen availability.
- Resuscitation efforts in settings without the access to supplemental oxygen should not be curtailed or limited.

INTRODUCTION

Since its discovery more than 2 centuries ago,[1] oxygen has been the most commonly used intervention in neonatal resuscitation and management.[2] Concentrated and hyperbaric oxygen administration was thought to be the key for the treatment of any neonatal respiratory compromise and resultant organ dysfunction as decreased oxygenation was attributed to be the causative factor.[3] In the mid-20th century it was found that positive-pressure ventilation with oxygen was more effective than hyperbaric oxygen in providing stabilization during neonatal resuscitation.[4] Subsequently multiple studies found short- and long-term multisystem organ affection secondary to oxidative damage caused by high oxygen exposure.[5–13] These findings led to studies comparing outcomes of term/late preterm neonates resuscitated with supplemental oxygen versus room air.

Disclosures: W.A. Carlo is on the Board of Mednax.
[a] Division of Neonatology, The University of Alabama at Birmingham, Suite 9380 WIC, 1700 6th Avenue South, Birmingham, AL 35249, USA; [b] Division of Neonatology, University and Polytechnic Hospital La Fe, Avenida Fernando Abril Martorell 106, Valencia 46026, Spain
* Corresponding author.
E-mail address: wcarlo@peds.uab.edu

Clin Perinatol 46 (2019) 475–491
https://doi.org/10.1016/j.clp.2019.05.014
0095-5108/19/© 2019 Elsevier Inc. All rights reserved.

Randomized controlled trials and metaanalyses have reported comparable or better outcomes in term/late preterm infants resuscitated with room air.[14–16] Resuscitation guidelines were modified subsequently to recommend starting resuscitation with room air in term/late preterm neonates whereas restrictive oxygen use with continuous pulse oximetry directed titration of oxygen concentrations was recommended for preterm neonates.[17–19]

HISTORICAL PERSPECTIVE

Since its discovery in early 17th century, oxygen has been a subject of intense attention and fascination by scientists and physicians alike. One of the first demonstrated benefits of oxygen during resuscitation was an increase in the survival of mice exposed to oxygen as compared with air,[20] which led to the notion that oxygen was a miracle molecule; the perfect antidote of hypoxia-related diseases. Chaussier in 1777 used oxygen for the resuscitation of neonates who failed to initiate normal respirations after birth, which led to its use in neonatal resuscitation, intrapartum asphyxia, and other illnesses that were ascribed to a lack of oxygenation.[3,21] Novel delivery methods including intermittent oxygen showers, intragastric oxygen administration, subcutaneous oxygen injections, and bassinet oxygen administration were tried without success.[20] Apnea/periodic breathing, commonly encountered in preterm neonates, was found to be responsive to oxygen therapy.[22] It was noted also that hypoxia could occur without cyanosis subcyanotic anoxia in neonates,[23] which was hypothesized to be a contributor in adverse events. Avoidance of hypoxia was thought to result in improvements in outcomes. These observations were used as a justification for the liberal and prolonged use of oxygen in neonatal resuscitation and several neonatal illnesses. Incubators with new designs that were efficient in maintaining high oxygen concentrations were introduced and widely adopted.[20] In subsequent years, retinopathy of prematurity (then known as retrolental fibroplasia) was identified as a potential complication of oxygen therapy.[1,24] Efforts to limit oxygen exposure were met with an increase in mortality and cerebral palsy. For every single baby in whom retinopathy of prematurity was prevented, there was a 16 times corresponding increase in mortality.[25]

With the advent of pulse oximetry and electrodes for measuring the partial pressure of oxygen in the blood, the focus shifted from targeting the concentration of inspired oxygen to targeting oxygenation. This change in practice resulted in several controlled trials aimed to determine the optimal oxygen saturation targets.[26–29] Even the short periods of hyperoxia encountered during resuscitation may have short- and long-term multisystem consequences.[30] However, several trials and their respective metaanalyses showed improved outcomes in the resuscitation of term and late preterm neonates initiated with room air, but using oxygen as needed.[16,31] The finding of improved outcomes with the initiation of resuscitation with room air rather than oxygen was followed by international recommendations for term/late preterm neonatal resuscitation to begin with room air and titration of Fio_2 to be based on oxygen saturations.[19] Clinical trials suggest that restricted Fio_2 ($Fio_2 = 0.21–0.30$) results in comparable outcomes as compared with liberal Fio_2 ($Fio_2 = 0.60–1$) in preterm neonates,[16,32,33] although the quality of this evidence is limited. Hence, the recommendation for preterm neonatal resuscitation consists of beginning with restricted Fio_2 and titration of Fio_2 based on oxygen saturation.[19] Current efforts are now focusing on enhancing the duration of time spent by neonates in target saturation ranges and optimizing responses to any deviations, starting from resuscitation and continuing during the neonatal period.

EXPERIMENTAL DATA ON SUPPLEMENTAL OXYGEN USE IN NEWBORN RESUSCITATION

Oxygen enjoyed a long and unquestioned status as the mainstay for neonatal resuscitation. The initial research efforts remained focused on improving the delivery rather than its safety and efficacy.[4,34] One of the earliest experiments that compared oxygen and air resuscitation found that positive-pressure ventilation with air had comparable outcomes with that of resuscitation with pure oxygen in a neonatal rabbit hypoxia model.[35] However, given the initial reports of increased mortality and worse neurologic outcomes associated with using restrictive oxygen,[25] resuscitation with air or restrictive Fio_2 was not adopted as a routine. Concerns were raised about the oxygen-induced free radical injury in neonates resuscitated with oxygen in the later part of the 20th century based on the work by McCord and Fridovich[36] and Saugstad and colleagues,[37,38] although oxygen-induced free radical injury was described earlier.[39] Experimental studies showed that there was no significant difference in the stabilization of vitals, normalization of metabolic derangements, or hypoxia-related brain injury in air versus 100% oxygen resuscitation groups.[40]

The results of the experimental findings and corresponding findings in human trials[16,32,33] led to an increased interest in research focusing on the adverse effects associated with high oxygen resuscitation. There has been increasing evidence of severe and persistent adverse effects after resuscitation with 100% oxygen, including increased pulmonary vasoreactivity and pulmonary hypertension,[41,42] organ damage and inflammation,[7,43] an increase in DNA mutations,[44,45] adverse effects on gene regulation and epigenetic changes,[46–49] and childhood cancers.[12,13]

CLINICAL DATA ON SUPPLEMENTAL OXYGEN USE IN NEWBORN RESUSCITATION

The initial trial of room air versus oxygen resuscitation of neonates with asphyxia[14] showed outcomes that did not differ between the 2 groups. This trial generated much interest and was followed by several trials with the similar aim of comparing room air with oxygen resuscitation. All subsequent trials also showed outcomes that did not differ in infants resuscitated with room air or oxygen.[5,15,50–53] The room air versus oxygen resuscitation trials were done in hospitals with backup oxygen availability and 14%[14] to 25%[15] of the neonates who were originally assigned to the room air group also received oxygen. The evidence in support of room air resuscitation led to changes in the recommendations by the World Health Organization in 1998[54] and the Neonatal Resuscitation Program (NRP)/International Liaison Committee on Resuscitation (ILCOR) in 2005[17,55] that room air could be used for neonatal resuscitation. However, these recommendations were not strong and left the decision of room air resuscitation at the discretion of the resuscitation team. A metaanalysis of the air versus oxygen trials in 2008 showed a significant risk reduction for death (risk ratio [RR], 0.69; 95% confidence interval [CI], 0.54–0.88) and a trend toward a reduction in severe hypoxic–ischemic encephalopathy risk (RR, 0.88; 95% CI, 0.72–1.08) in term neonates who received room air resuscitation.[56] These findings were reiterated in subsequent metaanalyses.[32,57] Oxygen saturations for healthy term and late preterm neonates not exposed to supplemental oxygen were documented[58–61] and subsequently used as targets for oxygen supplementation. Recommendations from NRP and ILCOR in 2010 included starting resuscitation of term neonates with room air with titration of the Fio_2 based on oxygen saturation targets.[18,62]

The fetus is in a state of relative hypoxia in utero[63] and the fetus is highly susceptible to fluctuations in maternal oxygenation.[64] The state of oxygen homeostasis in-utero is markedly different to that of the extrauterine survival necessities. After birth the Pao_2 level increases by 3 to 4 times of the in utero Pao_2 levels and the SpO_2, which is approximately 60% in utero[65] reaches greater than 85% in about 5 to 10 minutes in term neonates and 10 to 15 minutes in preterm neonates.[66] Increase in oxygen saturations after birth is inversely related to the gestational age in neonates who are not exposed to supplemental oxygen.[67] Oxygen saturation changes in healthy term neonates immediately after birth are well-documented.[58-61] However, given the difficulties in determining gestational age–specific oxygen saturation changes, ideal oxygen saturation targets in preterm neonates remain unclear. A recent metaanalysis of trials of resuscitation of preterm neonates with higher versus lower oxygen concentration has shown that an SpO_2 of less than 80% at 5 minutes was associated with higher risk of major intravascular hemorrhage (odds ratio [OR], 2.04; 95% CI, 1.01–4.11; $P<.05$) and death (OR 4.57; 95% CI, 1.62–13.98; $P<.05$).[68] So, term neonatal saturation targets ($SpO_2 > 80\%$ at 5 minutes) are adhered to in preterm neonatal resuscitation as well.[19,69]

The data regarding preterm neonatal resuscitation with room air are not as robust particularly. However, several trials comparing restrictive oxygen resuscitation (Fio_2 <0.30) versus liberal oxygen resuscitation (Fio_2 >0.65) reported no clear survival or morbidity benefits of restrictive oxygen for resuscitation.[11,70-74] The Fio_2 was quickly turned down to low Fio_2 ranges for most of the preterm neonates that were allocated to high oxygen groups using titration of oxygen based on saturation targets for term neonates. NRP and ILCOR (2015)[19,69] recommended that neonatal resuscitation should be initiated with room air in term and late preterm (>35 weeks gestation) using neonatal preductal saturation targets to guide the titration of supplemental oxygen as needed. For the resuscitation of preterm neonates (<35 weeks gestation), NRP and ILCOR (2015)[19,69] recommended to start resuscitation with restrictive oxygen ($Fio_2 = 0.21–0.30$) in the resuscitation of preterm neonates (<35 weeks gestation) and to use healthy term neonatal preductal saturation targets to guide the titration of supplemental oxygen as needed.

ROOM AIR RESUSCITATION TRIALS IN LOW- AND MIDDLE-INCOME COUNTRIES

The room air versus 100% oxygen resuscitation trials have shown the effectiveness and safety of room air resuscitation in low- and middle-income countries.[14,15,52,53] Room air resuscitation has been readily accepted and adopted in low- and middle-income countries based on data from randomized controlled trials and metaanalyses, but room air resuscitation has long been practiced in low- and middle-income countries because of limited resources.[75]

CLINICAL DATA ON NEWBORN RESUSCITATION IN LOW-RESOURCE SETTINGS WITHOUT SUPPLEMENTAL OXYGEN

The neonatal period (birth to 28 days) is the period in life with the highest risk for mortality. Neonatal mortality contributes to 40% of global annual mortality in 0- to 14-year age group and 47% of global annual mortality among those less than 5 years of age.[76] The average global neonatal mortality rate was 18 per 1000 live births in 2017 with a total of 2.5 million neonatal deaths in 2017. One million deaths occur on the day of birth globally.[77] Also, there are about 2.6 million stillbirths[78,79] with one-half of the deaths estimated to be occurring intrapartum.[80] Additionally, a large number of neonatal deaths are misclassified as fresh stillbirths.[81,82]

Estimates suggest that about 98% of all neonatal and perinatal deaths occur in low- and middle-income countries.[83] Global data show that neonatal mortality is about 52 times higher in low- and middle-income countries as compared with high-income countries.[84] Early neonatal death (0–7 days; 73%) and especially death within the first 12 hours (40.4%) after birth represents a substantial proportion of deaths in the neonatal period and has relatively increased in proportion to the mortality among those less than 5 years of age in recent decades.[85] The inability of initiating and continuing spontaneous respirations at birth, which is the underlying issue in a majority of neonatal deaths at fewer than 12 hours after birth is one of the foremost causes of perinatal mortality and subsequent hypoxia-related neurologic issues.[86–88] Because about 10% of all neonates need some degree of resuscitation for initiating and continuing spontaneous respirations, this finding indicates that about 13 million babies born each year need resuscitation.[84] Approximately 3 to 6 million neonates out of 13 million babies who require resuscitation each year globally need ventilation to initiate respirations.[89] Neonates who need ventilation to establish normal breathing contribute disproportionally to the global neonatal mortality burden, especially in low- and middle-income countries.[75]

Neonatal resuscitation in low- and middle-income countries poses a unique set of challenges.[84] Major factors contributing to high neonatal mortality in low- and middle-income countries include high rates of home births, a lack of trained birth attendants, and failure to provide prompt and effective basic neonatal resuscitation at birth.[84,90,91] It is estimated that about 60 million births occur outside health facilities (mainly at home) with rates of home births as high as 50% to 90% in some low- and middle-income countries.[84,92] Of those 60 million births, about 52 million are born without the presence of trained birth attendants.[93,94] The availability of trained birth attendants at birth is as low as 33% in some settings.[93,95] In addition, health care facilities are also poorly equipped and lack personnel trained in neonatal resuscitation.[84] The analysis of the hospital and health clinics where births were conducted in the First Breath trial showed that about 30% to 40% of the hospitals and 70% to 92% clinics lack oxygen supply.[77,96] The availability of neonatal resuscitation trained personals in birthing hospitals was only 2% to 12% in a national service provision assessment survey in 6 African countries, and resuscitation equipment, including that for respiratory support, was available in only 8% to 22% of the facilities.[86]

The delivery of prompt and optimal basic neonatal resuscitation is undeniably one of the foremost interventions to improve perinatal mortality in low- and middle-income countries.[26,97–103] In an observational study to determine the effect of basic neonatal resuscitation on outcomes, it was found that most of the neonates who required resuscitation were having primary apnea (94%). Of those neonates with primary apnea, about 50% responded to suction/stimulation and an additional 44% responded to simple bag and mask ventilation. The risk for death or prolonged admission was found to increase 16% for every 30-second delay in initiating bag and mask ventilation.[104] The finding of increasing death with delay in resuscitation indicates the importance of timely and prompt basic neonatal resuscitation.

SCALE UP OF NEONATAL RESUSCITATION WITH ROOM AIR IN LOW-RESOURCE SETTINGS

The scale up of neonatal resuscitation in low-resource settings has been done largely with room air resuscitation (**Table 1**). Large-scale studies on neonatal resuscitation and essential newborn care (ENC; which includes basic resuscitation) have shown the effectiveness of basic neonatal resuscitation. In a large (N = 71,689

Table 1
Major implementation trials of neonatal resuscitation from low- and middle-income countries with low-resource settings predominantly lacking oxygen availability

Sr. No	First Author, Year	N	Study Setting and Location	Study Design	Study Intervention	O$_2$ Availability
1	Carlo et al,[26] 2010	71,689	18 low-risk first level urban health centers in Zambia	Pre–post essential newborn care and followed by NRP	ENC followed by NRP	No O$_2$ available
2	Carlo et al,[97] 2010	120,009	Hospitals, clinics, and home in Argentina, Democratic Republic of Congo, Guatemala, India, Pakistan, and Zambia	Pre–post for ENC and followed by cluster RCT for NRP	ENC training followed by basic NRP training	>60% of births across all groups were at home where there was no O$_2$ available
3	Goudar et al,[105] 2012	24,870	Hospitals, clinics, and home in India	Pre–post for ENC and followed by cluster RCT for NRP	ENC training followed by basic NRP training	O$_2$ available in hospital, not at home; only 0.2% of total received O$_2$
4	Matendo et al,[106] 2011	13,595	Hospitals clinic and home in Democratic republic of Congo	Pre–post for ENC and followed by cluster RCT for NRP	ENC training followed by basic NRP training	No O$_2$ available
5	Carlo et al,[107] 2010	1096 VLBW neonates	Hospital, clinics, and home in Argentina, Democratic Republic of Congo, Guatemala, India, Pakistan, and Zambia	Pre–post for ENC and followed by cluster RCT for NRP	ENC training followed by basic NRP training	>50% of births across all groups were at home where there was no O$_2$ available
6	Msemo et al,[101] 2013	86,624	Unclear setting in Tanzania	Pre–post HBB	HBB training	Unclear, but likely no as HBB does not include O$_2$
7	Bellad et al,[108] 2016	70,704	Hospital and home in India and Kenya	Pre–post HBB	HBB training	Unclear, but likely no as HBB does not include O$_2$
8	Goudar et al,[109] 2013	9598	Clinics, hospital, and home in India	Pre–post HBB	HBB training	Unclear, but likely no as HBB does not include O$_2$
9	Bang et al,[110] 1999	10,191	Home in India	Intervention control	Home based neonatal care training	No O$_2$ available
10	Gill et al,[111] 2011	3497	Home in Zambia	Cluster RCT	Basic neonatal resuscitation and care training with facilitated referral	No O$_2$ available

Abbreviations: ENC, essential newborn care; HBB, helping babies breathe; RCT, randomized, controlled trial; VLBW, very low birth weight.

neonates) multicenter interventional study of basic neonatal resuscitation training of midwives and implementation in health clinics, early (7-day) neonatal mortality was decreased from 11.5 in 1000 live births to 6.8 in 1000 after basic neonatal resuscitation implementation (P<.001).[26] Because of the loss to follow-up of the highest risk infants (in part owing to early neonatal deaths), statistical modeling was used to developed the best estimates of the effect on deaths. Early neonatal mortality was estimated to be 36.2 in 1000 live births during the baseline period and decreased to 25.1 in 1000 after ENC training and to 15.9 in 1000 after further resuscitation training. Oxygen was not available in the health clinics where this study was conducted (**Fig. 1**).

In a large (N = 120,009 births; birthweight >1500 g) multicountry study (the First Breath trial) that tested ENC training (including basic neonatal resuscitation) with an active baseline before and after design, birth attendants were trained in ENC (including basic neonatal resuscitation) from rural communities from 6 countries (Argentina, Democratic Republic of Congo, Guatemala, India, Pakistan, and Zambia).[97] This was followed by a cluster randomized controlled trial of training the birth attendants from the same settings (except in Argentina) in a modified version of the NRP by American Academy of Pediatrics (including in-depth basic neonatal resuscitation). In this study most of the deliveries were home deliveries and there was no access to supplemental oxygen in the home settings. After implementation of ENC, there was a large reduction in the stillbirth rate (RR, 0.69; 95% CI, 0.54–0.88; P<.01). In the post NRP period there was no further significant decrease in mortality in clusters randomized to NRP training as compared with control clusters, although trends in reduction continued. The result of this study indicates that a large number of neonates who were stillborn before implementation of ENC could be effectively resuscitated and survive by the implementation of basic resuscitation techniques. The findings of no improvement in perinatal mortality after the implementation of NRP in a setting where ENC was introduced previously suggests that ENC (basic resuscitation without oxygen availability) was very effective as implemented in these low-resource settings.[97]

A subgroup (n = 24,870) analysis of the First Breath trial[97] for data from India[105] showed a significant decrease in stillbirth rate (RR, 0.62; 95% CI, 0.46–0.83) and perinatal mortality (RR, 0.69; 95% CI, 0.53–0.90) after implementation of ENC but

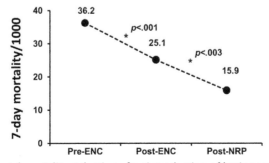

Fig. 1. Early neonatal mortality reduction after introduction of basic neonatal resuscitation at low-risk first-level community health centers in Zambia. (*From* Travers CP, Carlo WA. How to save 1 million lives in a year in low- and middle-income countries. Neonatology 2017;111(4):431–436. https://doi.org/10.1159/000460512. Epub 2017 May 25; with permission.)

no further reductions in stillbirth rate (RR, 1.31; 95% CI, 0.88–1.95) or perinatal mortality (RR, 1.10; 95% CI, 0.87–1.39) was found after NRP implementation. A subgroup (n = 13,595) analysis of First Breath trial data from the Democratic Republic of Congo[106] showed that initially there was no difference in the before and after ENC outcomes for perinatal (RR, 0.99; 95% CI, 0.77–1.27) and neonatal mortality (RR, 1.03; 95% CI–0.76,1.41) but after a period of use and reinforcement there was a significant decrease in perinatal (RR, 0.80; 95% CI, 0.66–0.97) and neonatal mortality (RR, 0.60; 95% CI, 0.39–0.93). Additional analysis of neonates with a birthweight of less than 1500 g (n = 1096) who were not included in the main trial because of requirements for advanced care showed no statistically significant difference in stillbirth rate, neonatal mortality, or perinatal mortality with either ENC or NRP introduction.[107]

In a large before and after study (N = 86,624)[101] to assess the impact of implementation of Helping Babies Breathe, which includes basic neonatal resuscitation, neonatal mortality (RR, = 0.53; 95% CI, 0.43–0.65; $P \leq .0001$) and stillbirth (RR, 0.76; 95% CI, 0.64–0.90; $P = .001$) rates were decreased. In a similar large before and after design trial (N = 70,704),[108] Helping Babies Breathe resulted in modest reductions in fresh stillbirth (11.0 vs 9.4/1000 births; $P = .17$), perinatal mortality (23.9 vs 22.9/1000 births; $P = .92$), and neonatal mortality (12.9 vs 13.6/1000 births; $P = .18$). In a relatively smaller study of similar before and after study design,[109] Helping Babies Breathe decreased stillbirths (OR, 0.76; 95% CI, 0.59–0.98) and fresh stillbirths (OR, 0.54; 95% CI, 0.37–0.78).

In a small (N = 10,191) home-based study, implementation of basic neonatal resuscitation with room air was associated with a 62.2% ($P<.001$) and 71% ($P<.001$) decease in neonatal and perinatal mortalities, respectively.[110] In a small cluster randomized design study (N = 3497) of training traditional birth attendants in neonatal resuscitation, neonatal mortality (RR, 0.55; 95% CI, 0.33–0.90) and birth asphyxia-related deaths (RR, 0.37; 95% CI, 0.17–0.81) were reduced.[111] All of these studies were done in low- and middle-income countries[26,97,101,105–111] and were done exclusively or largely in low-resource settings without the availability of supplemental oxygen.

A metaanalysis and systematic review of trials evaluating basic neonatal resuscitation implementation have also shown significant decreases in fresh stillbirths (RR, 0.74; 95% CI, 0.61–0.90), neonatal mortality (RR, 0.58%; 95% CI, 0.42–0.82), and perinatal mortality (RR, 0.82%; 95% CI, 0.74–0.91; **Fig. 2**).[112] It should be noted that, owing to the ethical challenges associated with undertaking randomized control trials for an intervention such as neonatal resuscitation, most of the studies on the subject have been observational or quasirandomized.

Focus should be directed to increase capacity for prompt and adequate basic neonatal resuscitation because the majority of the perinatal deaths in low-resource settings could be averted with the provision of basic resuscitation, which does not require expertise in advanced resuscitation and expensive equipment.[84] Advanced neonatal resuscitation (resuscitation involving intubation, medications or chest compressions) is necessary for only around 0.2% of all the neonates or 2.0% of neonates who do not establish spontaneous respirations at birth.[99,113] Thus, even in the face of resource limitation, it is possible to reduce neonatal mortality in health care facilities and even in the community through adherence and implementation of basic neonatal resuscitation.[84,101,114] Prompt transfer to a referral health care center with the availability of mechanical ventilation and other advanced life support modalities in resource-limited countries should be available after resuscitation for those neonates who require continued support.

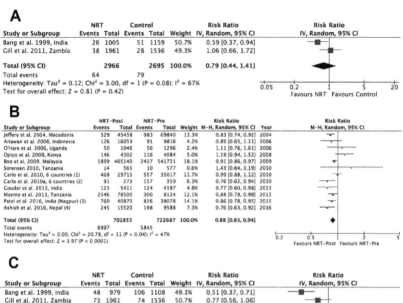

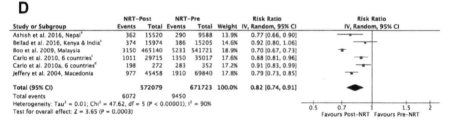

Fig. 2. (*A*) Neonatal resuscitation trials with intervention and control group. Forest plot comparing all SB between the NRT and the control groups. (*B*) Stillbirth. Neonatal resuscitation trials with pre–post implementation designs. Forest plot comparing all SB between the post-NRT and the pre-NRT groups. [a] Carlo et al. 2010. [b] Carlo et al. 2010. Data for very low birth weight infants. [c] Unpublished data obtained via personnel communication. [d] Unpublished data obtained via personnel communication. (*C*) Perinatal mortality. Neonatal resuscitation trials with intervention and control group. Forest plot comparing perinatal mortality between the NRT and the control groups. (*D*) Perinatal mortality. Neonatal resuscitation trials with pre-post implementation design. Forest plot comparing perinatal mortality between the post-NRT and the pre-NRT groups. [a] Unpublished data obtained via personnel communication. [b] Data for 2 sites: Kenya and India (Belgaum). [c] Carlo et al. 2010. [d] Carlo et al. 2010. Data for very low birth weight infants. (*E*) Early (0–7 days) neonatal mortality. Neonatal resuscitation trials with intervention and control group. Forest plot comparing all SB between the NRT and the control groups. (*F*) Early (0–7 days) neonatal mortality. Neonatal resuscitation trials with pre–post implementation designs. Forest plot comparing 7-day neonatal mortality between the post-NRT and the pre-NRT groups. [a] Data for 2 sites: Kenya and India (Belgaum). [b] Carlo et al. 2010. [c] Carlo et al. 2010. Data for very low birth weight infants. NRT, neonatal resuscitation training; SB, stillbirths. ([*A–F*] *From* Patel A, Khatib MN, Kurhe K, et al. Impact of neonatal resuscitation trainings on neonatal and perinatal mortality: a systematic review and meta-analysis. From BMJ Paediatr Open 2017 Nov 16;1(1):e000183. https://doi.org/10.1136/bmjpo-2017-000183. eCollection 2017.)

E

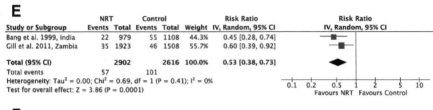

F

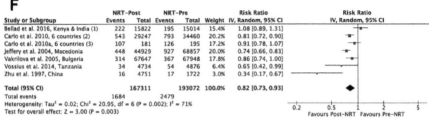

Fig. 2. (*continued*)

SUMMARY

Experimental and clinical studies have shown the effectiveness of stimulation and ventilation (lung expansion) with room air in newborn resuscitation. Therefore, resuscitation efforts in low-resource settings without the access to supplemental oxygen should not be curtailed or limited. Provision of effective and prompt resuscitation is the mainstay and is a key for reducing global neonatal mortality. Efforts should be made to improve training of neonatal resuscitation providers and health care facilities for the care of neonates requiring basic resuscitation including room air resuscitation. Neonatal resuscitation has the potential to reduce substantially fresh stillbirths and neonatal deaths.

Best Practices

What is the current practice for neonatal resuscitation in settings without access to supplemental oxygen?

Provision of effective and prompt resuscitation is key for reducing global neonatal mortality. Neonatal resuscitation has the potential to substantially reduce fresh stillbirths.

Efforts should be made to improve training of neonatal resuscitation providers and health care facilities for the care of neonates requiring basic resuscitation.

Resuscitation initiated with room air is the currently recommended practice worldwide.

Resuscitation efforts in settings without the access to supplemental oxygen should not be curtailed or limited.

What changes in current practice are likely to improve outcomes?

Resuscitation should be initiated in all newborns in whom it is indicated even when supplemental oxygen is not available.

Major recommendations

In low-resource settings, resuscitation at birth using room air is effective and should be provided when indicated as part of packages of interventions such as Helping Babies Breathe and Essential Newborn Care

Rating for the Strength of the Evidence

Bibliographic Source(s): This is important list current sources relevant to evidence.

Data from Refs.[31,97,115]

REFERENCES

1. Richmond S, Goldsmith JP. Refining the role of oxygen administration during delivery room resuscitation: what are the future goals? Semin Fetal Neonatal Med 2008;13(6):368–74.
2. Saugstad OD, Aune D. Optimal oxygenation of extremely low birth weight infants: a meta-analysis and systematic review of the oxygen saturation target studies. Neonatology 2014;105(1):55–63.
3. Kapadia V, Rabi Y, Oei JL. The Goldilocks principle. Oxygen in the delivery room: when is it too little, too much, and just right? Semin Fetal Neonatal Med 2018;23(5):347–54.
4. Cross K, Dawes G, Hyman A, et al. Hyperbaric oxygen and intermittent positive-pressure ventilation in resuscitation of asphyxiated newborn rabbits. Lancet 1964;284(7359):560–2.
5. Vento M, Sastre J, Asensi MA, et al. Room-air resuscitation causes less damage to heart and kidney than 100% oxygen. Am J Respir Crit Care Med 2005; 172(11):1393–8.
6. Kapadia VS, Chalak LF, DuPont TL, et al. Perinatal asphyxia with hyperoxemia within the first hour of life is associated with moderate to severe hypoxic-ischemic encephalopathy. J Pediatr 2013;163(4):949–54.
7. Koch JD, Miles DK, Gilley JA, et al. Brief exposure to hyperoxia depletes the glial progenitor pool and impairs functional recovery after hypoxic-ischemic brain injury. J Cereb Blood Flow Metab 2008;28(7):1294–306.
8. Munkeby BH, Borke WB, Bjornland K, et al. Resuscitation with 100% O2 increases cerebral injury in hypoxemic piglets. Pediatr Res 2004;56(5):783–90.
9. Vereczki V, Martin E, Rosenthal RE, et al. Normoxic resuscitation after cardiac arrest protects against hippocampal oxidative stress, metabolic dysfunction, and neuronal death. J Cereb Blood Flow Metab 2006;26(6):821–35.
10. Kapadia VS, Lal CV, Kakkilaya V, et al. Impact of the Neonatal Resuscitation Program-recommended low oxygen strategy on outcomes of infants born preterm. J Pediatr 2017;191:35–41.
11. Vento M, Moro M, Escrig R, et al. Preterm resuscitation with low oxygen causes less oxidative stress, inflammation, and chronic lung disease. Pediatrics 2009; 124(3):e439–49.
12. Naumburg E, Bellocco R, Cnattingius S, et al. Supplementary oxygen and risk of childhood lymphatic leukaemia. Acta Paediatr 2002;91(12):1328–33.
13. Spector LG, Klebanoff MA, Feusner JH, et al. Childhood cancer following neonatal oxygen supplementation. J Pediatr 2005;147(1):27–31.
14. Ramji S, Ahuja S, Thirupuram S, et al. Resuscitation of asphyxic newborn infants with room air or 100% oxygen. Pediatr Res 1993;34(6):809.
15. Saugstad OD, Rootwelt T, Aalen O. Resuscitation of asphyxiated newborn infants with room air or oxygen: an international controlled trial: the Resair 2 study. Pediatrics 1998;102(1):e1.
16. Tan A, Schulze A, O'Donnell CP, et al. Air versus oxygen for resuscitation of infants at birth. Cochrane Database Syst Rev 2005;(2):CD002273.
17. International Liaison Committee on Resuscitation. 2005 International consensus on cardiopulmonary resuscitation and emergency cardiovascular care science with treatment recommendations. Part 7: neonatal resuscitation. Resuscitation 2005;67(2–3):293–303.
18. Wyllie J, Perlman JM, Kattwinkel J, et al. Part 11: neonatal resuscitation: 2010 international consensus on cardiopulmonary resuscitation and emergency

cardiovascular care science with treatment recommendations. Resuscitation 2010;81(Suppl 1):e260–87.

19. Wyllie J, Perlman JM, Kattwinkel J, et al. Part 7: neonatal resuscitation: 2015 international consensus on cardiopulmonary resuscitation and emergency cardiovascular care science with treatment recommendations. Resuscitation 2015;95: e169–201.

20. Silverman WA. A cautionary tale about supplemental oxygen: the albatross of neonatal medicine. Pediatrics 2004;113(2):394–6.

21. Saugstad O. Oxygen supplementation in the newborn period: do we know the consequences?. Yearbook of Neonatal and Perinatal Medicine. Chicago: Year Book Medical Publishers; 2002.

22. Wilson JL, Long SB, Howard PJ. Respiration of premature infants: response to variations of oxygen and to increased carbon dioxide in inspired air. Am J Dis Child 1942;63(6):1080–5.

23. Smith CA, Kaplan E. Adjustment of blood oxygen levels in neonatal life. Am J Dis Child 1942;64(5):843–59.

24. Kinsey VE, Hemphill F. Etiology of retrolental fibroplasia: preliminary report of a cooperative study of retrolental fibroplasia. Am J Ophthalmol 1955;40(2):166–74.

25. Bolton D, Cross K. Further observations on cost of preventing retrolental fibroplasia. Lancet 1974;303(7855):445–8.

26. Carlo WA, McClure EM, Chomba E, et al. Newborn care training of midwives and neonatal and perinatal mortality rates in a developing country. Pediatrics 2010;126(5):e1064–71.

27. Schmidt B, Whyte RK, Asztalos EV, et al. Effects of targeting higher vs lower arterial oxygen saturations on death or disability in extremely preterm infants: a randomized clinical trial. JAMA 2013;309(20):2111–20.

28. Tarnow-Mordi W, Stenson B, Kirby A, et al. Outcomes of two trials of oxygen-saturation targets in preterm infants. N Engl J Med 2016;374(8):749–60.

29. Askie LM, Darlow BA, Finer N, et al. Association between oxygen saturation targeting and death or disability in extremely preterm infants in the neonatal oxygenation prospective meta-analysis collaboration. JAMA 2018;319(21): 2190–201.

30. van der Walt J. Oxygen - elixir of life or Trojan horse? Part 1: oxygen and neonatal resuscitation. Paediatr Anaesth 2006;16(11):1107–11.

31. Rabi Y, Rabi D, Yee W. Room air resuscitation of the depressed newborn: a systematic review and meta-analysis. Resuscitation 2007;72(3):353–63.

32. Lui K, Jones LJ, Foster JP, et al. Lower versus higher oxygen concentrations titrated to target oxygen saturations during resuscitation of preterm infants at birth. Cochrane Database Syst Rev 2018;(5):CD010239.

33. Oei JL, Vento M, Rabi Y, et al. Higher or lower oxygen for delivery room resuscitation of preterm infants below 28 completed weeks gestation: a meta-analysis. Arch Dis Child Fetal Neonatal Ed 2017;102(1):F24–30.

34. Hutchison J, Kerr M, Williams K, et al. Hyperbaric oxygen in the resuscitation of the newborn. Surv Anesthesiol 1964;8(6):600–1.

35. Campbell A, Cross K, Dawes G, et al. A comparison of air and O2, in a hyperbaric chamber or by positive pressure ventilation, in the resuscitation of newborn rabbits. J Pediatr 1966;68(2):153–63.

36. McCord JM, Fridovich I. The reduction of cytochrome c by milk xanthine oxidase. J Biol Chem 1968;243(21):5753–60.

37. Saugstad OD. Hypoxanthine as a measurement of hypoxia. Pediatr Res 1975; 9(4):158.

38. Saugstad O, Aasen A. Plasma hypoxanthine concentrations in pigs. Eur Surg Res 1980;12(2):123–9.
39. Gerschman R, Gilbert DL, Nye SW, et al. Oxygen poisoning and x-irradiation: a mechanism in common. Science 1954;119(3097):623–6.
40. Rootwelt T, Løberg EM, Moen A, et al. Hypoxemia and reoxygenation with 21% or 100% oxygen in newborn pigs: changes in blood pressure, base deficit, and hypoxanthine and brain morphology. Pediatr Res 1992;32(1):107.
41. Patel A, Lakshminrusimha S, Ryan RM, et al. Exposure to supplemental oxygen downregulates antioxidant enzymes and increases pulmonary arterial contractility in premature lambs. Neonatology 2009;96(3):182–92.
42. Lakshminrusimha S, Russell JA, Steinhorn RH, et al. Pulmonary arterial contractility in neonatal lambs increases with 100% oxygen resuscitation. Pediatr Res 2006;59(1):137.
43. Munkeby BH, Børke WB, Bjørnland K, et al. Resuscitation of hypoxic piglets with 100% O 2 increases pulmonary metalloproteinases and IL-8. Pediatr Res 2005; 58(3):542.
44. Sejersted Y, Aasland AL, Bjørås M, et al. Accumulation of 8-oxoguanine in liver DNA during hyperoxic resuscitation of newborn mice. Pediatr Res 2009; 66(5):533.
45. Solberg R, Andresen JH, Escrig R, et al. Resuscitation of hypoxic newborn piglets with oxygen induces a dose-dependent increase in markers of oxidation. Pediatr Res 2007;62(5):559.
46. Tyree MM, Dalgard C, O'Neill JT. Impact of room air resuscitation on early growth response gene-1 in a neonatal piglet model of cerebral hypoxic ischemia. Pediatr Res 2006;59(3):423.
47. Wollen EJ, Sejersted Y, Wright MS, et al. Transcriptome profiling of the newborn mouse lung after hypoxia and reoxygenation: hyperoxic reoxygenation affects mTOR signaling pathway, DNA repair, and JNK-pathway regulation. Pediatr Res 2013;74(5):536.
48. Rognlien AGW, Wollen EJ, Atneosen-Åsegg M, et al. Temporal patterns of gene expression profiles in the neonatal mouse lung after hypoxia-reoxygenation. Neonatology 2017;111(1):45–54.
49. Chen C-M, Liu Y-C, Chen Y-J, et al. Genome-wide analysis of DNA methylation in hyperoxia-exposed newborn rat lung. Lung 2017;195(5):661–9.
50. Vento M, Asensi M, Sastre J, et al. Six years of experience with the use of room air for the resuscitation of asphyxiated newly born term infants. Biol Neonate 2001;79(3–4):261–7.
51. Vento M, Asensi M, Sastre J, et al. Oxidative stress in asphyxiated term infants resuscitated with 100% oxygen. J Pediatr 2003;142(3):240–6.
52. Ramji S, Rasaily R, Mishra P, et al. Resuscitation of asphyxiated newborns with room air or 100% oxygen at birth: a multicentric clinical trial. Indian Pediatr 2003; 40(6):510–7.
53. Bajaj N, Udani RH, Nanavati RN. Room air vs. 100 per cent oxygen for neonatal resuscitation: a controlled clinical trial. J Trop Pediatr 2005;51(4):206–11.
54. World Health Organization. Basic newborn resuscitation: a practical guide. Geneva (Switzerland): World Health Organization; 1998.
55. American Heart Association, American Academy of Pediatrics. 2005 American Heart Association (AHA) guidelines for cardiopulmonary resuscitation (CPR) and emergency cardiovascular care (ECC) of pediatric and neonatal patients: neonatal resuscitation guidelines. Pediatrics 2006;117(5):e1029–38.

56. Saugstad OD, Ramji S, Soll RF, et al. Resuscitation of newborn infants with 21% or 100% oxygen: an updated systematic review and meta-analysis. Neonatology 2008;94(3):176–82.

57. Brown JV, Moe-Byrne T, Harden M, et al. Lower versus higher oxygen concentration for delivery room stabilisation of preterm neonates: systematic review. PLoS One 2012;7(12):e52033.

58. Harris AP, Sendak MJ, Donham RT. Changes in arterial oxygen saturation immediately after birth in the human neonate. J Pediatr 1986;109(1):117–9.

59. Reddy VK, Holzman IR, Wedgwood JF. Pulse oximetry saturations in the first 6 hours of life in normal term infants. Clin Pediatr (Phila) 1999;38(2):87–92.

60. Toth B, Becker A, Seelbach-Göbel B. Oxygen saturation in healthy newborn infants immediately after birth measured by pulse oximetry. Arch Gynecol Obstet 2002;266(2):105–7.

61. Altuncu E, Özek E, Bilgen H, et al. Percentiles of oxygen saturations in healthy term newborns in the first minutes of life. Eur J Pediatr 2008;167(6):687–8.

62. Kattwinkel J. Neonatal resuscitation: 2010 American Heart Association Guidelines for cardiopulmonary resuscitation and emergency cardiovascular care.(vol 126, pg e1400, 2010). Pediatrics 2011;128(1):176.

63. Gao Y, Raj JU. Regulation of the pulmonary circulation in the fetus and newborn. Physiol Rev 2010;90(4):1291–335.

64. Khaw K, Ngan Kee W, Chu C, et al. Effects of different inspired oxygen fractions on lipid peroxidation during general anaesthesia for elective Caesarean section. Br J Anaesth 2010;105(3):355–60.

65. Vento M, Aguar M, Brugada M, et al. Oxygen saturation targets for preterm infants in the delivery room. J Matern Fetal Neonatal Med 2012;25(sup1):45–6.

66. Vento M, Aguar M, Escobar J, et al. Antenatal steroids and antioxidant enzyme activity in preterm infants: influence of gender and timing. Antioxid Redox Signal 2009;11(12):2945–55.

67. Vento M, Saugstad O. Role of management in the delivery room and beyond in the evolution of bronchopulmonary dysplasia. In: Abman SH, editor. Bronchopulmonary dysplasia. New York: Informa Healthcare USA Inc; 2010. p. 292–313.

68. Oei JL, Finer NN, Saugstad OD, et al. Outcomes of oxygen saturation targeting during delivery room stabilisation of preterm infants. Arch Dis Child Fetal Neonatal Ed 2018;103(5):F446–54.

69. Wyckoff MH, Aziz K, Escobedo MB, et al. Part 13: neonatal resuscitation: 2015 American Heart Association guidelines update for cardiopulmonary resuscitation and emergency cardiovascular care. Circulation 2015;132(18 suppl 2):S543–60.

70. Armanian AM, Badiee Z. Resuscitation of preterm newborns with low concentration oxygen versus high concentration oxygen. J Res Pharm Pract 2012;1(1):25.

71. Kapadia VS, Chalak LF, Sparks JE, et al. Resuscitation of preterm neonates with limited versus high oxygen strategy. Pediatrics 2013;132(6):e1488–96.

72. Rabi Y, Singhal N, Nettel-Aguirre A. Room-air versus oxygen administration for resuscitation of preterm infants: the ROAR study. Pediatrics 2011;128(2):e374–81.

73. Rook D, Schierbeek H, Vento M, et al. Resuscitation of preterm infants with different inspired oxygen fractions. J Pediatr 2014;164(6):1322–6.e3.

74. Wang CL, Anderson C, Leone TA, et al. Resuscitation of preterm neonates by using room air or 100% oxygen. Pediatrics 2008;121(6):1083–9.

75. Berkelhamer SK, Kamath-Rayne BD, Niermeyer S. Neonatal resuscitation in low-resource settings. Clin Perinatol 2016;43(3):573–91.

76. Levels and trends in child mortality: UN Inter-agency group for child mortality estimation; 2018 [1-48]. Available at: https://data.unicef.org/wp-content/uploads/2018/10/Child-Mortality-Report-2018.pdf. Accessed June 17, 2019.
77. Manasyan A, Saleem S, Koso-Thomas M, et al. Assessment of obstetric and neonatal health services in developing country health facilities. Am J Perinatol 2013;30(9):787.
78. Blencowe H, Cousens S, Jassir FB, et al. National, regional, and worldwide estimates of stillbirth rates in 2015, with trends from 2000: a systematic analysis. Lancet Glob Health 2016;4(2):e98–108.
79. Liu L, Oza S, Hogan D, et al. Global, regional, and national causes of child mortality in 2000-13, with projections to inform post-2015 priorities: an updated systematic analysis. Lancet 2015;385(9966):430–40.
80. Leisher SH, Teoh Z, Reinebrant H, et al. Seeking order amidst chaos: a systematic review of classification systems for causes of stillbirth and neonatal death, 2009–2014. BMC Pregnancy Childbirth 2016;16(1):295.
81. Liu L, Kalter HD, Chu Y, et al. Understanding misclassification between neonatal deaths and stillbirths: empirical evidence from Malawi. PLoS One 2016;11(12): e0168743.
82. Lawn J, Shibuya K, Stein C. No cry at birth: global estimates of intrapartum stillbirths and intrapartum-related neonatal deaths. Bull World Health Organ 2005; 83:409–17.
83. Lawn JE, Cousens S, Zupan J, et al. 4 million neonatal deaths: when? Where? Why? Lancet 2005;365(9462):891–900.
84. Wall SN, Lee AC, Niermeyer S, et al. Neonatal resuscitation in low-resource settings: what, who, and how to overcome challenges to scale up? Int J Gynaecol Obstet 2009;107(Supplement):S47–64.
85. Lehtonen L, Gimeno A, Parra-Llorca A, et al. Early neonatal death: a challenge worldwide. Semin Fetal Neonatal Med 2017;22(3):153–60.
86. Pierrat V, Haouari N, Liska A, et al. Prevalence, causes, and outcome at 2 years of age of newborn encephalopathy: population based study. Arch Dis Child Fetal Neonatal Ed 2005;90(3):F257–61.
87. Al-Macki N, Miller SP, Hall N, et al. The spectrum of abnormal neurologic outcomes subsequent to term intrapartum asphyxia. Pediatr Neurol 2009;41(6): 399–405.
88. Van Lerberghe W. The world health report 2005: make every mother and child count. Geneva (Switzerland): World Health Organization; 2005.
89. Lee AC, Cousens S, Wall SN, et al. Neonatal resuscitation and immediate newborn assessment and stimulation for the prevention of neonatal deaths: a systematic review, meta-analysis and Delphi estimation of mortality effect. BMC Public Health 2011;11(3):S12.
90. Enweronu-Laryea C, Dickson KE, Moxon SG, et al. Basic newborn care and neonatal resuscitation: a multi-country analysis of health system bottlenecks and potential solutions. BMC Pregnancy Childbirth 2015;15(2):S4.
91. Kak L, Johnson J, McPherson R, et al. Helping babies breathe: lessons learned guiding the way forward. A 5-year report from the HBB global development alliance 2015. Available at: https://www.popline.org/node/627118. Accessed June 17, 2019.
92. Montagu D, Yamey G, Visconti A, et al. Where do poor women in developing countries give birth? A multi-country analysis of demographic and health survey data. PLoS One 2011;6(2):e17155.

93. United Nations Childrens Fund (UNICEF). State of the world's children: celebrating 20 years of the convention on the rights of the child. New York: UNICEF; 2009. ISBN: 978-92-806-4442-5.

94. Darmstadt GL, Lee AC, Cousens S, et al. 60 million non-facility births: who can deliver in community settings to reduce intrapartum-related deaths? Int J Gynaecol Obstet 2009;107(Suppl 1):S89–112.

95. World Health Organization. Postnatal care for mothers and newborns. Highlights from the World Health Organization 2013 guidelines. Geneva (Switzerland): World Health Organization; 2015.

96. Kouo-Ngamby M, Dissak-Delon FN, Feldhaus I, et al. A cross-sectional survey of emergency and essential surgical care capacity among hospitals with high trauma burden in a Central African country. BMC Health Serv Res 2015; 15(1):478.

97. Carlo WA, Goudar SS, Jehan I, et al. Newborn-care training and perinatal mortality in developing countries. N Engl J Med 2010;362(7):614–23.

98. Dickson KE, Kinney MV, Moxon SG, et al. Scaling up quality care for mothers and newborns around the time of birth: an overview of methods and analyses of intervention-specific bottlenecks and solutions. BMC Pregnancy Childbirth 2015;15(2):S1.

99. Deorari A, Paul V, Singh M, et al. Impact of education and training on neonatal resuscitation practices in 14 teaching hospitals in India. Ann Trop Paediatr 2001; 21(1):29–33.

100. Kamath-Rayne BD, Griffin JB, Moran K, et al. Resuscitation and obstetrical care to reduce intrapartum-related neonatal deaths: a MANDATE study. Matern Child Health J 2015;19(8):1853–63.

101. Msemo G, Massawe A, Mmbando D, et al. Newborn mortality and fresh stillbirth rates in Tanzania after helping babies breathe training. Pediatrics 2013;131(2): e353–60.

102. Dhaded SM, Somannavar MS, Vernekar SS, et al. Neonatal mortality and coverage of essential newborn interventions 2010-2013: a prospective, population-based study from low-middle income countries. Reprod Health 2015;12(2):S6.

103. Garces A, Mcclure EM, Hambidge M, et al. Training traditional birth attendants on the WHO Essential Newborn Care reduces perinatal mortality. Acta Obstet Gynecol Scand 2012;91(5):593–7.

104. Ersdal HL, Mduma E, Svensen E, et al. Early initiation of basic resuscitation interventions including face mask ventilation may reduce birth asphyxia related mortality in low-income countries: a prospective descriptive observational study. Resuscitation 2012;83(7):869–73.

105. Goudar SS, Dhaded SM, McClure EM, et al. ENC training reduces perinatal mortality in Karnataka, India. J Matern Fetal Neonatal Med 2012;25(6):568–74.

106. Matendo R, Engmann C, Ditekemena J, et al. Reduced perinatal mortality following enhanced training of birth attendants in the Democratic Republic of Congo: a time-dependent effect. BMC Med 2011;9(1):93.

107. Carlo WA, Goudar SS, Jehan I, et al. High mortality rates for very low birth weight infants in developing countries despite training. Pediatrics 2010;126(5): e1072–80.

108. Bellad RM, Bang A, Carlo WA, et al. A pre-post study of a multi-country scale up of resuscitation training of facility birth attendants: does helping babies breathe training save lives? BMC Pregnancy Childbirth 2016;16(1):222.

109. Goudar SS, Somannavar MS, Clark R, et al. Stillbirth and newborn mortality in India after helping babies breathe training. Pediatrics 2013;131(2):e344–52.

110. Bang AT, Bang RA, Baitule SB, et al. Effect of home-based neonatal care and management of sepsis on neonatal mortality: field trial in rural India. Lancet 1999;354(9194):1955–61.

111. Gill CJ, Phiri-Mazala G, Guerina NG, et al. Effect of training traditional birth attendants on neonatal mortality (Lufwanyama Neonatal Survival Project): randomised controlled study. BMJ 2011;342:d346.

112. Patel A, Khatib MN, Kurhe K, et al. Impact of neonatal resuscitation trainings on neonatal and perinatal mortality: a systematic review and meta-analysis. BMJ Paediatr Open 2017;1(1):e000183.

113. Zhu X, Fang H, Zeng S, et al. The impact of the Neonatal Resuscitation Program guidelines (NRPG) on the neonatal mortality in a hospital in Zhuhai, China. Singapore Med J 1997;38:485–7.

114. Newton O, English M. Newborn resuscitation: defining best practice for low-income settings. Trans R Soc Trop Med Hyg 2006;100(10):899–908.

115. Lassi ZS, Bhutta ZA. Community-based intervention packages for reducing maternal and neonatal morbidity and mortality and improving neonatal outcomes. Cochrane Database Syst Rev 2015;(3):CD007754.

Noninvasive Ventilation in the Age of Surfactant Administration

Roger F. Soll, MD*, Whittney Barkhuff, MD

KEYWORDS

- Newborn • Preterm • Continuous positive airway pressure • Surfactant

KEY POINTS

- Antenatal steroids, surfactant replacement therapy, and continuous positive airway pressure have revolutionized the care and outcomes of preterm infants.
- Antenatal steroid treatment of women at risk of preterm delivery has led to a reduction in neonatal death, respiratory distress syndrome, intraventricular hemorrhage, and necrotizing enterocolitis. There is no obvious benefit regarding chronic lung disease and limited evidence is available regarding neurodevelopment delay later in childhood.
- Continuous positive airway pressure has been used in the stabilization of preterm infants at risk of respiratory distress, in the treatment of respiratory distress, and in successful stabilization of preterm infants after extubation from assisted ventilation.
- Although surfactant replacement therapy improves the outcome of preterm infants, novel strategies combining adequate treatment with antenatal steroids, less invasive surfactant administration, and stabilization on nasal continuous positive airway pressure leads to further improvement in clinical outcome.

In 1972, 3 interventions that would change the face of neonatal-perinatal medicine were first reported: the use of antenatal corticosteroids in mothers at risk of preterm delivery,[1] the successful use of intratracheal surfactant replacement in an animal model,[2] and the successful use of nasal continuous positive airway pressure (CPAP) in infants with respiratory distress syndrome (RDS).[3]

In the decades since these original reports, the use of antenatal corticosteroids to promote lung maturation and the postnatal use of less invasive methods of respiratory support and surfactant replacement therapy have been extensively studied and have

Disclosure: Dr R.F. Soll is President of Vermont Oxford Network and Coordinating Editor of Cochrane Neonatal. Dr Soll has no other relevant conflicts of interest to disclose. Dr W. Barkhuff has no relevant conflicts of interest to disclose.
Department of Pediatrics, Neonatal-Perinatal Medicine, Larner College of Medicine, University of Vermont, 89 Beaumont Avenue, Burlington, VT 05405, USA
* Corresponding author.
E-mail address: Roger.Soll@uvmhealth.org

greatly improved the outcome of preterm newborns. However, the 2 postnatal interventions seem diametrically opposed; the successful use of less invasive ventilation demands that clinicians avoid intubating infants with respiratory distress in order to minimize complications of intubation and assisted ventilation, whereas the current approach to surfactant replacement therapy demands introduction of surfactant preparations into the trachea of these same infants. In addition, the greater use of antenatal corticosteroids forces clinicians to reevaluate the impact of both postnatal therapies in light of the benefits of this antenatal intervention.

The following article addresses the evolution of these therapies with specific focus on the evidence behind the use of less invasive ventilation practices (specifically CPAP) and the evidence supporting how and when surfactant should be used in conjunction with CPAP.

ANTENATAL STEROIDS

Antenatal administration of glucocorticoids enhances lung maturation and improves lung function by increasing production of phospholipids and surfactant-associated proteins.[4,5] Since the original trial by Liggins and Howie,[1] there have been more than 30 studies, including 7774 women and 8158 infants.[6] Meta-analysis of these studies shows significant improvement in clinical outcome of infants exposed to antenatal corticosteroids. The use of antenatal corticosteroids leads to a reduction in neonatal death (typical relative risk [RR] 0.69, 95% confidence interval [CI] 0.59–0.81), RDS (typical RR 0.66, 95% CI 0.56–0.77), intraventricular hemorrhage (IVH) (typical RR 0.55, 95% CI 0.40–0.76), and necrotizing enterocolitis (typical RR 0.50, 95% CI 0.32–0.78). There is no obvious benefit regarding chronic lung disease and limited evidence is available regarding neurodevelopment delay later in childhood.

Many have wondered why it took so long for antenatal corticosteroids to come into routine use. In the original trials of surfactant replacement therapy conducted in the late 1980s, fewer than 30% of infants received antenatal steroids. In 1995, Sinclair[7] showed that, as each result of randomized controlled trials of antenatal corticosteroids regarding mortality was added sequentially to a cumulative meta-analysis, the original positive results reported by Liggins and Howie[1] held and were only made more and more precise. Initial resistance to the use of antenatal steroids may in part have been caused by concerns regarding the balance of benefits and potential harms to treated mothers and in a variety of subgroups of infants, including the effect of antenatal steroids in twins or other multiples and the lack of benefit in ruptured or intact membranes. However, the meta-analysis does not support these concerns.[6]

It was not until the National Institutes of Health, informed by an up-to-date meta-analysis of randomized controlled trials[8,9] and analyses of observational data from large neonatal databases,[10] recommended the use of antenatal steroids that antenatal steroid use begin to take hold in the United States. Given the benefits seen in the data from the trials, the consensus panel concluded that "antenatal corticosteroid therapy is indicated for women at risk of premature delivery with few exceptions and will result in a substantial decrease in neonatal morbidity and mortality, as well as substantial savings in health care costs."[11] Since 1994, the use of antenatal corticosteroids in women at risk of premature delivery has steadily increased. At present, rates in most units are more than 80%.[12]

Despite the abundant evidence available on the efficacy of antenatal steroids, gaps in the evidence exist. Trials do not address the effect of antenatal steroids in the less mature infants now coming under care. Current guidelines recommend giving antenatal corticosteroids to infants at or greater than 24 weeks' gestation and only ask clinicians to "consider" antenatal steroid treatment in infants at 23 weeks' gestation. For infants at 22 weeks' gestation, corticosteroids are not recommended.[13] However, there is evidence from observational studies that antenatal steroids may benefit even these least mature infants.[14] In a multicenter observational cohort study of 29,932 live-born infants who received postnatal life support at 431 US Vermont Oxford Network member hospitals, survival to hospital discharge was higher for infants with antenatal steroid exposure (72.3%) compared with infants without antenatal steroid exposure (51.9%). This finding was particularly true for the most immature infants; the adjusted risk ratio for survival of infants at 22 weeks' gestation was 2.11 (95% CI, 1.68–2.65) and for 23 weeks' gestation was 1.54 (95% CI, 1.40–1.70). It is doubtful (although not unethical) that future trials will address the efficacy of steroids in this extremely immature population, despite the real need to further understand the downstream consequences on the development of these particularly fragile infants.

NASAL CONTINUOUS POSITIVE AIRWAY PRESSURE

Although CPAP was first introduced in the 1970s,[3] the utility and feasibility of nasal CPAP did not gain widespread recognition until the late 1980s. In part, the resurgent interest in CPAP began with a survey of centers who were recipients of SCORE (Support of Competitive Research) grants from the National Institute of Health for Lung Disease.[15] Avery and colleagues[15] noted variation in the incidence of bronchopulmonary dysplasia (BPD; then defined as oxygen at 28 days) among these elite centers, with the lowest rate of BPD seen in Columbia, the center with the most unusual approach to respiratory support of newborn infants. The policy at Columbia included stabilization on CPAP using short nasal prongs. Since then, there have been multiple reports regarding introduction of nasal CPAP and improvement in pulmonary outcomes. The Columbia experience was reproduced by the investigators at Boston Children's Hospital, again showing that their increased use of nasal CPAP was associated with a decrease in BPD and surfactant use.[16]

CPAP is thought to assist the breathing of preterm infants in several ways; CPAP improves oxygenation and reduces obstructive apnea by maintaining lung volume and reducing upper airway resistance.[17] If CPAP is successfully applied and intubation is avoided, less trauma to the airway occurs as a result of the intubation and as a result of long-term mechanical respiratory support.

Historically, randomized controlled trials have evaluated the use of CPAP in 2 clinical scenarios: (1) the treatment of infants with evolving RDS, and (2) supporting successful transition of infants extubated from mechanical ventilation. More recently, trials have addressed efforts to stabilize very preterm infants at risk for RDS.

CONTINUOUS POSITIVE AIRWAY PRESSURE FOR RESPIRATORY DISTRESS IN PRETERM INFANTS

The first studies of CPAP and other forms of continuous distending pressure (including continuous negative airway pressure) were conducted in infants with respiratory distress. Ho and colleagues[18] conducted a systematic review of randomized controlled trials of continuous distending pressure (CDP) in preterm infants with respiratory failure. Despite this being the most obvious use of nasal CPAP, few randomized trials address this approach to therapy. The review investigators identified 6 studies involving a total of only 355 infants: 2 using face mask CPAP[19,20], 2 continuous negative pressure (CNP),[21,22] 1 nasal CPAP,[23] and 1 both CNP (for less ill babies) and endotracheal CPAP (for sicker babies)[24] (**Table 1**).

Table 1
Randomized controlled trials of continuous distending pressure for respiratory distress in preterm infants

Study	Population/Setting	Intervention	Control	Comments
Belenky et al,[19] 1976	51 preterm infants (22 CPAP, 29 control) who were spontaneously breathing at trial entry. Clinical and radiograph evidence of RDS. Pao_2 50 mm Hg or less on Fio_2 of 0.6	Face mask CPAP or PEEP (6–14 cm H_2O)	Headbox oxygen or IPPV without PEEP	Endotracheal IPPV initiated in those on face mask IPPV with gastric distension or inadequate ventilation
Rhodes & Hall,[20] 1973	41 preterm infants (22 CPAP, 19 control) with clinical and radiograph features of RDS and Pao_2<60 mm Hg in Fio_2 0.5. Mean age for intervention group 10.1 h (SD = 1.8) and 12.4 h (SD = 2.0)	Tight-fitting mask CPAP (8–10 cm H_2O)	Headbox oxygen CPAP used on control patients failing headbox treatment	Assisted ventilation given for apnea requiring bag and mask ventilation, Pao_2<40 mm Hg in Fio_2 1.0 or Pco_2>80 mm Hg
Fanaroff et al,[21] 1973	29 preterm infants (15 CNP, 14 control) >1000 g with RDS with Po_2 <60 mm Hg in Fio_2 0.7. Total participants 19	CNP chamber (6–14 cm H_2O negative pressure)	Headbox oxygen	Study group failures received mechanical ventilation, and control group failures CPAP or mechanical ventilation
Samuels et al,[22] 1996	52 preterm infants with respiratory failure not caused by infection or congenital heart disease spontaneously breathing at 4 h in Fio_2 ≥ 0.4 to maintain Po_2 >60 mm Hg. Mean (SD) gestational age at birth 32.5 (1.8) vs 31.0 (1.9) wk, range 30–36 vs 29–36 wk	CNP chamber 4–6 cm H_2O	Headbox oxygen	Only 17% of the mothers of the 52 infants received prenatal corticosteroids (similar in each group) Neurodevelopmental assessment at 9 to 15 years of age was reported separately
Buckmaster et al,[23] 2007	Infants in nontertiary hospitals ≥31 and <37 wk weighing >1200 g, <24 h of age with respiratory distress who required >30% oxygen in a headbox to maintain oxygen saturation levels ≥94% for 30 min 300 infants were randomly assigned; of these, 158 were preterm infants with respiratory distress	Nasal CPAP using Hudson prong and bubble delivery circuit	Headbox oxygen	Surfactant not used before the time of transfer. Antenatal steroids used for 35% of infants
Durbin et al,[24] 1976	24 infants (12 CNP, 12 control) with severe RDS >1000 g, Pao_2<60 mm Hg in Fio_2>0.95 for 15 min. Mean age for control group 30.3 h (SD = 6.1), and for treatment group 28.2 (SD = 3.7)	8–12 cm H_2O CNP for less severe illness and endotracheal CPAP for more severe	Headbox oxygen	IPPV started if Pao_2<35 mm Hg

The authors identified 6 studies involving a total of only 355 infants: 2 using face mask CPAP (Belenky et al,[19] 1976; Rhodes & Hall,[20] 1973), 2 CNP (Fanaroff et al,[21] 1973; Samuels et al,[22] 1996), 1 nasal CPAP (Buckmaster et al,[23] 2007) and 1 both CNP (for less ill babies) and endotracheal CPAP (for sicker babies) (Durbin et al,[24] 1976).
Abbreviations: Fio_2, fraction of inspired oxygen; IPPV, intermittent positive pressure ventilation; PEEP, positive end-expiratory pressure; SD, standard deviation.

Three of these 6 trials were conducted in the 1970s[19–21]; even the most recently conducted trial[23] had a very low rate of antenatal steroid exposure (undoubtedly caused by the enrollment criteria for gestational age $\geq$31 and <37 weeks).

CDP is associated with lower risk of treatment failure (death or use of assisted ventilation) (typical RR 0.65, 95% CI 0.52–0.81; typical risk difference [RD] −0.20, 95% CI −0.29 to −0.10; number needed to treat for an additional beneficial outcome [NNTB] 5, 95% CI 4–10; 6 studies; 355 infants), lower overall mortality (typical RR 0.52, 95% CI 0.32–0.87; typical RD −0.15, 95% CI −0.26 to −0.04; NNTB 7, 95% CI 4–25; 6 studies; 355 infants), and lower mortality in infants with birth weight more than 1500 g (typical RR 0.24, 95% CI 0.07–0.84; typical RD −0.28, 95% CI −0.48 to −0.08; NNTB 4, 95% CI 2.00–13.00; 2 studies; 60 infants). Some harms were also reported with the use of nasal CPAP; the use of CDP was associated with an increased risk of pneumothorax (typical RR 2.64, 95% CI 1.39–5.04; typical RD 0.10, 95% CI 0.04–0.17; number needed to treat for an additional harmful outcome [NNTH] 17, 95% CI 17.00–25.00; 6 studies; 355 infants). This increased risk of pneumothorax is seen in many of the studies of nasal CPAP in which surfactant replacement therapy was not given. No difference in BPD (defined as oxygen use at 28 days) was seen in the few studies that reported this outcome (typical RR 1.22, 95% CI 0.44–3.39; 3 studies, 260 infants).

NASAL CONTINUOUS POSITIVE AIRWAY PRESSURE IMMEDIATELY AFTER EXTUBATION

In addition to the treatment of RDS, the other approach that was tested in early studies was the use of CPAP to facilitate extubation of infants from assisted ventilation. Davis and Ho[25] conducted a systematic review comparing the use of nasal CPAP with headbox oxygen in preterm infants being extubated following a period of intermittent positive pressure ventilation (IPPV).

Davis and Ho identified 9 trials[26–34] (**Table 2**). Most of the studies identified were conducted in the 1990s. Four studies[26,27,32,33] allowed crossover from headbox to nasal CPAP if an infant was deemed to have failed, either by showing respiratory insufficiency or by requiring reintubation.

Although results varied from trial to trial, there are clinically important improvements in outcome of infants extubated to nasal CPAP. In preterm infants being extubated following IPPV, nasal CPAP reduced the incidence of respiratory failure (defined as apnea, respiratory acidosis, and increased oxygen requirements) indicating the need for additional ventilator support (typical RR 0.62, 95% CI 0.51–0.76; typical RD −0.17, 95% CI −0.23 to −0.10; NNTB 6, 95% CI, 4–10). Fewer infants required nasal CPAP after extubation or required reintubation when nasal CPAP was used, a result that does not reach statistical significance (typical RR 0.93, 95% CI 0.72–1.19; typical RD −0.02, 95% CI −0.09–0.05). The use of nasal CPAP as rescue therapy for infants failing headbox in 4 trials dilutes the estimate of the effect for this outcome. There was no significant difference in rates of oxygen use at 28 days of age in patients allocated to nasal CPAP at the time of extubation from IPPV (typical RR 1.00, 95% CI 0.81–1.24; typical RD 0.00, 95% CI −0.09–0.09).

Similar effects of nasal CPAP on the risk of incidence of respiratory failure are seen in a subgroup analysis of preterm infants weighing less than 2000 g being extubated following IPPV. Infants managed on higher CPAP (>5 cm H_2O) showed the least risk of respiratory insufficiency and extubation failure, but the investigators caution against overinterpretation of this finding. The appropriate duration of treatment with nasal CPAP remains uncertain, as does the method of its weaning.

Table 2
Randomized controlled trials of nasal continuous positive airway pressure immediately after extubation

Study	Population/Setting	Intervention	Control	Comments
Allowed Crossover				
Higgins et al,[27] 1991	Infants weighing <1 kg at time of first elective extubation. Intubated at least 24 h, requiring <35% oxygen, MAP<7 cm H_2O, ventilator rate <20 breaths per minute, and weight at least 80% of birth weight. Number enrolled = 58	CPAP via binasal pharyngeal airway prongs using 4–6 cm H_2O	Headbox oxygen	Failure criteria: $Fio_2>0.60$ to maintain oxygen saturations >93%, $Pco_2>60$ or pH<7.23, or moderate to severe apnea
Engelke et al,[26] 1982	Neonates intubated for more than 72 h but <14 d. Birth weight >1000 g. Number enrolled = 18	Nasal CPAP at 6 cm H_2O	Headbox oxygen	Extubation failure defined as (1) progressive atelectasis and respiratory distress, (2) $Pco_2>60$ mm Hg with pH<7.20, or Fio_2 increased by >0.15–0.20
Davis et al,[32] 1998	1. Birth weight 600–1250 g 2. Endotracheal tube for >12 h 3. Stable or improving respiratory status: ventilator rate <20/min and inspired oxygen requirement <50%. Number enrolled = 92	CPAP 7 cm H_2O via a Portex tube inserted 2.5 cm into 1 nostril and connected to a Bear Cub ventilator	Headbox oxygen	Extubation failure criteria comprised apnea (recurrent minor or 1 major), increased Fio_2 (>15% absolute increase above that required preextubation) or respiratory acidosis (pH<7.25 with $Pco_2>50$ mm Hg)
Dimitriou et al,[33] 2000	Gestational age ≤34 wk and postnatal age ≤14 d. Methylxanthines were commenced universally before extubation. Number enrolled = 150	Nasal CPAP 3–5 cm H_2O. CPAP provided either by single prong (n = 40), Argyle prongs (n = 22), or Flow Driver prongs (n = 13) depending on availability in individual units	Headbox oxygen	Extubation failure criteria comprised $Fio_2>0.60$, respiratory acidosis (pH<7.25), and 1 major or frequent minor apneic episodes
Did Not Allow Crossover				
Chan & Greenough,[28] 1993	Ventilated infants <1800 g with no congenital abnormalities. Number enrolled = 120	Nasal CPAP of 3 cm H_2O	Headbox oxygen	Criteria for reintubation pH<7.25 with $Pco_2 >6.67$ kPa $Fio_2 >0.60$ or recurrent minor or 1 major apnea

Study	Population	Intervention	Control	Failure/reintubation criteria
So et al,[29] 1995	Birth weight <1500 g, GA<34 wk, mechanical ventilation within first few hours of life, weaning started within 7 d of life. Number enrolled = 50	Single-prong nasal CPAP at 5 cm H_2O	Headbox oxygen	Reintubation if Po_2<50 mm Hg with Fio_2≥0.70, pH<7.25, and Pco_2>60 mm Hg, severe or frequent apnea. Aminophylline load given. Extubation from ETT CPAP
Annibale et al,[30] 1994	Birth weight 600–1500 g, endotracheal intubation within 48 h of life, eligible for extubation by day 14 of life, and stable or improving clinical course. Number enrolled = 82	1. Nasopharyngeal CPAP at 6 cm H_2O until reached (defined) goal criteria 2. Nasopharyngeal CPAP for 6 h then headbox oxygen	Headbox oxygen	Failure defined as an Fio_2≥0.80, pH<7.20, severe apnea and bradycardia, or clinical deterioration
Tapia et al,[31] 1995	Preterm infants <1500 g requiring ventilation for more than 48 h. Criteria for entry: Fio_2<0.40, rate<20/min, peak pressure <15 cm H_2O. Number enrolled = 59	1. Preextubation ETT CPAP (3–4 cm H_2O) for 12–24 h 2. Postextubation nasopharyngeal CPAP (3–4 cm H_2O) for 12–24 h	Headbox oxygen	Failure defined as need to return to mechanical ventilation within 72 h of extubation because of either (1) frequent or severe apnea, (2) pH<7.25 and Pco_2>60 mm Hg. or (3) Fio_2>0.60. Extubated from low-rate ventilation. Loaded with aminophylline
Peake et al,[34] 2005	Gestational age <32 wk, ventilated via an ETT during the first 28 d of life, and being extubated for the first time. Median (range) birth weights: CPAP 1012 g (640–1474 g), headbox 1105 g (574–1670 g)	Nasal CPAP: level set at 4–6 cm water via Infant Flow Driver CPAP stopped after 24 h and interrupted every 6–8 h for a 1-h break off CPAP	Headbox oxygen: humidified oxygen delivered to keep saturations in a prescribed (not specified) range	Failure criteria were any of pH<7.25 on 2 consecutive blood gases, Pco_2>55 mm Hg on 2 consecutive blood gases, Fio_2 ≥ 0.7, and 3 or more episodes of apnea requiring stimulation or 1 requiring IPPV. All infants received at least 1 dose of surfactant. All infants were commenced on methylxanthine therapy when the ventilator rate was <40/min

Davis and Ho[25] identified 9 trials (Engelke et al,[26] 1982; Higgins et al,[27] 1991; Chan& Greenough,[28] 1993; So et al,[29] 1995; Annibale et al,[30] 1994; Tapia et al,[31] 1995; Davis et al,[32] 1998; Dimitriou et al,[33] 1998; and Peake et al,[34] 2005). Four studies (Higgins et al,[27] 1991; Engelke et al,[26] 1982; Davis et al,[32] 1998; and Dimitriou 2000 et al[33]) allowed crossover from headbox to nasal CPAP if an infant was deemed to have failed, either by showing respiratory insufficiency or by requiring reintubation.

Abbreviations: ETT, endotracheal tube; GA, gestational age; MAP, mean arterial pressure.

PROPHYLACTIC NASAL CONTINUOUS POSITIVE AIRWAY PRESSURE FOR PREVENTING MORBIDITY AND MORTALITY IN VERY PRETERM INFANTS

Most of the recent studies on CPAP have dealt with the early stabilization of preterm infants at high risk for, or having early signs and symptoms of, respiratory distress. These studies are discussed in greater detail later because they address the question most interesting to caregivers and are conducted in a more generalizable population regarding both gestational age and antenatal steroid exposure.

Seven trials recruiting 3123 babies were included in the meta-analysis by Subramaniam and colleagues.[35] Four trials recruiting 765 babies compared CPAP with supportive care,[36-39] and 3 trials (2364 infants) compared CPAP with mechanical ventilation.[40-42] Apart from a lack of blinding of the intervention, all studies were thought to be low risk for bias. These studies are discussed in detail later and in **Table 3**.

RANDOMIZED CONTROLLED TRIALS COMPARING CONTINUOUS POSITIVE AIRWAY PRESSURE WITH SUPPORTIVE CARE

Four randomized controlled trials comparing CPAP with supportive care are discussed here.[36-39] The 1 study of more historical interest is the study of Han and colleagues.[36] Han and colleagues[36] studied 82 spontaneously breathing infants who were less than 33 weeks' gestation and less than 2 hours old. No mother received antenatal corticosteroids, and surfactant therapy was not available. The other 3 studies were conducted in a more contemporary context. Sandri and colleagues[37] studied 230 infants of 28 to 31 weeks' gestation who did not require intubation in the delivery room. Infants were randomly assigned to prophylactic or rescue CPAP within 30 minutes of life irrespective of oxygen requirement and clinical status. Rescue CPAP was started when the fraction of inspired oxygen (Fio_2) requirement was greater than 0.4 for more than 30 minutes to maintain transcutaneous oxygen saturation between 93% and 96%. Exogenous surfactant was given when Fio_2 requirement was greater than 0.4 on CPAP in the presence of radiological signs of RDS. Prenatal corticosteroids steroids were given to the mothers of 83.3% of the infants in the CPAP group and 82.4% of the infants in the control group. Tapia and colleagues[31,38] studied 256 spontaneously breathing infants with birth weights of 800 to 1500 g at 5 minutes of life. The investigators compared a complex management strategy; infants were randomized to initial support with nasal CPAP and selective use of surfactant via the INSURE (intubation, surfactant, and extubation to CPAP; CPAP/INSURE) protocol (n = 131) or supplemental oxygen, surfactant, and mechanical ventilation (oxygen/ MV) if required (n = 125). In the CPAP/INSURE group, CPAP was discontinued after 3 to 6 hours if RDS did not occur. If RDS developed and the Fio_2 was greater than 0.35, the INSURE protocol was indicated. Failure criteria included Fio_2 greater than 0.60, severe apnea or respiratory acidosis, and receipt of more than 2 doses of surfactant. In the oxygen/MV group, in the presence of RDS, supplemental oxygen without CPAP was given, and, if Fio_2 was greater than 0.35, surfactant and mechanical ventilation were provided. Antenatal steroid was used in 90.8% of the CPAP group and 88.0% of the control group.

Gonçalves-Ferri and colleagues[39] conducted a multicenter randomized clinical trial in 5 public university hospitals in Brazil. One-hundred and ninety-seven preterm infants with birth weights of 1000 to 1500 g who were spontaneously breathing at 15 minutes of life were randomized to receive routine treatment (n = 99) or nasal CPAP (n = 98). Antenatal steroids were administered to the mothers of 66 (67%) infants in the CPAP group and 63 (64%) infants in the control group. When randomized to

Table 3
Randomized controlled trials of prophylactic or very early initiation of continuous positive airway pressure for preterm infants

Study	Population/Setting	Intervention	Control	Comments
Randomized Controlled Trials Comparing CPAP with Supportive Care				
Han et al,[36] 1987	87 infants were eligible. Preterm infants (n = 82) of 32 wk gestation or less and stratified by sex	Nasopharyngeal CPAP of 6 cm H_2O pressure applied at birth. Infants who failed to improve (Pao_2<50 mm Hg in Fio_2>0.8, apnea) were managed with endotracheal CPAP and then IPPV as indicated by Pao_2<50 mm Hg in Fio_2>0.9, or pH<7.2 mainly caused by $Paco_2$>60 mm Hg, apnea Subsequent management similar to treatment group	Oxygen in a headbox. Nasal CPAP given when Pao_2<50 mm Hg in Fio_2>0.5, or apnea (given to 33%)	No mother received antenatal corticosteroids and postnatal surfactant therapy was not available Both groups of infants received an initial Fio_2 ranging from 0.3 to 0.6
Sandri et al,[37] 2004	Preterm infants (n = 230) between 28 and 31 + 6 wk gestation	Prophylactic nasal CPAP of 4–6 cm H_2O applied within 30 min of birth (n = 115) Nasal CPAP was given through nasal prongs using the Infant Flow Driver system (n = 115)	Control: received nasal CPAP when the Fio_2 in the hood was >0.4 for more than 30 min, to maintain transcutaneous oxygen saturation (Spo_2) between 93% and 96% Nasal CPAP was given through nasal prongs using the Infant Flow Driver system (n = 115)	Newborns receiving nasal CPAP at a pressure of 6 cm H_2O, requiring an Fio_2>0.4 for more than 30 min to maintain Spo_2 in the range 93% to 96%, radiological signs of RDS were intubated, treated with surfactant, and manually ventilated for 2–5 min. The infants were then extubated and placed on nasal CPAP if they had a good respiratory drive and maintained a satisfactory Spo_2 value

(continued on next page)

Table 3
(continued)

Study	Population/Setting	Intervention	Control	Comments
Tapia et al,[38] 2012	265 preterm infants with birth weight 800–1500 g who were spontaneously breathing at 5 min of life but needing respiratory support because of increased respiratory effort, grunting respiration, or cyanosis 131 infants were given CPAP (as soon as possible after allocation) 125 infants randomized to the oxygen/MV group	CPAP (as soon as possible after allocation) using a bubble CPAP system (Fisher & Paykel Healthcare) with a distending pressure of 5 cm H_2O. The short binasal prongs included with the CPAP system were used. Before the nasal prongs were inserted, CPAP was maintained at 5 cm H_2O through a mask connected to a T-piece resuscitator, ensuring that the infants in this group were maintained on CPAP from the time of enrollment. Infants with an $Fio_2>0.35$ to maintain Spo_2 in the target range and radiograph findings compatible with RDS were intubated and given surfactant following the INSURE protocol	Oxygen/MV group were initially managed with oxygen via low-flow nasal cannula and transferred to an oxyhood. In infants with RDS on chest radiograph and an $Fio_2>0.35$ on oxyhood therapy, surfactant was administered followed by mechanical ventilation	—
Gonçalves-Ferri et al,[39] 2014	250 infants were eligible for the study. Premature infants with a birth weight of 1000–1500 g without major malformations or fetal hydrops These infants were not intubated or extubated in <15 min after birth	Positive pressure was applied using a Neopuff manual ventilator with a PEEP at 5 cm H_2O and 100% oxygen. After stabilization, ventilation institutional protocols. The CPAP group was maintained with positive pressure for at least 48 h	Infants who presented with central cyanosis, oxygen was started according to the techniques recommended by the guidelines of the AAP and AHA. According to the study protocol, infants in the control group who failed supportive therapy were to be administered CPAP before the use of mechanical ventilation	—

Study	Inclusion/Exclusion criteria	CPAP group	Intubation group	Comments
Morley et al,[40] 2008	Inclusion criteria: infants (n = 616) with a gestational age at delivery between 25 wk and 28 wk 6 d with no known condition that might adversely affect breathing after birth apart from prematurity. Ability to breath at 5 min after birth but needing respiratory support because of increased respiratory effort, grunting respiration, or cyanosis. Exclusion criteria: infants who were intubated before randomization. Infants who did not require any respiratory support or oxygen	Nasal CPAP started at 8 cm H_2O with short single or double prong and continued until met criteria for extubation according to local protocol or until met criteria for intubation (pH<7.25, Pco_2>60 mm Hg, Fio_2>0.6 or apnea)	Intubated and ventilated at 5 min of age	The allocated treatment was started within 5 min of life in both groups
Finer et al,[41] 2010	1316 infants with a gestational age at delivery between 24 wk and 27 wk 6 d without known malformations	Nasal CPAP via a T-piece resuscitator, a neonatal ventilator or an equivalent device with a recommended pressure of 5 cm H_2O in the delivery room irrespective of respiratory status. Infants were intubated if they met any of the following criteria for intubation: pH<7.25, Pco_2>65 mm Hg, Fio_2>0.5 or hemodynamic instability. The allocated treatment was commenced soon after birth (n = 663)	Intubated within 1 h of life in the delivery room and received surfactant. They could be extubated within 24 h for: $Paco_2$ of <50 mm Hg, pH>7.30, $Fio_2 \geq 0.35$, $Spo_2 \geq 88\%$, a mean arterial pressure of 8 cm H_2O or less, a ventilator rate $\geq$20 breaths/min, amplitude less than twice the mean arterial pressure if on high-frequency ventilation, hemodynamic stability, without clinically significant patent ductus arteriosus (n = 653)	—

(continued on next page)

Table 3
(continued)

Study	Population/Setting	Intervention	Control	Comments
Dunn et al,[42] 2011	Neonates born between 26 wk gestation and 29 wk 6 d gestation were enrolled at participating Vermont Oxford Network centers Experimental group: n = 224 Control group: n = 219	Infants were supported with nasal CPAP within 15 min after birth and intubated only if meeting 1 or more of the following criteria: (1) >12 episodes of apnea that required stimulation or >1 episode that required bagging in a 6-h period; (2) P_{CO_2}>65 mm Hg on arterial or capillary blood gas; or (3) requirement for Fio_2 of >0.4 to maintain oxygen saturation of 86% to 94%. Intubation was discretionary if Fio_2 was 0.4–0.6 and mandatory if Fio_2>0.6	Infants were intubated 5–15 min after birth. These infants were then given surfactant and stabilized on mechanical ventilation for a minimum of 6 h	—

Abbreviations: AAP, American Academy of Pediatrics; AHA, American Heart Association; INSURE, intubation, surfactant, and extubation to CPAP; MV, mechanical ventilation.

CPAP, positive pressure was applied using a Neopuff manual ventilator with positive end-expiratory pressure (PEEP) at 5 cm H_2O and 100% oxygen.

RESULTS OF META-ANALYSIS: RANDOMIZED CONTROLLED TRIALS COMPARING CONTINUOUS POSITIVE AIRWAY PRESSURE WITH SUPPORTIVE CARE

In the meta-analysis of trials of comparing CPAP with supportive care, there was a marginal and imprecise reduction in the need for assisted ventilation (typical RR 0.66, 95% CI 0.45–0.98; typical RD −0.16, 95% CI −0.34–0.02; 4 studies, 765 infants, very low quality evidence). There was no significant difference between CPAP and supportive care in the incidence of BPD defined at 28 days (typical RR 1.02, 95% CI 0.77–1.36, 3 studies, 535 participants)[36,38,39] or when defined at 36 weeks' postmenstrual age (typical RR 0.79, 95% CI 0.50–1.24; 3 studies, 683 participants).[37–39]

RANDOMIZED CONTROLLED TRIALS COMPARING CONTINUOUS POSITIVE AIRWAY PRESSURE WITH MECHANICAL VENTILATION

The systematic review and meta-analysis of prophylactic or extremely early application of CPAP by Subramaniam and colleagues[35] also includes 3 of the larger and more recent trials comparing CPAP with mechanical ventilation.[40–42] Morley and colleagues[40] conducted the COIN (CPAP or Intubation) Trial within the Australasian Trial Network. The COIN Trial compared the effectiveness of nasal CPAP (8 cm H_2O) with intubation and mechanical ventilation in preterm infants who were breathing spontaneously at 5 minutes after birth. The COIN Trial enrolled 616 infants 25 weeks to 28 weeks 6 days' gestational age who were judged to require respiratory support at 5 minutes of age. As with many of these recent trials, there was an extremely high rate of antenatal corticosteroid treatment; antenatal corticosteroids were given to the mothers of 94% of infants in both groups. Surfactant was given to 38% of infants in the CPAP group and 77% in the control group. Infants who were randomized to stabilization on CPAP had a statistically nonsignificant reduction in the rate of death or BPD. The mean duration of ventilation was shorter in the CPAP group (3 days in the CPAP group and 4 days in the ventilator group). However, the CPAP group had a higher rate of pneumothorax than the ventilator group (9% vs 3%). Surfactant therapy was not required by protocol for intubated infants, and only three-quarters of the intubation cohort received surfactant, in contrast with infants in the CPAP group in which 46% of infants required ventilator support and 50% received surfactant.

The largest CPAP trial (n = 1316), the Surfactant Positive Pressure and Pulse Oximetry Randomized Trial (SUPPORT) was conducted by Finer and colleagues[41] through the Eunice Kennedy Shriver National Institutes of Health and Human Development Neonatal Research Network. The SUPPORT trial was designed to evaluate nasal CPAP started immediately after birth compared with prophylactic surfactant therapy and ventilator support started within 60 minutes after birth in infants born at 24 to 27 weeks' gestation.[41] This comparison was one part of a 2-by-2 factorial design that also assigned infants to 1 of 2 oxygen saturation target ranges (85%–89% or 91%–95%). As seen in the COIN Trial, antenatal corticosteroids were given to most of the infants in both groups; 96.8% in the CPAP group, of which 73.6% received a full course, and 95.6% in the ventilated group, of which 69.8% received a full course. Surfactant was given to 67.1% of the CPAP group and 98.9% of the ventilated group. The overall rate of death or BPD in the CPAP group was 48% compared with 51% in the surfactant group (RR 0.91, 95% CI 0.83–1.01). In the least mature infants, those born between 24 and 25 weeks' gestation, the death rate was lower in the CPAP group than in the surfactant group (20% vs 29%; RR 0.68, 95% CI 0.50–0.92). In addition, duration of mechanical ventilation was shorter (25 vs 28 days) and use of postnatal corticosteroid therapy was reduced in the CPAP group (7% vs 13%). The rate of air leaks did not differ between the groups and there were no adverse effects of the CPAP strategy despite a reduction in the use of surfactant. Follow-up at 18 to 22 months' corrected age showed no difference in the risk of death or neurodevelopmental impairment (27.9% of the infants in the CPAP group vs 29.9% of those in the surfactant/ventilation group; RR 0.93, 95% CI 0.78–1.10).[43]

Dunn and colleagues[42] conducted the Vermont Oxford Network Delivery Room Management (VON DRM) Trial, in which 656 infants born at 26 to 29 weeks' gestation were randomly assigned to 1 of 3 treatment groups: prophylactic surfactant and continued ventilation (the PS group, n = 213), prophylactic surfactant and extubation to CPAP (the ISX group, n = 219; identical to the INSURE approach), or CPAP (without surfactant) (the CPAP group, n = 224). Prenatal corticosteroids were given to 98.7% of the CPAP group and 98.6% of the intubated group. Surfactant was given to 45.1% of the CPAP group, and more than 98% of the ISX group and prophylactic surfactant group. Both the CPAP group and the ISX group fared better than infants receiving prophylactic surfactant administration and continued mechanical ventilation regarding the primary outcome of BPD or death (CPAP vs PS: RR 0.83, 95% CI 0.64–1.09. ISX vs PS: RR 0.78, 95% CI: 0.59–1.03) (discussed in more detail later).

RESULTS OF META-ANALYSIS: RANDOMIZED CONTROLLED TRIALS COMPARING CONTINUOUS POSITIVE AIRWAY PRESSURE WITH MECHANICAL VENTILATION

In the meta-analysis of trials comparing CPAP with assisted ventilation with or without surfactant, application of CPAP resulted in a significant reduction in the incidence of BPD at 36 weeks' postmenstrual age (typical RR 0.89, 95% CI 0.79–0.99; typical RD −0.04, 95% CI −0.08–0.00; 3 studies, 772 infants) and death or BPD at 36 weeks' postmenstrual age (typical RR 0.89, 95% CI 0.81–0.97; typical RD −0.05, 95% CI −0.09–0.01; 3 studies, 1042 infants). There was also a clinically important reduction in the need for mechanical ventilation (typical RR 0.50, 95% CI 0.42–0.59; typical RD −0.49, 95% CI −0.59 to −0.39; 2 studies, 760 infants) and the use of surfactant in the CPAP group (typical RR 0.54, 95% CI 0.40–0.73; typical RD −0.41, 95% CI −0.54 to −0.28; 3 studies, 1744 infants).

Based on these analyses, as well as on other trials of selective early use of surfactant versus CPAP not included in the meta-analysis, the early use of CPAP with subsequent selective surfactant administration is currently the recommended approach to management of extremely preterm infants at risk or having early signs of RDS.[44]

DEVICES AND PRESSURE SOURCES FOR ADMINISTRATION OF NASAL CONTINUOUS POSITIVE AIRWAY PRESSURE

De Paoli and colleagues[45] conducted a systematic review of devices and pressure sources for administration of nasal CPAP. CPAP has been delivered by a variety of devices and a variety of interfaces. Currently available CPAP systems include variable-flow systems (using a fast-moving jet of compressed gas to accelerate an air mass) and constant-flow systems.[46] Constant-flow systems are either ventilator derived or use the classic underwater bubble CPAP system. Bubble CPAP systems have captured the world's imagination in that they are inexpensive can be used in a variety of care settings.

Limited data are available to help determine which technique of pressure generation and which type of nasal interface for nasal CPAP delivery most effectively reduces the need for additional respiratory support in preterm infants extubated to nasal CPAP following IPPV for RDS or in those treated with nasal CPAP soon after birth. De Paoli and colleagues identified 7 randomized controlled trials[47-53] that addressed different aspects of this question.

Preterm Infants Being Extubated to Nasal Continuous Positive Airway Pressure Following a Period of Intermittent Positive Pressure Ventilation for Respiratory Distress Syndrome

Four studies[48,51-53] compared the use of different nasal CPAP devices in the period following endotracheal intubation and ventilation for RDS. Meta-analysis of the results from Davis and colleages[48] and Roukema and colleagues[51] showed that short binasal prongs are more effective at preventing reintubation than single nasal or nasopharyngeal prongs (typical RR 0.59, CI 0.41-0.85; typical RD -0.21, CI -0.35 to -0.07; NNTB 5, 95% CI 3-14). In one study comparing short binasal prong devices,[53] the reintubation rate was significantly lower with the Infant Flow Driver than with the Medicorp prong (RR 0.33, 95% CI 0.17-0.67; RD -0.32, 95% CI -0.49 to -0.15; NNTB 3, 95% CI 2-7). The other study comparing short binasal prong devices (Infant Flow Driver vs INCA prongs) showed no significant difference in the reintubation rate but did show a significant reduction in the total days in hospital in the Infant Flow Driver group (MD -12.60, 95% CI -22.81 to -2.39 days).[52]

Preterm Infants Primarily Treated with Nasal Continuous Positive Airway Pressure Soon after Birth

The Mazzella and colleagues[49] trial was the only study published in full that randomized preterm infants with early RDS to different nasal CPAP devices. In the 1 trial identified, Mazzella and colleagues[49] found a significantly lower oxygen requirement and respiratory rate in infants randomized to short binasal prongs compared with CPAP delivered via nasopharyngeal prong. The requirement for intubation beyond 48 hours from randomization was not assessed.

Studies Randomizing Preterm Infants to Different Nasal Continuous Positive Airway Pressure Systems Using Broad Inclusion Criteria

Two studies randomized preterm infants to different nasal CPAP systems using inclusion criteria that resulted in significant heterogeneity in the clinical conditions of those randomized.[47,50] Limited data are reported by either of these studies. Rego and Martinez[50] showed a significantly higher incidence of nasal hyperemia with the use of the Argyle prong compared with Hudson prongs (RR 2.39, 95% CI 1.27-4.50; RD 0.28, 95% CI, 0.10-0.46).

INCIDENCE AND OUTCOME OF CONTINUOUS POSITIVE AIRWAY PRESSURE FAILURE IN PRETERM INFANTS

CPAP does have drawbacks. It requires a growing nursing expertise and, even with the best care, may result in traumatic nasal injury. Despite clinicians' best efforts, infants fail nasal CPAP for a variety of reasons, including lung immaturity, chest wall instability, upper airway obstruction, and poor respiratory drive.

Several publications highlight the difficulties and the consequences of administering CPAP, particularly in the less mature infants. As a lead up to the SUPPORT trial, Finer and colleagues[54] conducted a feasibility study of initiating CPAP in the delivery room and continuing CPAP therapy once in the neonatal intensive care unit (NICU) without resorting to intubation for surfactant. Infants who were of less than28 weeks' gestation, who were born in 5 National Institute of Child Health and Human Development Neonatal Research Network NICUs were randomized to receive either CPAP/PEEP or no pressure support using a neonatal T-piece resuscitator (Neopuff). Infants were not to be intubated for the sole purpose of surfactant administration in the delivery room. A total of 104 infants were enrolled over a 6-month period: 55 CPAP and 49 control infants. Despite the intention to avoid intubation in the delivery room for the purpose of surfactant administration, 27 (49%) infants randomized to the delivery room CPAP arm were intubated as part of their initial resuscitation. After admission to the NICU, all nonintubated infants were placed on CPAP and were to be intubated for surfactant administration only after they met a prespecified definition of respiratory insufficiency (Fio_2>0.3 with an oxygen saturation by pulse oximeter of <90% and/or an arterial oxygen pressure of <45 mm Hg, an arterial partial pressure of carbon dioxide of >55 mm Hg, or apnea requiring bag and mask ventilation). Of the infants initially randomized to stabilization on CPAP, 16 more were subsequently intubated in the NICU by the seventh day of life. Overall, 80% of the studied infants required intubation within the first 7 days of life.

Dargaville and colleagues[55] reported on outcomes of CPAP failure in Australian and New Zealand Neonatal Network data from 2007 to 2013. Within the cohort of 19,103 infants, 11,684 were initially managed on CPAP. Failure of CPAP occurred in 863 (43%) of 1989 infants starting on CPAP at 25 to 28 weeks' gestation and 2061 (21%) of 9695 infants at 29 to 32 weeks. CPAP failure was associated with a substantially higher rate of pneumothorax, and a heightened risk of death, BPD, and other morbidities compared with those managed successfully on CPAP. The incidence of death or BPD was also increased (25–28 weeks: 39% vs 20%, adjusted odds ratio 2.30, 99% CI 1.71–3.10. At 29–32 weeks: 12% vs 3.1%, adjusted odds ratio 3.62; 99% CI 2.76–4.74). The CPAP failure group had longer durations of respiratory support and hospitalization. Given the serious consequences associated with CPAP failure, Dargaville and colleagues[55] suggest the strategies to promote successful CPAP application should be pursued vigorously.

CONTINUOUS POSITIVE AIRWAY PRESSURE AND PULMONARY SURFACTANT

Administration of pulmonary surfactant has been proved to be effective in both the prevention and treatment of RDS. Compared with management of RDS with assisted ventilation, pulmonary surfactant administration leads to a decrease in the immediate need for respiratory support and supplemental oxygen as well as a decrease in the risk of pneumothorax, mortality, and the combined outcome of death or BPD.[56–60] Widespread use of surfactant therapy has been credited with significant improvements in survival in preterm infants without increasing the incidence of neurologic or developmental disability.[61]

Trials done in the early 1980s suggested that prophylactic use of pulmonary surfactant would lead to further improvements in pneumothorax and mortality.[62] Although both prophylactic surfactant administration and surfactant treatment of infants with established RDS are successful treatment strategies, there are theoretic advantages and disadvantages of each approach. Prophylactic administration offers the advantage of replacing surfactant before the onset of respiratory failure, decreasing the need for ventilator support, and avoiding the barotrauma that may result from even short periods of assisted ventilation.[63] Surfactant may distribute more homogeneously when given immediately at birth into lungs still filled with fluid, leading to an improvement in response and decreasing the risk of lung injury.[64] However, surfactant treatment reserved for infants with established RDS offers the advantage of treating only infants with clinical disease, eliminating the potential risks and costs of treating surfactant-insufficient infants who receive no benefit of treatment.

In the shifting landscape of neonatal care, with increased use of antenatal steroids and successful application of the less invasive approaches previously discussed, the use of aggressive prophylactic surfactant has been questioned. Surfactant administration can be expensive, particularly in low-resource settings. In addition, intubation and mechanical ventilation may not be possible or desirable in institutions with limited resources. Surfactant may not have the same degree of benefit in infants who have received antenatal steroids, and those same infants may be best suited for CPAP treatment.[65] The introduction of these therapies may have changed the risk/benefit analysis of aggressive universal prophylactic intubation and treatment of infants at high risk for RDS.

An updated analysis of trials comparing prophylactic surfactant administration with selective surfactant treatment identified 11 studies (9 without routine application of CPAP in the selective group and 2 with routine application of CPAP in the selective treatment group).[66] The meta-analysis of studies conducted before the routine application of CPAP showed a decrease in the risk of air leak and neonatal mortality associated with prophylactic administrations of surfactant. However, the analyses of studies that allowed for routine stabilization on CPAP showed a decrease in the risk of chronic lung disease in infants stabilized on nasal CPAP. This finding has shifted the evidence base such that, seen in aggregate, there is no longer a proven benefit of prophylactic surfactant, and the more recent studies suggest improved outcome with a less aggressive treatment. This suggestion is reflected in changes of practice, with a decrease in intubation in the delivery room being seen through the first decade of the twenty-first century.[12,60]

LESS INVASIVE SURFACTANT ADMINISTRATION

The push toward stabilizing more infants on nasal CPAP has led to tension regarding when or whether to intubate these infants to give surfactant therapy. Both the use of less invasive ventilation by CPAP as well as surfactant are proved to improve outcome. However, they seem to be opposite approaches: surfactant administration requires early intubation and surfactant treatment, whereas stabilization on CPAP requires that clinicians avoid intubation if possible. Therefore, an approach that combines the benefits of surfactant administration and the benefits of early CPAP without the drawbacks associated with mechanical ventilation has great appeal. Less invasive means of administering surfactant have been developed to couple the theoretic advantages of both of these approaches.

INTUBATION, SURFACTANT ADMINISTRATION, AND EXTUBATION

The first less invasive approach to surfactant administration was the INSURE approach, in which spontaneously breathing infants are intubated, received surfactant, and are then rapidly extubated back to nasal CPAP. In 1994, Verder and colleagues[67] first reported the use of INSURE. In this unblinded trial, 35 infants with moderate to severe RDS were randomized to surfactant therapy plus nasal CPAP (INSURE) and compared with 33 infants given nasal continuous positive airway pressure alone. The need for subsequent mechanical ventilation was reduced with surfactant therapy (43% INSURE vs 85% controls). The same Scandinavian group went on to perform 2 additional unblinded studies in the 1990s, enrolling infants born at less than30 weeks' gestation and stabilized on CPAP.[68] When infants showed signs of RDS, they were randomized to intubation, surfactant administration, and rapid extubation to CPAP or to continued CPAP with rescue surfactant only if needed as shown by clinical deterioration. The results of these studies are encouraging. Infants had a decreased need for repeat dosing of surfactant, decreased oxygen requirement, and decreased subsequent need for mechanical ventilation.

Other randomized controlled trials followed. Stevens and colleagues[69] performed a systematic review comparing randomized controlled trials that used early surfactant administration within less than1 hour of mechanical ventilation followed by extubation versus selective surfactant administration, continued mechanical ventilation, and extubation from low respiratory support. Six randomized controlled clinical trials met selection criteria and were included in this review. In these studies of infants with signs and symptoms of RDS, intubation and early surfactant therapy followed by extubation to nasal CPAP compared with later selective surfactant administration was associated with a lower incidence of mechanical ventilation (typical RR 0.67, 95% CI 0.57, 0.79), air leak syndromes (typical RR 0.52, 95% CI 0.28, 0.96), and BPD (typical RR 0.51, 95% CI 0.26, 0.99). A larger proportion of infants in the early surfactant group received surfactant than in the selective surfactant group (typical RR 1.62, 95% CI 1.41, 1.86). In stratified analysis by Fio_2 at study entry, a lower threshold for treatment ($Fio_2<0.45$) resulted in lower incidence of air leak (typical RR 0.46 and 95% CI 0.23, 0.93) and BPD (typical RR 0.43, 95% CI 0.20, 0.92). A higher treatment threshold ($Fio_2>0.45$) at study entry was associated with a higher incidence of patent ductus arteriosus requiring treatment (typical RR 2.15, 95% CI 1.09, 4.13).

Other large trials have addressed the use of INSURE in the early stabilization of even less mature infants. The third arm of previously discussed VON DRM Trial used this approach and showed it to be as effective as prophylactic surfactant administration.[42] The multicenter VON DRM Trial used an INSURE arm, in which infants were given prophylactic surfactant and rapidly extubated to CPAP. Termed ISX (intubation, surfactant, and extubation) in this study, these infants were compared with infants who were intubated, given prophylactic surfactant, and maintained on mechanical ventilation. The ISX (INSURE) group was intubated at 5 to 15 minutes after birth, administered surfactant, and extubated to CPAP 15 to 30 minutes later if the Fio_2 was less than0.6 and the infant did not have severe respiratory distress or apnea. There was no difference in the primary outcome of death or chronic lung disease at 36 weeks' postmenstrual age.

THIN CATHETER ADMINISTRATION

Multiple trials have used an even less invasive method of surfactant administration. The thin catheter administration (TCA) technique is a method of surfactant administration by which a thin catheter (feeding tube or flexible angiocatheter) is inserted into the trachea of a spontaneously breathing infant stabilized on nasal CPAP allowing for surfactant administration. TCA is not strictly noninvasive; laryngoscopy is still needed to visualize the vocal cords and place the catheter for surfactant administration. However, they do prevent the operators from giving positive pressure ventilation or leaving the endotracheal tube in for a period of time after surfactant administration.

Seven randomized controlled trials have evaluated the effectiveness and safety of TCA of surfactant by endotracheal tube. Of these trials, 4 directly compared surfactant administration by TCA with INSURE, using the same treatment criteria for both groups. The remaining 3 trials compared surfactant administration by TCA with other administration methods (primarily intubation, mechanical ventilation, and surfactant administration) at varying treatment thresholds. Previous meta-analyses have been performed with the data from these studies.[70] However, these analyses did not distinguish between those studies, which compared TCA with INSURE (using the same administration criteria) and those that compared TCA to intubation followed by mechanical ventilation, some at different thresholds of administration. In our reanalysis of the data, it is clear that there are some benefits to TCA of surfactant. Although the meta-analysis does not support an effect on mortality (typical RR 0.85, 95% CI 0.56–1.28; typical risk difference −0.02, 95% CI −0.05–0.02). A marginal effect is seen on BPD (typical RR 0.73, 95% CI 0.53–1.01; typical risk difference −0.04–0.09 to 0.00) and pneumothorax (typical RR 0.61, 95% CI 0.37–1.00; typical risk difference −0.05, 95% CI −0.10 to −0.01). However, there is an impact on the combined outcome of BPD or death (typical RR 0.74, 95% CI 0.59–0.94; typical risk difference −0.07 to −0.12 to −0.02) as well as the need for mechanical ventilation in the first 72 hours (typical RR 0.74, 95% CI 0.65–0.85; typical risk difference 0.14, 95% CI −0.21–0.08).

ALTERNATIVES TO NASAL CONTINUOUS POSITIVE AIRWAY PRESSURE

Although clinicians are increasingly trying to manage preterm infants without mechanical ventilation, the reality is that many preterm infants stabilized on CPAP will fail, requiring intubation stabilization on mechanical ventilation.[54,55] Nasal IPPV represents an attempt to improve these failure rates. Nasal IPPV is a method of noninvasive respiratory support in which intermittent ventilator-generated breaths via a nasal interface are used to augment CPAP alone. It is discussed in greater detail in companion articles in this publication. Meta-analysis of trials of the early use nasal IPPV compared with early use of nasal CPAP in preterm infants reported significantly reduced risk of respiratory failure (typical RR 0.65, 95% CI 0.51–0.82; typical RD −0.09, 95% CI −0.13 to −0.04) and intubation (typical RR 0.78, 95% CI 0.64–0.94; typical RD −0.07, 95% CI −0.12 to −0.02) among infants treated with early nasal IPPV compared with early nasal CPAP.[71] The meta-analysis did not show a reduction in the risk of chronic lung disease among infants randomized to nasal IPPV (typical RR 0.78, 95% CI 0.58–1.06). Similar positive results are reported in the meta-analysis of trials of nasal IPPV compared with nasal CPAP in preterm neonates after extubation.[72]

Five trials used the synchronized form of NIPPV; 4 used the nonsynchronized form and 1 used both methods. Eight studies used NIPPV delivered by a ventilator, 1 used a bilevel device, and 1 used both methods. The use of nasal IPPV after extubation reduced respiratory failure (typical RR 0.70, 95% CI 0.60–0.80; typical RD −0.13, 95% CI −0.17 to −0.08; NNTB 8, 95% CI 6–13; 10 trials, 1431 infants) and the need for reintubation (typical RR 0.76, 95% CI 0.65–0.88; typical RD −0.10, 95% CI −0.15 to −0.05; NNTB 10, 95% CI 7–20; 10 trials, 1431 infants).

SUMMARY

Nasal CPAP represents one of the simplest but most important advances in neonatal care in the past 30 years. Growing expertise by caregivers worldwide will allow this technique to be one of the greatest lifesaving therapies ever introduced in neonatal care. Early use of CPAP with subsequent selective surfactant administration is currently the recommended approach to management of extremely preterm infants at risk of, or having, early signs of RDS.[44] However, the exact approach to the use of CPAP versus exogenous surfactant administration is evolving because of the trials of the less invasive surfactant treatment, including INSURE and thin catheter surfactant administration. In addition, many technical aspects of how best to deliver CPAP, including the role of IPPV, require further exploration.

Best Practices

What is the current practice?

CPAP has proved to be effective in the prevention and treatment of infants with RDS. CPAP is also effective in stabilization of infants extubated from assisted ventilation.

What changes in current practice are likely to improve outcomes?

Use of CPAP coupled with timely use of surfactant replacement therapy leads to optimal neonatal outcomes.

Major recommendations

Preterm infants at high risk for or having respiratory distress should be initially stabilized on CPAP.

Clear protocols for when (or whether) these infant should receive surfactant replacement therapy should be in place. Centers should consider less invasive approaches to surfactant administration so that exposure to assisted ventilation is minimized.

Rating for the strength of the evidence: moderate level of certainty

Summary statement

Preterm infants at high risk for or having respiratory distress should be initially stabilized on CPAP.

REFERENCES

1. Liggins GC, Howie RN. A controlled trial of antepartum glucocorticoid treatment for prevention of the respiratory distress syndrome in premature infants. Pediatrics 1972;50(4):515–25.
2. Enhörning G, Robertson B. Lung expansion in the premature rabbit fetus after tracheal deposition of surfactant. Pediatrics 1972;50(1):58–66.
3. Gregory GA, Kitterman JA, Phibbs RH, et al. Treatment of the idiopathic respiratory-distress syndrome with continuous positive airway pressure. N Engl J Med 1971;284(24):1333–40.
4. Ballard PL, Ballard R. Scientific basis and therapeutic regimens for use of antenatal glucocorticoids. Am J Obstet Gynecol 1995;173(1):254–62.
5. Bolt RJ, van Weissenbruch MM, Lafeber HN, et al. Glucocorticoids and lung development in the fetus and preterm infant. Pediatr Pulmonol 2001;32(1):76–91.
6. Roberts D, Brown J, Medley N, et al. Antenatal corticosteroids for accelerating fetal lung maturation for women at risk of preterm birth. Cochrane Database Syst Rev 2017;(3):CD004454.
7. Sinclair JC. Meta-analysis of randomized controlled trials of antenatal corticosteroid for the prevention of respiratory distress syndrome: discussion. Am J Obstet Gynecol 1995;173(1):335–44.
8. Crowley P, Chalmers I, Keirse MJ. The effects of corticosteroid administration before preterm delivery: an overview of the evidence from controlled trials. Br J Obstet Gynaecol 1990;97(1):11–25.
9. Crowley PA. Antenatal corticosteroid therapy: a meta-analysis of the randomized trials, 1972 to 1994. Am J Obstet Gynecol 1995;173(1):322–35.
10. Wright LL, Horbar JD, Gunkel H, et al. Evidence from multicenter networks on the current use and effectiveness of antenatal corticosteroids in low birth weight infants. Am J Obstet Gynecol 1995;173(1):263–9.

11. The effect of antenatal steroids for fetal maturation on perinatal outcomes. NIH Consens Statement 1994;12(2):1–24.
12. Soll RF, Edwards EM, Badger GJ, et al. Obstetric and neonatal care practices for infants 501 to 1500 g from 2000 to 2009. Pediatrics 2013;132(2):222–8.
13. Antenatal corticosteroid therapy for fetal maturation. Committee Opinion No. 713. American College of Obstetricians and Gynecologists. Obstet Gynecol 2017;130: e102–9.
14. Ehret DEY, Edwards EM, Greenberg LT, et al. Association of antenatal steroid exposure with survival among infants receiving postnatal life support at 22 to 25 weeks' gestation. JAMA Netw Open 2018;1(6):e183235.
15. Avery ME, Tooley WH, Keller JB, et al. Is chronic lung disease in low birth weight infants preventable? A survey of eight centers. Pediatrics 1987;79:26–30.
16. Van Marter LJ, Allred EN, Pagano M, et al. Do clinical markers of barotrauma and oxygen toxicity explain interhospital variation in rates of chronic lung disease? The Neonatology Committee for the Developmental Network. Pediatrics 2000; 105(6):1194–201.
17. De Paoli AG, Morley C, Davis PG. Nasal CPAP for neonates: what do we know in 2003? Arch Dis Child Fetal Neonatal Ed 2003;88:F168–72.
18. Ho JJ, Subramaniam P, Davis PG. Continuous distending pressure for respiratory distress in preterm infants. Cochrane Database Syst Rev 2015;(7):CD002271.
19. Belenky DA, Orr RJ, Woodrum DE, et al. Is continuous transpulmonary pressure better than conventional respiratory management of hyaline membrane disease? A controlled study. Pediatrics 1976;58(6):800–8.
20. Rhodes PG, Hall RT. Continuous positive airway pressure delivered by face mask in infants with the idiopathic respiratory distress syndrome: a controlled study. Pediatrics 1973;52(1):1–5.
21. Fanaroff AA, Cha CC, Sosa R, et al. Controlled trial of continuous negative external pressure in the treatment of severe respiratory distress syndrome. J Pediatr 1973;82(6):921–8.
22. Samuels MP, Raine J, Wright T, et al. Continuous negative extrathoracic pressure in neonatal respiratory failure. Pediatrics 1996;98(6 Pt 1):1154–60.
23. Buckmaster AG, Gaston A, Wright IMR, et al. Continuous positive airway pressure therapy for infants with respiratory distress in non tertiary care centers: a randomized controlled trial. Pediatrics 2007;120(3):509–18.
24. Durbin GM, Hunter NJ, McIntosh N, et al. Controlled trial of continuous inflating pressure for hyaline membrane disease. Arch Dis Child 1976;51(3):163–9.
25. Davis PG, Ho JJ. Nasal continuous positive airway pressure immediately after extubation for preventing morbidity in preterm infants. Cochrane Database Syst Rev 2003;(2):CD000143.
26. Engelke SC, Roloff DW, Kuhns LR. Postextubation nasal continuous positive airway pressure. Am J Dis Child 1982;136:359–61.
27. Higgins RD, Richter SE, Davis JM. Nasal continuous positive pressure facilitates extubation of very low birthweight neonates. Pediatrics 1991;88:999–1003.
28. Chan V, Greenough A. Randomised trial of methods of extubation in acute and chronic respiratory distress. Arch Dis Child 1993;68:570–2.
29. So B-H, Tamura M, Mishina J, et al. Application of nasal continuous positive airway pressure to early extubation in very low birthweight infants. Arch Dis Child 1995;72:F191–3.
30. Annibale D, Hulsey T, Engstrom P, et al. Randomised, controlled trial of nasopharyngeal continuous positive airways pressure in the extubation of very low birthweight infants. J Pediatr 1994;124:455–60.

31. Tapia J, Bancalari A, Gonzalez A, et al. Does continuous positive airways pressure (CPAP) during weaning from intermittent mandatory ventilation in very low birthweight infants have risks or benefits? A controlled trial. Pediatr Pulmonol 1995;19:269–79.

32. Davis P, Jankov R, Doyle L, et al. Randomised, controlled trial of nasal continuous positive airway pressure in the extubation of infants weighing 600 to 1250g. Arch Dis Child Fetal Neonatal Ed 1998;79:F54–7.

33. Dimitriou G, Greenough A, Kavvadia V, et al. Elective use of nasal continuous positive airways pressure following extubation of preterm infants. Eur J Pediatr 2000;159:434–9.

34. Peake M, Dillon P, Shaw NJ. Randomized trial of continuous positive airways pressure to prevent reventilation in preterm infants. Pediatr Pulmonol 2005;39: 247–50.

35. Subramaniam P, Ho JJ, Davis PG. Prophylactic or very early initiation of continuous distending pressure for preterm infants. Cochrane Database Syst Rev 2016;(6):CD001243.

36. Han VKM, Beverley DW, Clarson C, et al. Randomized controlled trial of very early continuous distending pressure in the management of preterm infants. Early Hum Dev 1987;15:21–32.

37. Sandri F, Ancora G, Lanzoni A, et al. Prophylactic nasal continuous positive airway pressure in newborns of 28-31 weeks gestation: multicentre randomised controlled clinical trial. Arch Dis Child Fetal Neonatal Ed 2004;89:F394–8.

38. Tapia JL, Urzua S, Bancalari A, et al, The South American Neocosur Network. Randomized trial of early bubble continuous positive airway pressure for very low birth weight infants. J Pediatr 2012;161:75–80.

39. Gonçalves-Ferri WA, Martinez FE, Caldas JPS, et al. Application of continuous positive airway pressure in the delivery room: a multicenter randomized clinical trial. Braz J Med Biol Res 2014;47(3):259–64.

40. Morley CJ, Davis PG, Doyle LW, et al, COIN Trial Investigators. Nasal CPAP or intubation at birth for very preterm infants. N Engl J Med 2008;358(7):700–8.

41. Finer NN, Carlo WA, Walsh MC, et al, SUPPORT Study Group of the Eunice Kennedy Shriver NICHD Neonatal Research Network. Early CPAP versus surfactant in extremely preterm infants. N Engl J Med 2010;362(21):1970–9.

42. Dunn MS, Kaempf J, de Klerk A, et al, The Vermont Oxford Network DRM Study Group. Randomized trial comparing 3 approaches to the initial respiratory management of preterm neonates. Pediatrics 2011;128:e1069–76.

43. Vaucher YE, Peralta-Carcelen M, Finer NN, et al. Neurodevelopmental outcomes in the early CPAP and pulse oximetry trial. N Engl J Med 2012;367(26):2495–504.

44. Committee on Fetus and Newborn, American Academy of Pediatrics. Respiratory support in preterm infants at birth. Pediatrics 2014;133(1):171–4.

45. De Paoli AG, Davis PG, Faber B, et al. Devices and pressure sources for administration of nasal continuous positive airway pressure (NCPAP) in preterm neonates. Cochrane Database Syst Rev 2008;(1):CD002977.

46. Verder H, Bohlin K, Kamper J, et al. Nasal CPAP and surfactant for treatment of respiratory distress syndrome and prevention of bronchopulmonary dysplasia. Acta Paediatr 2009;98:1400–8.

47. Buettiker V, Hug MI, Baenziger O, et al. Advantages and disadvantages of different nasal CPAP systems in newborns. Intensive Care Med 2004;30:926–30.

48. Davis P, Davies M, Faber B. A randomised controlled trial of two methods of delivering nasal continuous positive airway pressure after extubation to infants

weighing less than 1000g: binasal (Hudson) versus single nasal prongs. Arch Dis Child Fetal Neonatal Ed 2001;85:F82–5.

49. Mazzella M, Bellini C, Calevo MG, et al. A randomised control study comparing the Infant Flow Driver with nasal continuous positive airway pressure in preterm infants. Arch Dis Child Fetal Neonatal Ed 2001;85:F86–90.

50. Rego MAC, Martinez FE. Comparison of two nasal prongs for application of continuous positive airway pressure in neonates. Pediatr Crit Care Med 2002;3:239–43.

51. Roukema H, O'Brien K, Nesbitt K, et al. A randomized controlled trial of Infant Flow continuous positive airway pressure (CPAP) versus nasopharyngeal CPAP in the extubation of babies <=1250g (abstract). Pediatr Res 1999;45:318A.

52. Stefanescu BM, Murphy WP, Hansell BJ, et al. A randomized, controlled trial comparing two different continuous positive airway pressure systems for the successful extubation of extremely low birth weight infants. Pediatrics 2003;112:1031–8.

53. Sun SC, Tien HC. Randomized controlled trial of two methods of nasal CPAP (NCPAP): flow driver vs conventional NCPAP (abstract). Pediatr Res 1999;45:322A.

54. Finer NN, Carlo WA, Duara S, et al. Delivery room continuous positive airway pressure/positive end-expiratory pressure in extremely low birth weight infants: a feasibility trial. Pediatrics 2004;114(3):651–7.

55. Dargaville PA, Gerber A, Johansson S, et al, Australian and New Zealand Neonatal Network. Incidence and outcome of CPAP failure in preterm infants. Pediatrics 2016;138(1). https://doi.org/10.1542/peds.2015-3985.

56. Soll R, Ozek E. Prophylactic protein free synthetic surfactant for preventing morbidity and mortality in preterm infants. Cochrane Database Syst Rev 2010;(1):CD001079.

57. Soll RF. Prophylactic natural surfactant extract for preventing morbidity and mortality in preterm infants. Cochrane Database Syst Rev 2000;(2):CD000511.

58. Soll RF. Synthetic surfactant for respiratory distress syndrome in preterm infants. Cochrane Database Syst Rev 2000;2:CD001149.

59. Seger N, Soll R. Animal derived surfactant extract for treatment of respiratory distress syndrome. Cochrane Database Syst Rev 2009;(2):CD007836.

60. Polin RA, Carlo WA, Committee on Fetus and Newborn, American Academy of Pediatrics. Surfactant replacement therapy for preterm and term neonates with respiratory distress. Pediatrics 2014;133(1):156–63.

61. Schwartz RM, Luby AM, Scanlon JW, et al. Effect of surfactant on morbidity, mortality and resource use in newborn infants weighing 500-1500 gms. N Engl J Med 1994;330:1476–80.

62. Soll RF, Morley CJ. Prophylactic versus selective use of surfactant in preventing morbidity and mortality in preterm infants [review]. Cochrane Database Syst Rev 2001;(2):CD000510. [Update in: Cochrane Database Syst Rev 2012;(3):CD000510].

63. Nilsson R, Grossman G, Robertson B. Lung surfactant and the pathogenesis of neonatal bronchiolar lesions induced by artificial ventilation. Pediatr Res 1978;12:249–55.

64. Jobe A, Ikegami M, Jacobs H, et al. Surfactant and pulmonary blood flow distributions following treatment of premature lambs with natural surfactant. J Clin Invest 1984;73:848–56.

65. Jobe AH, Mitchell BR, Gunkel JH. Beneficial effects of the combined use of prenatal corticosteroids and postnatal surfactant on preterm infants. Am J Obstet Gynecol 1993;168(2):508–13.

66. Rojas-Reyes MX, Morley CJ, Soll R. Prophylactic versus selective use of surfactant in preventing morbidity and mortality in preterm infants. Cochrane Database Syst Rev 2012;(3):CD000510.

67. Verder H, Robertson B, Greisen G, et al. Surfactant therapy and nasal continuous positive airway pressure for newborns with respiratory distress syndrome. N Engl J Med 1994;331:1051–5.

68. Verder H, Albertsen P, Ebbesen F, et al. Nasal continuous positive airway pressure and early surfactant therapy for respiratory distress syndrome in newborns less than 30 weeks's gestation. Pediatrics 1999;(103):1–6.

69. Stevens TP, Harrington EW, Blennow M, et al. Early surfactant administration with brief ventilation vs. s elective surfactant and continued mechanical ventilation for preterm infants with or at risk for respiratory distress syndrome. Cochrane Database Syst Rev 2007;(4):CD003063.

70. Aldana-Aguirre JC, Pinto M, Featherstone RM, et al. Less invasive surfactant administration versus intubation for surfactant delivery in preterm infants with respiratory distress syndrome: a systematic review and meta-analysis. Arch Dis Child Fetal Neonatal Ed 2017;102(1):F17–23.

71. Lemyre B, Laughon M, Bose C, et al. Early nasal intermittent positive pressure ventilation (NIPPV) versus early nasal continuous positive airway pressure (NCPAP) for preterm infants. Cochrane Database Syst Rev 2016;(12):CD005384.

72. Lemyre B, Davis PG, De Paoli AG, et al. Nasal intermittent positive pressure ventilation (NIPPV) versus nasal continuous positive airway pressure (NCPAP) for preterm neonates after extubation. Cochrane Database Syst Rev 2017;(2):CD003212.

Nasal Intermittent Mandatory Ventilation Versus Nasal Continuous Positive Airway Pressure Before and After Invasive Ventilatory Support

Osayame Ekhaguere, MBBS, MPH[a],*, Shama Patel, MD[a],
Haresh Kirpalani, BM, MSc[b]

KEYWORDS

- Noninvasive respiratory support • Continuous positive airway pressure
- Noninvasive intermittent positive pressure ventilation • Respiratory failure
- Premature infants • Intubation • Heated humidified high-flow nasal cannula

KEY POINTS

- Continuous positive airway pressure (CPAP), noninvasive intermittent positive pressure ventilation (NIPPV), and heated humidified high-flow nasal cannula (HHFNC) are the mainstays of primary and postextubation respiratory support in preterm infants.
- The physiologic basis and practical application of CPAP and HHFNC are well delineated, whereas those of NIPPV remain unsubstantiated and varied in the literature.
- Available evidence suggests that NIPPV is superior to CPAP for primary and postextubation respiratory support in preterm infants.
- Guidelines are needed on the practical application of NIPPV for preterm infants.

INTRODUCTION

In current neonatal practice, a consensus now exists that avoidance or limitation of invasive positive pressure ventilation in preterm infants when possible is of benefit.[1] Clinical trials on noninvasive respiratory support for newborns began in the late 1960s.[2,3] However, inadequate devices and interfaces and, serious complications

Disclosures: None.
[a] Department of Pediatrics, Section of Neonatal-Perinatal Medicine, Indiana University, Riley Hospital for Children at Indiana University Health, 1030 West Michigan Street, C4600, Indianapolis, IN 46202, USA; [b] Department of Pediatrics, Division of Neonatology, The Children's Hospital of Philadelphia, 3401 Civic Center Boulevard, Philadelphia, PA 19104, USA
* Corresponding author.
E-mail address: osaekhag@iu.edu

limited their adoption.[4,5] Because invasive mechanical ventilation significantly reduced neonatal mortality, focus on noninvasive support was limited. However, the association of invasive mechanical ventilation with bronchopulmonary dysplasia (BPD),[6] poor neurodevelopment,[7] later mortality, and impacts on health care costs[8] became more widely appreciated and stimulated further work to improve devices and interfaces. Investigations into noninvasive respiratory support expanded in the late 1980s after early observations raised hope of decreasing the incidence of BPD.[9] More systematic work then began on whether it would (1) obviate mechanical ventilation, (2) prevent extubation failure, and (3) reduce the incidence of BPD. There has been a significant increase in the use of noninvasive respiratory support in the last 2 decades.[10] However, there is emerging evidence that the incidence of BPD has remained unchanged in the same time period.[10] Noninvasive respiratory support is now available as continuous positive airway pressure (CPAP), nasal intermittent positive pressure ventilation (NIPPV), and heated humidified high-flow nasal cannula (HHFNC).

This article focuses on 2 of the most extensively studied modes of noninvasive respiratory support: CPAP and NIPPV. It reviews their mechanisms of action and physiologic effects, and summarizes the evidence comparing their clinical use. Evidence is drawn primarily from randomized controlled trials (RCTs). In brief, it also discusses HHFNC and a newer form of noninvasive support: noninvasive high-frequency ventilation.

CONTINUOUS POSITIVE AIRWAY PRESSURE
Brief History

The physiologic consequences of laryngeal braking (grunting) sparked interest in CPAP respiratory support.[2,11] Teleologically, the goal seemed to be to overcome atelectasis in spontaneously breathing newborns. Could this be used therapeutically? In the earliest publication of its use, there was an astonishing 55% increase in the expected survival.[2]

Physiologic Principles of Continuous Positive Airway Pressure

Continuous positive airway pressure generates distending pressure that maintains functional residual capacity.[12] CPAP reduces elastic, flow-resistive, and inertial resistance properties of the respiratory system and stabilizes the compliant premature chest wall.[13–15] Ultimately this reduces ventilation-perfusion mismatch and improves oxygenation, work of breathing, and thoracoabdominal synchrony.[16,17] Because atelectasis leads to inflammation, unsurprisingly, CPAP reduces the inflammatory response in the lower respiratory tract.[18] In lamb studies, CPAP compared with mechanical ventilation reduced alveolar neutrophil influx, hydrogen peroxide production, and protein accumulation,[18,19] the hallmarks of lung injury that predispose preterm infants to BPD.[19]

Continuous Positive Airway Pressure Generating Devices

CPAP generating devices can be broadly classified into variable or continuous-flow systems.

Variable-flow continuous positive airway pressure
These devices vary CPAP levels predominantly by varying gas flow rate. They entrain gas flow and generate pressure during inspiration by the Bernoulli effect with the presence of an adaptive flip valve at the nasal interface[20]. The Infant Flow LP CPAP system (Care Fusion, Yorba Linda, CA) is an example of a variable-flow CPAP device.

Continuous-flow continuous positive airway pressure

These devices generate pressure by preventing gas egress from the circuit, which is accomplished by an expiratory limb resistance or a titratable positive end-expiratory pressure (PEEP) valve, depending on the specific device.[20] Ventilator-derived CPAP, and bubble CPAP (bCPAP) are both continuous-flow CPAP devices. The submerged expiratory limb of the bCPAP system generates its pressure. Varying the submersion depth changes the pressure (**Fig. 1**). Some observational studies suggest that bubbling from bCPAP further improves gas exchange by delivering low-amplitude, high-frequency oscillations to the lungs, [21,22] but this is unsubstantiated in observational studies.[23]

Continuous Positive Airway Pressure Delivery Interfaces

Earlier CPAP systems used head and face chambers or endotracheal tubes to transmit CPAP.[24] In current practice, soft and less irritant binasal prongs and nasal masks often made of silicone-based material are used. There is evidence of superiority of short binasal compared with single nasal and nasopharyngeal prongs in preventing reintubation and improving oxygenation.[25] Long nasopharyngeal tubes, which sit over the pharynx, are also used but are prone to obstruction. Binasal prongs and masks may also result in complications. The major reported complication is nasal septal injury, some requiring surgical intervention.[26,27] However, dedicated nursing care and barrier dressings (hydrocolloid and silicone gel sheeting) have been shown to reduce significantly the risk of nasal injury.[26,28-30]

Comparative Studies

Continuous positive airway pressure versus supportive care for initial respiratory support for preterm infants

Most trials in this category were in an era when antenatal steroids and surfactant were still emerging therapies, which makes extrapolating their results to medically advanced neonatal practice difficult. However, they still provide insight for low-resource settings.

Two Cochrane meta-analyses examined CPAP versus supportive care for primary respiratory support.[31,32] Supportive care included head-box oxygen or regular nasal

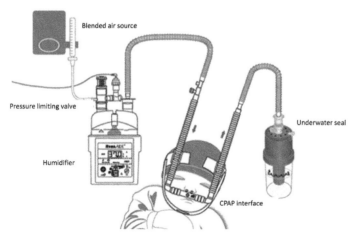

Fig. 1. Bubble CPAP setup showing blended air source, heater humidification system, underwater seal, and CPAP interface. (*Courtesy of* GaleMedCorporation, I-Lan, Taiwan)

cannula with thermoregulation and intravenous fluids. The first meta-analysis included premature infants treated within the first 15 minutes of life, regardless of the respiratory status of the infant.[31] Four trials that recruited 765 subjects were included. Failure was determined as need for mechanical ventilation in 3 trials and need for CPAP in 1 trial. Individually, the older trials did not show any difference. However, in newer trials dating from 2012, CPAP significantly decreased the failure rates. In the meta-analysis, CPAP was superior to supportive care in reducing treatment failure (typical risk ratio [RR] 0.66, 95% confidence interval [CI] 0.45 to 0.98; typical risk difference [RD] −0.16, 95% CI −0.34 to −0.02).[31] There was no reduction in BPD or mortality.[31]

The second meta-analysis evaluated continuous distending pressure compared with supportive care in infants diagnosed with respiratory distress syndrome at any time after birth.[32] It included 6 trials with a total of 355 infants. The interventions included CPAP or continuous negative pressure via a chamber. The outcome measure was composite death or use of assisted ventilation. Distending pressure significantly reduced respiratory failure and mortality compared with standard care (RR 0.65, 95% CI 0.52–0.81; RD −0.20, 95% CI −0.29 to −0.10; number needed to treat [NNT] 5, 95% CI 4–10).[32] However, there was an increased incidence of pneumothorax in the continuous distending pressure group (RR 2.64, 95% CI 1.39–5.04).[32]

Continuous positive airway pressure versus supportive care for preventing extubation failure in preterm infants

A Cochrane meta-analysis examined 9 RCTs comparing CPAP versus supportive care in preventing extubation failure within 7 days.[33] Head-box oxygen or low-flow nasal cannula constituted supportive care. In a meta-analysis of these trials, nasal CPAP reduced the incidence of respiratory failure (apnea, respiratory acidosis, and increased oxygen requirement) indicating the need for additional ventilatory support (RR 0.62, 95% CI 0.51–0.76; RD −0.17, 95% CI −0.24 to −0.10, NNT 6).[33] The use of head-box oxygen is uncommon in current practice, limiting generalization. However, the trials have had a great impact on the use of CPAP for postextubation respiratory support.

Comparisons of different continuous positive airway pressure generating devices

There have been remarkably few head-to-head comparisons between devices

Various continuous positive airway pressure devices for primary respiratory support Four RCTs have compared variable with continuous CPAP devices for initial respiratory support.[34–37] Three used bubble CPAP and 1 used a ventilator-derived system[37] as the continuous-flow device. The IFD system was used in 3[34,35,37] and the Jet CPAP (Hamilton Medical AG, Switzerland) in the fourh study.[36] There was no difference in need for mechanical ventilation in these trials. It is worth noting that 1 of these trials enrolled infants at less than 37 and 1 at less than 36 weeks' gestation.[34,35] Extrapolating these results to more premature infants is problematic.

Various continuous positive airway pressure devices for postextubation management of premature infants Five trials compared variable (IFD) with continuous-flow CPAP devices.[37–41] Bubble CPAP was used in 1 study.[38] Two studies are only available in abstract form.[39,41] Results from these trials indicate that variable CPAP is either superior to ventilator CPAP (2 trials: 16% vs 54% failure rate in one[39] and 38% vs 60% in the other[41]) or has similar efficacy to continuous-flow CPAP when used after extubation.[37,38,40]

NASAL INTERMITTENT POSITIVE PRESSURE VENTILATION

NIPPV is the application of CPAP throughout the respiratory cycle with superimposed cycled intermittent peak inspiratory pressures (PIP) without an endotracheal tube.[20]

The cycled PIPs may be synchronized (S-NIPPV) or nonsynchronized (NS-NIPPV) with the infant's spontaneous breathing.[20,42] Bilevel CPAP (also referred to as bi-NIPPV or biphasic CPAP) is a form of NIPPV but should be distinguished. The maximal PIP and cycling times differentiate bilevel CPAP from conventional NIPPV. The former has a smaller PIP range (typically 9–11 cm H_2O, and usually limited by the device) and longer cycling time (typically 0.5–1.0 seconds).[43] There is debate over whether bilevel CPAP is a different mode and strategy of noninvasive respiratory support or a spectrum of NIPPV.[43]

Brief History

NIPPV has been in use since the 1970s. In early observational reports, NIPPV resulted in favorable blood gas values.[44] A small clinical trial followed in 1970, which found that NIPPV reduced need for, and increased time to, mechanical ventilation compared with head box but with unacceptable side effects when using the available interfaces.[3] Reports of significant head molding, cerebellar hemorrhage, and gastric perforation stymied wide adoption of NIPPV.[3–5] NIPPV resurfaced in the late 1990s when trials comparing it with CPAP revealed no increased risk of complications.[45–47]

Physiologic Principles of Noninvasive Intermittent Positive Pressure Ventilation

The baseline distending pressure of NIPPV offers the same physiologic advantages as CPAP. However, the effects of the superimposed PIP remain uncertain.[43] The premise is that the generated PIP transmits to the lungs[45] and results in increased lung volumes, improved gas exchange, and decreased work of breathing.[48–50] However, studies show substantially less pressure delivered to the lung than proximally measured.[51,52] Compared with CPAP, some investigators have shown that NIPPV improves tidal volume and minute ventilation,[50,53] whereas others have shown no difference.[49,54,55] Of the 6 studies investigating carbon dioxide clearance between NIPPV and CPAP, only 2 reported lower carbon dioxide during NIPPV.[50,56]

NIPPV may also induce the Head paradoxic reflex and be of benefit in apnea of prematurity management.[20] Again, the evidence is conflicting on its effect on apnea.[52,57] One consistent physiologic consequence of NIPPV compared with CPAP is reduced work of breathing.[49,50,54,55,58]

Noninvasive Intermittent Positive Pressure Ventilation Generating Devices

Conventional NIPPV is ventilator generated, whereas bilevel CPAP is CPAP-driver generated. Any conventional ventilator can deliver NS-NIPPV. However, synchronization requires special adaptations.[43] These either are fitted with the ventilator or are an accessory. The 2 methods mainly used in trials are[1] the pneumatic capsule (Graseby Medical, Watford, United Kingdom) or other European variants of this, as in the Sophie-Respirator (Stephan Medizintechnik GmbH, Gackenbach, Germany), which detect abdominal wall movements to trigger the ventilator; and[2] flow sensors at the airway opening that use flow signals to trigger spontaneous breaths. The Giulia (Giulia Neonatal Nasal Ventilator, Ginevri Medical Technologies, Rome, Italy) is an example of a flow-sensor system.[59] Other techniques not widely available or extensively studied include pressure sensors seen in the SLE2000 ventilator (Specialized Laboratory Equipment Ltd, South Croydon, United Kingdom) and respiratory inductance plethysmography.[60] More recently, the invasive diaphragmatic electromyogram, by neutrally adjusted ventilator assist, has become popular but remains untested in an RCT.[61]

Devices for bilevel CPAP at present are limited to the Infant Flow SiPAP (synchronized inspiratory positive airway pressure) device (Care Fusion, Yorba Linda, CA), which is also used to generate CPAP.[37] This device can be adapted to simulate the

PIP seen with conventional NIPPV.[53,62] The Graseby capsule has also been incorporated into the SiPAP device to produce synchronized bilevel CPAP.[53]

Nasal mask or prongs, which may be short or long, single or binasal, are interfaces commonly used with NIPPV and bilevel CPAP.

The degrees of pressures and rates given during NIPPV parallel those given in conventional mechanical ventilation. Typical pressure settings are PIP of 14 to 24 cm H_2O and PEEP of 3 to 6 cm H_2O, with rate of 20 to 30 cycles/min and inspiratory time less than 0.5 seconds. These values differ from bilevel CPAP, in which high PEEP ranges between 9 and 11 cm H_2O and low PEEP 5 to 7 cm H_2O. Cycled rates are similar to ventilator-generated NIPPV; however, inspiratory times are typically longer (>0.5 seconds).[43]

Comparative Studies

Noninvasive intermittent positive pressure ventilation versus supportive care for primary respiratory support

Only 1 trial has compared NIPPV with head box. It randomized 44 infants with mean gestational age and birth weight of 33 weeks and 1892 g, respectively. Treatment failure, defined as partial pressure of oxygen less than 45 mm Hg in 100% oxygen, occurred in 13 of 22 infants (59%) and 20 of 22 infants (91%) in the NIPPV and head box group, respectively (RR 0.65, 95% CI 0.45–0.94; RD −0.32, 95% CI −0.56 to −0.08). There was no difference in survival (54% vs 36%).[3]

Noninvasive intermittent positive pressure ventilation versus supportive care for postextubation management of premature infants

A single trial compared NIPPV and head box, randomizing 95 infants with birth weight less than 2 kg. Infants received mechanical ventilation for at least 24 hours and were less than 28 days of age. The outcome measure was need for reintubation within 72 hours. Extubation failure occurred in 16% versus 62% in the NIPPV and head box groups, respectively (RR 0.25, 95% CI 0.12–0.51; RD −0.47, 95%CI −0.64 to −0.29).[63]

Comparing Noninvasive Intermittent Positive Pressure Ventilation Generating Devices

Comparing noninvasive intermittent positive pressure ventilation devices for primary respiratory support

One hundred and twenty-four infants less than 1500 g and less than 32 weeks of gestational age were randomized in a trial of S-NIPPV versus bilevel CPAP.[64] Randomization was after 2 hours of life, if mechanical ventilation was not required. Resuscitation included sustained inflation and infants less than 26 weeks' gestation received INSURE (intubation-surfactant-extubation) therapy. Respiratory failure occurred in 10 (16%) and 8 (13%) of the S-NIPPV and bilevel CPAP group, respectively (RR 1.25, 95% CI 0.52–2.96; RD 0.03, 95%CI −0.09–0.16). Duration of noninvasive support did not differ between groups.[64]

As primary respiratory support for preterm infants with or without respiratory distress syndrome, there are no RCTs directly comparing NS-NIPPV with S-NIPPV.

Comparing noninvasive intermittent positive pressure ventilation devices for postextubation management of premature infants

No RCTs directly compare NS-NIPPV with S-NIPPV; neither are there trials of NS-NIPPV or S-NIPPV versus bilevel CPAP for the prevention of extubation failure. The only comparison comes from a large pragmatic RCT that evaluated NIPPV (NS-NIPPV and bilevel CPAP) as primary (49%) or postextubation support (51%) versus CPAP on preventing death and BPD in preterm infants less than 30 weeks' gestation.[65] Subgroup analysis of the 241 and 215 infants who received ventilator-generated or flow driver NIPPV found no difference in the composite death or BPD outcome. Mortality in the flow driver NIPPV group was higher.[65]

Comparative Studies of the Modality of Noninvasive Intermittent Positive Pressure Ventilation and Continuous Positive Airway Pressure

Any form of noninvasive intermittent positive pressure ventilation versus continuous positive airway pressure for primary respiratory support

To ensure inclusion of all new trials since the 2016 Cochrane meta-analysis were included, the authors performed a new search and meta-analysis of updated trial information. We excluded 1 study from the 2016 Cochrane Review as it is only available as an abstract.[62] We also included a study that was excluded from the Cochrane Review.[66] This study used DuoPap (Hamilton Medical, Bonaduz, Switzerland), which alternates 2 different levels of PEEP, as seen with other bilevel CPAP devices.[66]

Using a fixed effect model, we pooled data from all 16 trials of 2014 infants.[56,60,65–78] The incidence of respiratory failure was reduced significantly by NIPPV (RR 0.55, 95% CI 0.46–0.65; RD −0.12, 95% CI −0.16 to −0.09, NNT 8) **(Fig. 2)**. These findings are similar to those reported in the 2016 Cochrane Review.

Nonsynchronized noninvasive intermittent positive pressure ventilation versus continuous positive airway pressure for primary respiratory support

Seven studies, which included 1077 infants, tested NS-NIPPV.[56,68,71,72,75,77,78] When pooled, the incidence respiratory failure was significantly reduced with use of NS-NIPPV (RR 0.57, 95% CI 0.44–0.73; RD −0.12, 95% CI −0.17 to −0.07. NNT 8).

Synchronized noninvasive intermittent positive pressure ventilation versus continuous positive airway pressure for primary respiratory support

There were 4 studies testing S-NIPPV, which, when pooled, included 338 infants.[60,69,73,76] S-NIPPV was superior to CPAP in the prevention of respiratory failure (RR 0.40, 95% CI 0.26–0.62; RD −0.20, 95% CI −0.29 to −0.12, NNT 5).

Bilevel continuous positive airway pressure (bilevel noninvasive intermittent positive pressure ventilation) versus continuous positive airway pressure for primary respiratory support

The authors identified 4 eligible studies that included 415 infants.[66,67,70,74] When pooled, bilevel CPAP was superior in preventing primary respiratory failure compared with CPAP (RR 0.59, 95% CI 0.38–0.94; RD −0.08, 95% CI −0.15 to −0.01, NNT 12).

Study or Subgroup	NIPPV Events	NIPPV Total	CPAP Events	CPAP Total	Weight	Risk Ratio M-H, Fixed, 95% CI	Year
Kugelman et al, 2007	11	43	20	41		Not estimable	2007
Bisceglia et al, 2007	1	42	1	46		Not estimable	2007
Sai Sunil Kishore, 2009	7	37	16	39	7.0%	0.46 [0.21, 0.99]	2009
Lista et al, 2010	2	20	3	20	1.3%	0.67 [0.12, 3.57]	2010
Meneses et al, 2011	25	100	34	100	15.2%	0.74 [0.48, 1.14]	2011
Ramanathan et al, 2012	4	53	14	57	6.0%	0.31 [0.11, 0.87]	2012
Kirpalani et al, 2013	20	94	26	90	11.9%	0.74 [0.44, 1.22]	2013
Armanina et al, 2014	2	44	1	54	0.4%	2.45 [0.23, 26.18]	2014
Shi et al, 2014	7	71	14	73	6.2%	0.51 [0.22, 1.20]	2014
Zhou et al, 2015	2	45	9	40	4.3%	0.20 [0.05, 0.86]	2015
Aguiar et al, 2015	16	111	20	109	9.0%	0.79 [0.43, 1.43]	2015
Salama et al, 2015	3	30	6	30	2.7%	0.50 [0.14, 1.82]	2015
Silvera et al, 2015	12	40	25	40	11.2%	0.48 [0.28, 0.82]	2015
Oncel et al, 2016	13	100	29	100	13.0%	0.45 [0.25, 0.81]	2016
Sadeghnia et al, 2016	5	35	9	35	4.0%	0.56 [0.21, 1.49]	2016
Dursun et al, 2018	5	42	17	42	7.8%	0.29 [0.12, 0.72]	2018
Total (95% CI)		**822**		**829**	**100.0%**	**0.55 [0.46, 0.67]**	
Total events	123		223				

Heterogeneity: Chi² = 11.77, df = 13 (P = .55); I² = 0%
Test for overall effect: Z = 6.01 (P<.00001)

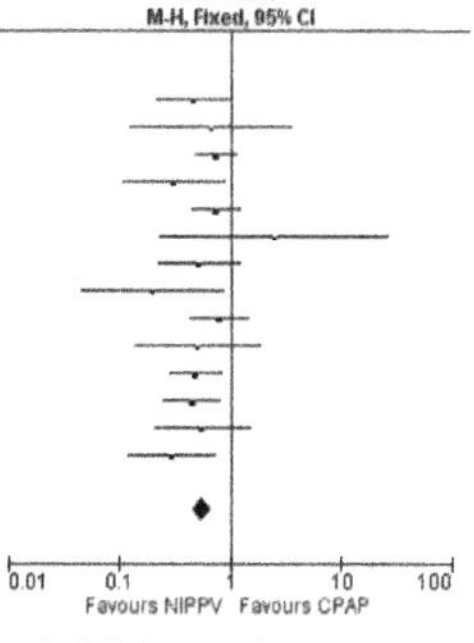

Favours NIPPV   Favours CPAP

Fig. 2. Forrest plot of NIPPV (all types) versus CPAP as initial respiratory support. M-H, Mantel-Haenszel.

Noninvasive intermittent positive pressure ventilation versus continuous positive airway pressure for postextubation respiratory support

In a 2017 Cochrane Review, the investigators analyzed 10 trials comparing NIPPV with CPAP for postextubation respiratory support.[79] The authors identified 2 additional studies[80,81] including 641 more infants to the 2017 Cochrane Review. Of the 12 trials included in this review, 5 used S-NIPPV,[45–47,82,83] 4 used ventilator-derived NS-NIPPV,[81,84–86] 2 used bilevel CPAP-derived NS-NIPPV,[80,87] and 1 used mixed therapies.[65] Compared with CPAP, NIPPV significantly reduced the rate of postextubation failure (RR 0.60, 95% CI 0.45–0.81; RD −0.15, 95% CI −0.23 to −0.08, NNT 7) **(Fig. 3)**. These findings are similar to those in the 2017 Cochrane Review.[79]

Nonsynchronized noninvasive intermittent positive pressure ventilation versus continuous positive airway pressure for postextubation respiratory support

Four studies in this category were identified, which included 279 infants.[81,84–86] When pooled, extubation failure was also significantly reduced in the NS-NIPPV compared with the CPAP group (RR 0.53, 95% CI 0.32–0.88; RD −0.12, 95% CI −0.22 to −0.03; NNT, 8).

Synchronized noninvasive intermittent positive pressure ventilation versus continuous positive airway pressure for postextubation respiratory support

The authors identified 5 studies in this category, which included 272 infants.[45–47,82,83] Three used a trigger sensor applied to the subject's abdomen (Star Sync Abdominal Sensor, Infrasonics Inc.)[45–47] and 1 used pneumotachograph (Giulia, Ginevri, Rome, Italy).[82] When pooled, extubation failure incidence was significantly reduced with NIPPV compared with CPAP (RR 0.26, 95% CI 0.16–0.44; RD −0.31, 95% CI −0.40 to −0.21, NNT 3).

Bilevel continuous positive airway pressure versus continuous positive airway pressure postextubation respiratory support

The 2 trials that used bilevel CPAP, when pooled, included 679 infants.[80,87] When pooled, the incidence of postextubation respiratory failure did not differ between groups (RR 1.01, 95% CI 0.81–1.24; RD 0.00, 95% CI −0.07–0.07).

No RCT has directly examined differences between ventilator-generated and flow driver–generated NIPPV or between S-NIPPV and NS-NIPPV.[43]

In summary, as more patients have accumulated in trials, the evidence supports NIPPV rather than CPAP for initial and postextubation respiratory support in preterm infants. The most benefit may remain for synchronized methods of applying NIPPV. Future trials are needed to refine methods of synchronization.

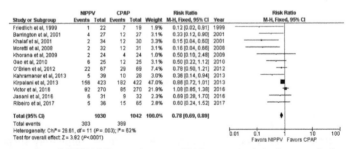

Fig. 3. Forrest plot of NIPPV (all types) versus CPAP as postextubation respiratory support.

HEATED HUMIDIFIED HIGH-FLOW NASAL CANNULA
Brief History

This form of noninvasive respiratory support delivers heated, humidified air flow at rates greater than 1 L/min through a specialized nasal prong. Interest in HHFNC began in the late 1990s. It was premised on the hypothesis that the clinical response of the regular nasal cannula was caused by inadvertently generated PEEP.[88] This hypothesis was subsequently verified in clinical studies.[89]

Physiologic Effect

Similar to CPAP, the high flow of oxygen or air creates continuous distending pressure, which maintains functional residual capacity. Other putative benefits of HHFNC include improved airway conductance, washout of nasopharyngeal dead space, and reduction of inspiratory resistance.[90]

Humidified High-flow Nasal Cannula Generating Devices

HHFNC requires an oxygen and medical air source, a heating and humidification system, a flow meter, and a patient interface. Unlike CPAP and NIPPV generating devices, the basic functional theories behind HHFNC devices are the same. Two commonly available systems are the Vapotherm 2000 (Vapotherm Inc., Stevensville, MD) and Optiflow Junior (Fisher & Paykel Healthcare, Auckland, New Zealand) (**Fig. 4**).[91] Any nasal cannula can be used to apply HHFNC. However, the most commonly used are soft, malleable, silicone-based nasal cannulae.

Comparative Studies

Humidified high-flow nasal cannula versus continuous positive airway pressure for primary respiratory support

A Cochrane Review in 2016, including 4 RCTs and 439 patients, found no difference between HHFNC and CPAP as primary respiratory support.[92] However, there have been 4 additional trials published in the intervening period.[93–96] The authors excluded 1 study from the Cochrane Review that is only available as an abstract.[97] There are now more than 1500 preterm infants randomized in trials of HHFNC as primary respiratory support for preterm infants. Using a random effect model, we pooled the data from newer trials with those of the 2016 meta-analysis. Our findings indicate that CPAP is superior to HHFNC in preventing respiratory failure (RR 1.86, 95% CI 1.46–2.37; RD 0.10, 95% CI 0.06–0.13, NNT 17) (**Fig. 5**).

The investigators of the largest pragmatic trials comparing HHFNC with CPAP evaluated the demographic and clinical factors that predict HHFNC success as primary respiratory support.[98] Of the 278 infants with gestational age 28 to 36 weeks randomized to the HHFNC, 207 (74.5%) were successful and 71 (25.5%) had treatment failure. Birth gestational age greater than or equal to 30 weeks and prerandomization fraction of inspired oxygen less than 0.30 were independent predictors of treatment success.[98]

Humidified high-flow nasal cannula versus noninvasive intermittent positive pressure ventilation for primary respiratory support

There are 3 trials that have compared HHFNC with NIPPV for primary respiratory support.[99–101] Synchronization was used in 1 trial, which was a pilot study,[99] whereas synchronization was not specified in the others. There was no difference in respiratory failure between NIPPV and HHFNC in all 3 trials.

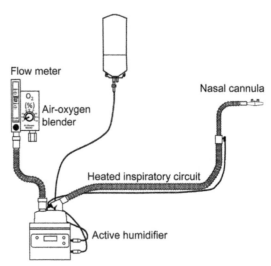

Fig. 4. Basic setup for high-flow nasal cannula oxygen delivery, showing flow meter, blended air source, heater humidifier system, heated inspiratory circuit, and nasal cannula interference. (*Adapted from* Nishimura M. High-flow nasal cannula oxygen therapy in adults. J Intensive Care. 2015 Mar 31;3(1):15. https://doi.org/10.1186/s40560-015-0084-5. eCollection 2015.)

Humidified high-flow nasal cannula versus continuous positive airway pressure for preventing postextubation failure

A Cochrane meta-analysis of 6 published studies including 934 infants compared HHFNC with CPAP for preventing postextubation failure.[92] HHFNC conferred no additional risk of treatment failure (RR 1.21, 95% CI, 0.95–1.55) or reintubation (RR 0.91, 95% CI, 0.68–1.20). Three trials have been published since then, 2 indicating no difference between HHFNC and CPAP[102,103] and 1 indicating higher failure rates with HHFNC.[104]

NONINVASIVE HIGH-FREQUENCY VENTILATION
Brief History

In noninvasive high-frequency ventilation (NIHFV), high-frequency oscillatory pressure waveforms are superimposed on constant positive airway pressure through a nasal prong, mask, or pharyngeal tube.[105] First described in 1998,[106] NIHFV is gaining attention in neonatal practice. Among surveyed clinicians in Europe and Canada, 17% and 18% reported the use of NIHFV.[107,108] However, there remains a paucity of randomized data.

Physiologic Effect

The theoretic rationale for the use of NIHFV is based on 2 factors: (1) that the effect of low tidal volumes and optimal distending pressure seen in conventional high-

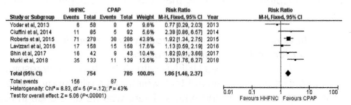

Fig. 5. Forrest plot of HHFNC versus CPAP as initial respiratory support.

frequency ventilation (HFV) can be achieved noninvasively, and (2) its nondependence on synchronization to ventilate.[105] However, as with high-frequency ventilation, there is poor understanding of how it results in physiologic change. Observational and small crossover studies in preterm infants indicate that NIHFV is effective in eliminating carbon dioxide.[106,109–111] However, in a recent larger crossover trial involving 26 premature infants that alternated between NIHFV and CPAP for 4 hours, there was no difference in carbon dioxide clearance.[112]

Noninvasive High-frequency Ventilation Generating Device

In theory, any ventilator able to generate HFV can be used for NIHFV. There is great variation in those reported in the literature. Examples include the Infant Star ventilator (Infrasonics, San Diego, CA), Babylog 8000 (Drager, Lubeck, Germany), and the high-frequency percussive ventilator VDR3 (Percussionaire Corp, Sagle, ID). Nasopharyngeal endotracheal tubes, short binasal prongs, and heated humidified nasal probes are interphases used to administer NIHFV.

As with HFV, a mean airway pressure, amplitude, and frequency are set. Wide variation in NIHFV setting exists from the observational and small RCTs published. Mean airway pressure ranges from 4 to 13, amplitude 20 to 60, and frequency range from 5 to 10 Hz have been used.[105] The amplitude is adjusted to yield adequate chest oscillation.

Comparative Studies

Trials comparing NIHFV with other forms of noninvasive respiratory support in preterm infants are sparse. Of the 3 trials available, NIHFV was compared with CPAP in 2 and bilevel CPAP in the third as primary respiratory support. Two trials assessed respiratory failure within 72 hours.

In the first trial involving CPAP, the investigators randomized 81 preterm infants with a gestational age of 28 to 30 weeks who had received INSURE. The need for mechanical ventilation was significantly greater with the CPAP (56%) compared with the NIHFV (24%) ($P = .004$).[113] There were no differences in mortality, BPD, or intraventricular hemorrhage. In the second trial, 124 infants with a gestational age of 28 to 34 weeks were randomized.[114] No difference was seen in the rate of respiratory failure within 72 hours between the two groups. The third was a feasibility trial. Preterm infants with birth weight less than 1250 g who failed CPAP were randomized to NIHFV (n = 16) versus bilevel CPAP (n = 23) as rescue. Respiratory failure tended to occur less often with the NIHFV compared with the bilevel CPAP (38% vs 65%), HYPE[115] but this was not statistically significant ($P = .09$). There were no differences in the rates of BPD or the use of invasive mechanical ventilation at 72 hours and 7 days postrandomization.

SUMMARY

CPAP and NIPPV are integral to current neonatal practice. Both are effective as primary respiratory support and in postextubation management in preterm infants. The available evidence indicates that NIPPV is superior to CPAP in both instances. However, their effect on mortality and the incidence of BPD is similar, and there is limited evidence to assess their effect on neurodevelopment. Although the application of CPAP is fairly similar across studies, there are wide variations in definition, mode of generation, and method of application of NIPPV in studies. As primary respiratory support, CPAP is superior to HHFNC and superior or equivalent to HHFNC for postextubation failure. The limited available evidence

Table 1
Comparative advantages and disadvantages of continuous positive airway pressure, noninvasive intermittent positive pressure ventilation, and humidified high-flow nasal cannula

Feature	Nasal CPAP	NIPPV	HHFNC
Device generator	Two broad groups: variable and continuous-flow devices	Two broad groups: ventilator and SiPAP (bilevel CPAP)	Two common available devices: Fisher & Paykel and Vapotherm device
Mode of delivery	Single mode of delivery	Variable modes: synchronization and nonsynchronization. Also, high peak pressures and bilevel CPAP	Single mode of delivery
Generated pressure	CPAP pressure is predictable and regulated	CPAP and peak inspiratory pressure are predictable and regulated. Peak pressure can be high or low depending on device generator/delivery mode	Flow rate is set and generates an unmeasured pressure. The pressure generated is not predictable or regulated
Effect of leak (eg, poorly positioned interface, or open mouth) on delivered pressure	Pressure loss. Can be minimize by positioning, placement of soother, or chin strapping (the latter not recommended)	Pressure loss. Can be minimize by positioning, placement of soother, or chin strapping (the latter not recommended)	Flow and resultant pressure loss. Can be minimize by positioning, placement of soother, or chin strapping (the latter not recommended)
Pressure alarm	Present	Present	Absent in Fisher & Paykel devices but present in the Vapotherm device[116]
Risk of nasal injury[92]	Comparable with NIPPV and higher than HHFNC; can be mitigated by barrier (eg, silicone gel) dressing	Comparable with NIPPV and higher than HHFNC; can be mitigated by barrier (eg, silicone gel) dressing	Less than CPAP and NIPPV. However, not absent
Precipitation of humidity rain out[117]	Present. May be less with nasal prongs	Present	Present. May be less with the Vapotherm device
Nursing perception[118]	Requires vigilant attention and nursing time to avoid leak or undue pressure. Similar application process, maintenance, and comfort to NIPPV but different from HHFNC	Requires vigilant attention and nursing time to avoid leak or undue pressure. Similar application process, maintenance, and comfort to CPAP but different from HHFNC	Perception of increased infant comfort and easy application, maintenance compared with CPAP and NIPPV

(continued on next page)

Table 1
(continued)

Feature	Nasal CPAP	NIPPV	HHFNC
Parental perception[119]	Perception that infants were less satisfied compared with HHFNC and allowed for less contact, interaction, and parents ability to care for infant compared with HHFNC	Not assessed in any study but presumed to be similar to CPAP	Increased perception of infant being satisfied, increased contact, interaction, and parental ability to care for child compared with CPAP
Optimal patient population to use	Small infants may benefit more compared with HHFNC	Small infants, postextubation support; likely better outcomes with synchronization	Better for larger infants who struggle more with the interface

suggests that NIPPV is equivalent to HHFNC as primary respiratory support for preterm infants. NIHFV is a newer mode of noninvasive ventilation that requires further rigorous evaluation of efficacy and safety before adoption into practice (**Table 1**).

REFERENCES

1. Carlo WA, Polin RAJP. Respiratory support in preterm infants at birth. Pediatrics 2014;133(1):171–4.
2. Gregory GA, Kitterman JA, Phibbs RH, et al. Treatment of the idiopathic respiratory-distress syndrome with continuous positive airway pressure. New England Journal of Medicine 1971;284(24):1333–40.
3. Llewellyn M, Tilak K, Swyer PJ. A controlled trial of assisted ventilation using an oro-nasal mask. Arch Dis Child 1970;45(242):453–9.
4. Pape KE, Armstrong DL, Fitzhardinge PM. CNS pathology associated with mask ventilation. Pediatrics 1977;60(5):787–8.
5. Garland JS, Nelson DB, Rice T, et al. Increased risk of gastrointestinal perforations in neonates mechanically ventilated with either face mask or nasal prongs. Pediatrics 1985;76(3):406–10.
6. Jobe AH, Bancalari E. Bronchopulmonary dysplasia. Am J Respir Crit Care Med 2001;163(7):1723–9.
7. Schmidt B, Asztalos EV, Roberts RS, et al. Impact of bronchopulmonary dysplasia, brain injury, and severe retinopathy on the outcome of extremely low-birth-weight infants at 18 months: results from the trial of indomethacin prophylaxis in preterms. JAMA 2003;289(9):1124–9.
8. Stroustrup A, Trasande L. Epidemiological characteristics and resource use in neonates with bronchopulmonary dysplasia: 1993-2006. Pediatrics 2010; 126(2):291–7.
9. Avery ME, Tooley WH, Keller JB, et al. Is chronic lung disease in low birth weight infants preventable? A survey of eight centers. Pediatrics 1987;79(1):26–30.
10. Doyle LW, Carse E, Adams AM, et al. Ventilation in extremely preterm infants and respiratory function at 8 years. N Engl J Med 2017;377(4):329–37.

11. Harrison VC, Heese Hde V, Klein M. The significance of grunting in hyaline membrane disease. Pediatrics 1968;41(3):549–59.
12. Morley C. Continuous distending pressure. Arch Dis Child Fetal Neonatal Ed 1999;81(2):F152–6.
13. da Silva WJ, Abbasi S, Pereira G, et al. Role of positive end-expiratory pressure changes on functional residual capacity in surfactant treated preterm infants. Pediatr Pulmonol 1994;18(2):89–92.
14. Saunders RA, Milner AD, Hopkin IE. The effects of continuous positive airway pressure on lung mechanics and lung volumes in the neonate. Biol Neonate 1976;29(3–4):178–86.
15. Miller MJ, DiFiore JM, Strohl KP, et al. Effects of nasal CPAP on supraglottic and total pulmonary resistance in preterm infants. J Appl Physiol (1985) 1990;68(1):141–6.
16. Agostoni E, Mead J. Statics of the respiratory system. In: Fenn WO, Rahn H, editors. Handbook of Physiology. Washington, DC: American Physiological Society; 1964. p. 387–409.
17. Chernick V. Hyaline-membrane disease: therapy with constant lung-distending pressure. N Engl J Med 1973;289(6):302–4.
18. Jobe AJ. The new BPD: an arrest of lung development. Pediatr Res 1999;46(6):641–3.
19. Groneck P, Speer CP. Inflammatory mediators and bronchopulmonary dysplasia. Arch Dis Child Fetal Neonatal Ed 1995;73(1):F1–3.
20. Courtney SE, Barrington KJ. Continuous positive airway pressure and noninvasive ventilation 2007;34(1):73–92.
21. Lee KS, Dunn MS, Fenwick M, et al. A comparison of underwater bubble continuous positive airway pressure with ventilator-derived continuous positive airway pressure in premature neonates ready for extubation. Biol Neonate 1998;73(2):69–75.
22. Pillow JJ, Hillman N, Moss TJ, et al. Bubble continuous positive airway pressure enhances lung volume and gas exchange in preterm lambs. Am J Respir Crit Care Med 2007;176(1):63–9.
23. Morley CJ, Lau R, De Paoli A, et al. Nasal continuous positive airway pressure: does bubbling improve gas exchange? Arch Dis Child Fetal Neonatal Ed 2005;90(4):F343–4.
24. DiBlasi RM. Nasal continuous positive airway pressure (CPAP) for the respiratory care of the newborn infant. Respir Care 2009;54(9):1209–35.
25. De Paoli AG, Davis PG, Faber B, et al. Devices and pressure sources for administration of nasal continuous positive airway pressure (NCPAP) in preterm neonates. Cochrane Database Syst Rev 2008;(1):CD002977.
26. Gupta S, Donn SM. Continuous positive airway pressure: physiology and comparison of devices. Semin Fetal Neonatal Med 2016;21(3):204–11.
27. Robertson NJ, McCarthy LS, Hamilton PA, et al. Nasal deformities resulting from flow driver continuous positive airway pressure. Arch Dis Child Fetal Neonatal Ed 1996;75(3):F209–12.
28. Imbulana DI, Owen LS, Dawson JA, et al. A randomized controlled trial of a barrier dressing to reduce nasal injury in preterm infants receiving binasal noninvasive respiratory support. J Pediatr 2018;201:34–9.e3.
29. Gunlemez A, Isken T, Gokalp AS, et al. Effect of silicon gel sheeting in nasal injury associated with nasal CPAP in preterm infants. Indian Pediatr 2010;47(3):265–7.
30. Xie LH. Hydrocolloid dressing in preventing nasal trauma secondary to nasal continuous positive airway pressure in preterm infants. World J Emerg Med 2014;5(3):218–22.

31. Subramaniam P, Ho JJ, Davis PG. Prophylactic nasal continuous positive airway pressure for preventing morbidity and mortality in very preterm infants. Cochrane Database Syst Rev 2016;(6):CD001243.

32. Ho JJ, Subramaniam P, Davis PG. Continuous distending pressure for respiratory distress in preterm infants. Cochrane Database Syst Rev 2015;(7):CD002271.

33. Davis PG, Henderson-Smart DJ. Nasal continuous positive airways pressure immediately after extubation for preventing morbidity in preterm infants. Cochrane Database Syst Rev 2003;(2):CD000143.

34. Mazzella M, Bellini C, Calevo MG, et al. A randomised control study comparing the Infant Flow Driver with nasal continuous positive airway pressure in preterm infants. Arch Dis Child Fetal Neonatal Ed 2001;85(2):F86–90.

35. Mazmanyan P, Mellor K, Doré CJ, et al. A randomised controlled trial of flow driver and bubble continuous positive airway pressure in preterm infants in a resource-limited setting. Arch Dis Child Fetal Neonatal Ed 2016;101(1):16–20.

36. Bhatti A, Khan J, Murki S, et al. Nasal Jet-CPAP (variable flow) versus Bubble-CPAP in preterm infants with respiratory distress: an open label, randomized controlled trial. J Perinatol 2015;35(11):935–40.

37. Bober K, Swietlinski J, Zejda J, et al. A multicenter randomized controlled trial comparing effectiveness of two nasal continuous positive airway pressure devices in very-low-birth-weight infants. Pediatr Crit Care Med 2012;13(2):191–6.

38. Gupta S, Sinha SK, Tin W, et al. A randomized controlled trial of post-extubation bubble continuous positive airway pressure versus Infant Flow Driver continuous positive airway pressure in preterm infants with respiratory distress syndrome. J Pediatr 2009;154(5):645–50.

39. Sun SC, Tien HC. Randomized controlled trial of two methods of nasal CPAP(NCPAP): flow driver Vs conventional NCPAP. Pediatr Res 1999;45(7):322.

40. Stefanescu BM, Murphy WP, Hansell BJ, et al. A randomized, controlled trial comparing two different continuous positive airway pressure systems for the successful extubation of extremely low birth weight infants. Pediatrics 2003; 112(5):1031–8.

41. Roukema H, O'Brien K, Nesbitt K, et al. A randomized controlled trial of infant flow continuous positive airway pressure (CPAP) versus nasopharyngeal CPAP in the extubation of babies ≤ 1250 grams. Pediatr Res 1999;45(7):318.

42. Ferguson KN, Roberts CT, Manley BJ, et al. Interventions to improve rates of successful extubation in preterm infants: a systematic review and meta-analysis. JAMA Pediatr 2017;171(2):165–74.

43. Owen LS, Manley BJ. Nasal intermittent positive pressure ventilation in preterm infants: equipment, evidence, and synchronization. Semin Fetal Neonatal Med 2016;21(3):146–53.

44. Helmrath TA, Hodson WA, Oliver TK Jr. Positive pressure ventilation in the newborn infant: the use of a face mask. J Pediatr 1970;76(2):202–7.

45. Friedlich P, Lecart C, Posen R, et al. A randomized trial of nasopharyngeal-synchronized intermittent mandatory ventilation versus nasopharyngeal continuous positive airway pressure in very low birth weight infants after extubation. J Perinatol 1999;19(6 Pt 1):413–8.

46. Khalaf MN, Brodsky N, Hurley J, et al. A prospective randomized, controlled trial comparing synchronized nasal intermittent positive pressure ventilation versus nasal continuous positive airway pressure as modes of extubation. Pediatrics 2001;108(1):13–7.

47. Barrington KJ, Bull D, Finer NN. Randomized trial of nasal synchronized intermittent mandatory ventilation compared with continuous positive airway pressure after extubation of very low birth weight infants. Pediatrics 2001;107(4):638–41.

48. Kiciman NM, Andréasson B, Bernstein G, et al. Thoracoabdominal motion in newborns during ventilation delivered by endotracheal tube or nasal prongs. Pediatr Pulmonol 1998;25(3):175–81.

49. Aghai ZH, Saslow JG, Nakhla T, et al. Synchronized nasal intermittent positive pressure ventilation (SNIPPV) decreases work of breathing (WOB) in premature infants with respiratory distress syndrome (RDS) compared to nasal continuous positive airway pressure (NCPAP). Pediatr Pulmonol 2006;41(9):875–81.

50. Moretti C, Gizzi C, Papoff P, et al. Comparing the effects of nasal synchronized intermittent positive pressure ventilation (nSIPPV) and nasal continuous positive airway pressure (nCPAP) after extubation in very low birth weight infants. Early Hum Dev 1999;56(2–3):167–77.

51. Owen LS, Morley CJ, Davis PG. Pressure variation during ventilator generated nasal intermittent positive pressure ventilation in preterm infants. Arch Dis Child Fetal Neonatal Ed 2010;95(5):F359–64.

52. Ryan CA, Finer NN, Peters KL. Nasal intermittent positive-pressure ventilation offers no advantages over nasal continuous positive airway pressure in apnea of prematurity. Am J Dis Child 1989;143(10):1196–8.

53. Miedema M, van der Burg PS, Beuger S, et al. Effect of nasal continuous and biphasic positive airway pressure on lung volume in preterm infants. J Pediatr 2013;162(4):691–7.

54. Ali N, Claure N, Alegria X, et al. Effects of non-invasive pressure support ventilation (NI-PSV) on ventilation and respiratory effort in very low birth weight infants. Pediatr Pulmonol 2007;42(8):704–10.

55. Chang HY, Claure N, D'Ugard C, et al. Effects of synchronization during nasal ventilation in clinically stable preterm infants. Pediatr Res 2011;69(1):84–9.

56. Bisceglia M, Belcastro A, Poerio V, et al. A comparison of nasal intermittent versus continuous positive pressure delivery for the treatment of moderate respiratory syndrome in preterm infants. Minerva Pediatr 2007;59(2):91–5.

57. Pantalitschka T, Sievers J, Urschitz MS, et al. Randomised crossover trial of four nasal respiratory support systems for apnoea of prematurity in very low birthweight infants. Arch Dis Child Fetal Neonatal Ed 2009;94(4):F245–8.

58. Huang L, Mendler MR, Waitz M, et al. Effects of synchronization during noninvasive intermittent mandatory ventilation in preterm infants with respiratory distress syndrome immediately after extubation. Neonatology 2015;108(2):108–14.

59. Wright CJ, Polin RA. Noninvasive support: does it really decrease bronchopulmonary dysplasia? Clin Perinatol 2016;43(4):783–98.

60. Kugelman A, Feferkorn I, Riskin A, et al. Nasal intermittent mandatory ventilation versus nasal continuous positive airway pressure for respiratory distress syndrome: a randomized, controlled, prospective study. J Pediatr 2007;150(5): 521–6, 526.e1.

61. Stein H, Firestone K. Application of neurally adjusted ventilatory assist in neonates. Semin Fetal Neonatal Med 2014;19(1):60–9.

62. Wood F, Gupta S, Tin W, et al. G170 randomised controlled trial of synchronised intermittent positive airway pressure (SiPAP™) versus continuous positive airway pressure (CPAP) as a primary mode of respiratory support in preterm infants with respiratory distress syndrome. Arch Dis Child 2013;98(Suppl 1):A78.

63. Kumar M, Avasthi S, Ahuja S, et al. Unsynchronized nasal intermittent positive pressure ventilation to prevent extubation failure in neonates: a randomized controlled trial. Indian J Pediatr 2011;78(7):801–6.

64. Salvo V, Lista G, Lupo E, et al. Noninvasive ventilation strategies for early treatment of RDS in preterm infants: an RCT. Pediatrics 2015;135(3):444–51.

65. Kirpalani H, Millar D, Lemyre B, et al. A trial comparing noninvasive ventilation strategies in preterm infants. N Engl J Med 2013;369(7):611–20.

66. Zhou B, Zhai J, Jiang H, et al. Usefulness of DuoPAP in the treatment of very low birth weight preterm infants with neonatal respiratory distress syndrome. Eur Rev Med Pharmacol Sci 2015;19(4):573–7.

67. Aguiar T, Macedo I, Voutsen O, et al. Nasal bilevel versus continuous positive airway pressure in preterm infants: a randomized controlled trial. J Clin Trials 2015;5(3):221.

68. Armanian A-m, Badiee Z, Heidari G, et al. Initial treatment of respiratory distress syndrome with nasal intermittent mandatory ventilation versus nasal continuous positive airway pressure: a randomized controlled trial. Int J Prev Med 2014; 5(12):1543.

69. Dursun M, Uslu S, Bulbul A, et al. Comparison of early nasal intermittent positive pressure ventilation and nasal continuous positive airway pressure in preterm infants with respiratory distress syndrome. J Trop Pediatr 2018. https://doi.org/10.1093/tropej/fmy058.

70. Lista G, Castoldi F, Fontana P, et al. Nasal continuous positive airway pressure (CPAP) versus bi-level nasal CPAP in preterm babies with respiratory distress syndrome: a randomised control trial. Arch Dis Child Fetal Neonatal Ed 2010; 95(2):F85–9.

71. Meneses J, Bhandari V, Alves JG, et al. Noninvasive ventilation for respiratory distress syndrome: a randomized controlled trial. Pediatrics 2011;127(2):300–7.

72. Oncel MY, Arayici S, Uras N, et al. Nasal continuous positive airway pressure versus nasal intermittent positive-pressure ventilation within the minimally invasive surfactant therapy approach in preterm infants: a randomised controlled trial. Arch Dis Child Fetal Neonatal Ed 2016;101(4):F323–8.

73. Ramanathan R, Sekar K, Rasmussen M, et al. Nasal intermittent positive pressure ventilation after surfactant treatment for respiratory distress syndrome in preterm infants< 30 weeks' gestation: a randomized, controlled trial. J Perinatol 2012;32(5):336.

74. Sadeghnia A, Barekateyn B, Badiei Z, et al. Analysis and comparison of the effects of N-BiPAP and Bubble-CPAP in treatment of preterm newborns with the weight of below 1500 grams affiliated with respiratory distress syndrome: a randomised clinical trial. Adv Biomed Res 2016;5:3.

75. Sai Sunil Kishore M, Dutta S, Kumar P. Early nasal intermittent positive pressure ventilation versus continuous positive airway pressure for respiratory distress syndrome. Acta Paediatr 2009;98(9):1412–5.

76. Salama GSA, Ayyash FF, Al-Rabadi AJ, et al. Nasal -IMV versus Nasal-CPAP as an initial mode of respiratory support for premature infants with RD: a prospective randomized clinical trial. Rawal Medical Journal 2015;40(2):197–202.

77. Shi Y, Tang S, Zhao J, et al. A prospective, randomized, controlled study of NIPPV versus nCPAP in preterm and term infants with respiratory distress syndrome. Pediatr Pulmonol 2014;49(7):673–8.

78. Silveira CST, Leonardi KM, Melo APCF, et al. Response of preterm infants to 2 noninvasive ventilatory support systems: nasal CPAP and nasal intermittent positive-pressure ventilation. Respir Care 2015;60(12):1772–6.

79. Lemyre B, Davis PG, De Paoli AG, et al. Nasal intermittent positive pressure ventilation (NIPPV) versus nasal continuous positive airway pressure (NCPAP) for preterm neonates after extubation. Cochrane Database Syst Rev 2017;(2):CD003212.

80. Victor S, Roberts SA, Mitchell S, et al. Biphasic positive airway pressure or continuous positive airway pressure: a randomized trial. Pediatrics 2016; 138(2):e20154095.

81. Ribeiro SNS, Fontes MJF, Bhandari V, et al. Noninvasive ventilation in New-borns≤ 1,500 g after tracheal extubation: randomized clinical trial. Am J Perina-tol 2017;34(12):1190–8.

82. Moretti C, Giannini L, Fassi C, et al. Nasal flow-synchronized intermittent positive pressure ventilation to facilitate weaning in very low-birthweight infants: un-masked randomized controlled trial. Pediatr Int 2008;50(1):85–91.

83. Gao WW, Tan SZ, Chen YB, et al. Randomized trail of nasal synchronized inter-mittent mandatory ventilation compared with nasal continuous positive airway pressure in preterm infants with respiratory distress syndrome. Zhongguo Dang Dai Er Ke Za Zhi 2010;12(7):524–6 [in Chinese].

84. Khorana M, Paradeevisut H, Sangtawesin V, et al. A randomized trial of non-synchronized Nasopharyngeal Intermittent Mandatory Ventilation (nsNIMV) vs. Nasal Continuous Positive Airway Pressure (NCPAP) in the prevention of extuba-tion failure in pre-term < 1,500 grams. J Med Assoc Thai 2008;91(Suppl 3): S136–42.

85. Kahramaner Z, Erdemir A, Turkoglu E, et al. Unsynchronized nasal intermittent positive pressure versus nasal continuous positive airway pressure in preterm infants after extubation. J Matern Fetal Neonatal Med 2014;27(9):926–9.

86. Jasani B, Nanavati R, Kabra N, et al. Comparison of non-synchronized nasal intermittent positive pressure ventilation versus nasal continuous positive airway pressure as post-extubation respiratory support in preterm infants with respira-tory distress syndrome: a randomized controlled trial. J Matern Fetal Neonatal Med 2016;29(10):1546–51.

87. O'Brien K, Campbell C, Brown L, et al. Infant flow biphasic nasal continuous positive airway pressure (BP- NCPAP) vs. infant flow NCPAP for the facilitation of extubation in infants' </= 1,250 grams: a randomized controlled trial. BMC Pediatr 2012;12:43.

88. Locke RG, Wolfson MR, Shaffer TH, et al. Inadvertent administration of positive end-distending pressure during nasal cannula flow. Pediatrics 1993;91(1): 135–8.

89. Courtney SE, Pyon KH, Saslow JG, et al. Lung recruitment and breathing pattern during variable versus continuous flow nasal continuous positive airway pres-sure in premature infants: an evaluation of three devices. Pediatrics 2001; 107(2):304–8.

90. Mikalsen IB, Davis P, Oymar K. High flow nasal cannula in children: a literature review. Scand J Trauma Resusc Emerg Med 2016;24:93.

91. Nishimura M. High-flow nasal cannula oxygen therapy in adults: physiological benefits, indication, clinical benefits, and adverse effects. Respir Care 2016; 61(4):529–41.

92. Wilkinson D, Andersen C, O'Donnell CP, et al. High flow nasal cannula for respira-tory support in preterm infants. Cochrane Database Syst Rev 2016;(2):CD006405.

93. Lavizzari A, Colnaghi M, Ciuffini F, et al. Heated, humidified high-flow nasal can-nula vs nasal continuous positive airway pressure for respiratory distress

syndrome of prematurity: a randomized clinical noninferiority trial. JAMA Pediatr 2016. https://doi.org/10.1001/jamapediatrics.2016.1243.

94. Roberts CT, Owen LS, Manley BJ, et al. Nasal high-flow therapy for primary respiratory support in preterm infants. N Engl J Med 2016;375(12):1142–51.

95. Shin J, Park K, Lee EH, et al. Humidified high flow nasal cannula versus nasal continuous positive airway pressure as an initial respiratory support in preterm infants with respiratory distress: a randomized, controlled non-inferiority trial. J Korean Med Sci 2017;32(4):650–5.

96. Murki S, Singh J, Khant C, et al. High-flow nasal cannula versus nasal continuous positive airway pressure for primary respiratory support in preterm infants with respiratory distress: a randomized controlled trial. Neonatology 2018; 113(3):235–41.

97. Nair G, Karna P. Comparison of the effects of Vapotherm and nasal CPAP in respiratory distress. Presented at the Pediatric Academic Societies Meeting, Baltimore, May 14–17, 2005. abstract (http://www.abstracts2view.com/pas/).

98. Manley BJ, Roberts CT, Froisland DH, et al. Refining the use of nasal high-flow therapy as primary respiratory support for preterm infants. J Pediatr 2018;196: 65–70.e1.

99. Kugelman A, Riskin A, Said W, et al. A randomized pilot study comparing heated humidified high-flow nasal cannulae with NIPPV for RDS. Pediatr Pulmonol 2015;50(6):576–83.

100. Wang Z, Xiang J, Gao W, et al. Comparison of clinical efficacy of two noninvasive respiratory support therapies for respiratory distress syndrome in very low birth weight preterm infants. Zhongguo Dang Dai Er Ke Za Zhi 2018;20(8): 603–7.

101. Iranpour R, Sadeghnia A, Abari SS. High flow nasal cannula in the treatment of respiratory distress syndrome in one day-old neonate. Br J Med Res 2016;15(4).

102. Soonsawad S, Swatesutipun B, Limrungsikul A, et al. Heated humidified high-flow nasal cannula for prevention of extubation failure in preterm infants. Indian J Pediatr 2017;84(4):262–6.

103. Kang WQ, Xu BL, Liu DP, et al. Efficacy of heated humidified high-flow nasal cannula in preterm infants aged less than 32 weeks after ventilator weaning. Zhongguo Dang Dai Er Ke Za Zhi 2016;18(6):488–91 [in Chinese].

104. Kadivar M, Mosayebi Z, Razi N, et al. High flow nasal cannulae versus nasal continuous positive airway pressure in neonates with respiratory distress syndrome managed with Insure method: a randomized clinical trial. Iran J Med Sci 2016;41(6):494.

105. Mukerji A, Dunn M. High-frequency ventilation as a mode of noninvasive respiratory support. Clin Perinatol 2016;43(4):725–40.

106. van der Hoeven M, Brouwer E, Blanco CE. Nasal high frequency ventilation in neonates with moderate respiratory insufficiency. Arch Dis Child Fetal Neonatal Ed 1998;79(1):F61–3.

107. Fischer HS, Bohlin K, Buhrer C, et al. Nasal high-frequency oscillation ventilation in neonates: a survey in five European countries. Eur J Pediatr 2015;174(4): 465–71.

108. Mukerji A, Shah PS, Shivananda S, et al. Survey of noninvasive respiratory support practices in Canadian neonatal intensive care units. Acta Paediatr 2017; 106(3):387–93.

109. Colaizy TT, Younis UM, Bell EF, et al. Nasal high-frequency ventilation for premature infants. Acta Paediatr 2008;97(11):1518–22.

110. Mukerji A, Finelli M, Belik J. Nasal high-frequency oscillation for lung carbon dioxide clearance in the newborn. Neonatology 2013;103(3):161–5.

111. Bottino R, Pontiggia F, Ricci C, et al. Nasal high-frequency oscillatory ventilation and CO2 removal: a randomized controlled crossover trial. Pediatr Pulmonol 2018;53(9):1245–51.

112. Klotz D, Schneider H, Schumann S, et al. Non-invasive high-frequency oscillatory ventilation in preterm infants: a randomised controlled cross-over trial. Arch Dis Child Fetal Neonatal Ed 2018;103(4):F1–f5.

113. Zhu XW, Zhao JN, Tang SF, et al. Noninvasive high-frequency oscillatory ventilation versus nasal continuous positive airway pressure in preterm infants with moderate-severe respiratory distress syndrome: a preliminary report. Pediatr Pulmonol 2017;52(8):1038–42.

114. Malakian A, Bashirnezhadkhabaz S, Aramesh MR, et al. Noninvasive high-frequency oscillatory ventilation versus nasal continuous positive airway pressure in preterm infants with respiratory distress syndrome: a randomized controlled trial. J Matern Fetal Neonatal Med 2018;1–151. https://doi.org/10.1080/14767058.2018.1555810.

115. Mukerji A, Sarmiento K, Lee B, et al. Non-invasive high-frequency ventilation versus bi-phasic continuous positive airway pressure (BP-CPAP) following CPAP failure in infants< 1250 g: a pilot randomized controlled trial. J Perinatol 2017;37(1):49.

116. Walsh M, Engle W, Laptook A, et al. National Institute of Child Health and Human Development Neonatal Research Network. Oxygen delivery through nasal cannulae to preterm infants: can practice be improved? Pediatrics 2005;116(4):857–61.

117. Klerk A. Humidification during noninvasive respiratory support of the newborn: continuous positive airway pressure, nasal intermittent positive pressure ventilation, and humidified high-flow nasal cannula. In: Esquinas AM, editor. Humidification in the Intensive Care Unit. 2012. p. 271–84.

118. Roberts CT, Manley BJ, Dawson JA, et al. Nursing perceptions of high-flow nasal cannulae treatment for very preterm infants. J Paediatr Child Health 2014;50(10):806–10.

119. Klingenberg C, Pettersen M, Hansen EA, et al. Patient comfort during treatment with heated humidified high flow nasal cannulae versus nasal continuous positive airway pressure: a randomised cross-over trial. Arch Dis Child Fetal Neonatal Ed 2014;99(2):F134–7.

Is Nasal High Flow Inferior to Continuous Positive Airway Pressure for Neonates?

Kate A. Hodgson, MBBS (Hons), BMedSci[a,b,*],
Brett J. Manley, MBBS (Hons), PhD[a,c], Peter G. Davis, MBBS, MD[a,c]

KEYWORDS

- Newborn • High flow • CPAP • Ventilation

KEY POINTS

- Evidence suggests that CPAP is superior to nasal high flow for initial noninvasive support of preterm infants with respiratory distress syndrome.
- Nasal high flow is noninferior to CPAP for postextubation support of preterm infants ≥28 weeks' gestation.
- Limited data are available for nasal high flow use in extremely preterm infants born less than 28 weeks' gestation, or term infants.
- Compared with CPAP, nasal high flow use does not increase the risk of bronchopulmonary dysplasia in very preterm infants.

BACKGROUND

Rates of preterm birth are increasing,[1] and many preterm infants require respiratory support. The ultimate goal of treatment is to maintain adequate gas exchange, while minimizing short- and long-term respiratory and neurodevelopmental sequelae. In 1971, Kitchen and Campbell[2] published a landmark trial of neonatal intensive care, demonstrating that supportive care, including mechanical ventilation, of very low birth weight infants improved their chances of survival. This earliest phase of modern neonatal intensive care was characterized by poor survival rates and frequent short- and long-term complications related to mechanical ventilation.

Disclosure Statement: No conflicts of interest to disclose.
[a] Neonatal Services, Newborn Research Centre, The Royal Women's Hospital, Level 7, 20 Flemington Road, Parkville, Victoria 3052, Australia; [b] Department of Obstetrics and Gynaecology, The University of Melbourne, Australia; [c] Department of Obstetrics and Gynaecology, The University of Melbourne, Murdoch Children's Research Institute, Australia
* Corresponding author. Newborn Research Centre, The Royal Women's Hospital, Level 7, 20 Flemington Road, Parkville, Victoria 3052, Australia.
E-mail address: Kate.Hodgson@thewomens.org.au

Clin Perinatol 46 (2019) 537–551
https://doi.org/10.1016/j.clp.2019.05.005
0095-5108/19/© 2019 Elsevier Inc. All rights reserved.

Several advances in neonatal intensive care greatly improved survival rates. Most important were the widespread use of antenatal corticosteroids from the 1980s[3] and the development and application of exogenous surfactant in the 1990s.[4] Although survival rates increased, even for the most premature infants, the major morbidities of prematurity, including bronchopulmonary dysplasia (BPD), remained high. The risk of BPD is inversely proportional to birth weight, with most infants with BPD born less than 1000 g.[5] Use of mechanical ventilation and supplemental oxygen, for even brief periods, are independent risk factors for BPD.[6] Noninvasive respiratory support (without the need for endotracheal intubation) was developed to mitigate this risk. Three landmark randomized controlled trials (RCTs) from 2008 to 2011 demonstrated that even very preterm infants are successfully managed with continuous positive airway pressure (CPAP) from birth.[7–9] Subsequently, CPAP has become the mainstay of initial respiratory treatment of preterm infants.

CPAP is not without disadvantages. The interface is bulky, skilled nursing care is required to optimally manage infants, and CPAP use is associated with nasal trauma[10] and pneumothorax.[9] The best approach to noninvasive respiratory support that minimizes the risk of BPD in preterm infants is yet to be established. These issues, and the ongoing search for less invasive therapies for preterm infants, have led to the increased use of nasal high flow therapy (nHF). nHF uses smaller prongs and a set flow, not pressure, to deliver heated, humidified gas. nHF was used in many neonatal units worldwide before robust evidence of its safety and efficacy was available. This was caused by several perceived benefits of nHF compared with CPAP: improved patient comfort,[11] reduced rates of nasal trauma,[12] and the preference of parents[13] and nursing staff.[12] Over the last 5 years, the evidence base for nHF use has expanded. Retrospective and observational studies, followed by RCTs comparing nHF with CPAP, have provided guidance for clinicians. Several of the RCTs have had a noninferiority design, because of the postulated advantages of nHF for the clinician, patient, and parents. From these trials, there is evidence to support the use of nHF in some clinical settings, depending on the patient population and clinician preference. In other settings CPAP is the superior modality. Several factors must be considered by units choosing between CPAP and nHF, for the unit as a whole, and on an individual patient basis.

This review addresses the question: "Is nHF inferior to CPAP?" To answer this question, one must determine which outcomes are deemed important, what is considered inferior (or noninferior), which patients are being cared for, and in which setting. This review outlines the evidence for nHF use, potential future research, and recommendations for practice.

CONTINUOUS POSITIVE AIRWAY PRESSURE FOR PRIMARY RESPIRATORY SUPPORT IN PRETERM INFANTS

Three large RCTs have examined the use of CPAP as an alternative to endotracheal intubation and mechanical ventilation in very preterm infants. In the COIN trial, 610 infants born 25 to 28 weeks' gestation were randomized to CPAP or intubation and ventilation at 5 minutes of life.[9] CPAP use did not significantly reduce the primary outcome of death or BPD at 36 weeks' corrected gestation, compared with intubation. However, fewer infants randomized to CPAP received surfactant and these infants had fewer days of mechanical ventilation. In a trial comparing three approaches to initial respiratory management, Dunn and colleagues[7] found similar results for infants 26 to 29 + 6 weeks' gestation: 48% of infants managed with CPAP did not require mechanical ventilation and there were no significant differences in the relative risk of death or BPD or any other secondary outcomes. A third RCT randomly assigned 1316 infants 24 to 28 weeks' gestation to receive CPAP, initiated in the delivery room, or intubation and surfactant within 1 hour of birth, with subsequent protocol-guided respiratory support management.[8] The authors found no difference in the primary outcome of death or BPD. Infants managed with CPAP were less likely to be treated with postnatal corticosteroids and received fewer days of mechanical ventilation. Subsequent meta-analysis has shown that CPAP use is associated with lower rates of death and BPD, compared with routine intubation at birth.[14] With no clear evidence of increased adverse events, and possible benefit, CPAP is now generally recommended as first-line respiratory support for preterm infants.[15]

THE EVIDENCE FOR CONTINUOUS POSITIVE AIRWAY PRESSURE AS POSTEXTUBATION SUPPORT

Early and successful extubation from mechanical ventilation is important in limiting the risk of BPD. Use of CPAP following extubation improves the likelihood of extubation success,[16] and is the most commonly used form of postextubation respiratory support for extremely preterm infants.[17] There is also some evidence that higher set CPAP pressure (7–9 cm H_2O vs 4–6 cm H_2O) may further improve extubation success.[18]

COMPLICATIONS OF CONTINUOUS POSITIVE AIRWAY PRESSURE

Although CPAP provides effective noninvasive respiratory support for preterm infants, the inherent difficulties of delivering CPAP, along with nursing and parental preferences, have led to the use of alternative noninvasive therapies, such as nHF.

Nasal trauma is a recognized complication of nasal CPAP use in preterm infants, with a reported incidence of 20% to 100%, depending on the classification system used and gestational age of the population studied.[10] Several factors increase the risk of severe nasal trauma in very preterm infants: lower gestational age, lower birth weight, incorrect sizing and positioning of CPAP prongs, and prolonged use.[10] The risk of nasal trauma is reduced by careful nursing care to ensure appropriate positioning of nasal prongs and the prophylactic use of a hydrocolloid nasal barrier dressing.[19]

Pneumothorax is another recognized complication of CPAP, with an incidence in extremely preterm infants of 5% to 9%.[7–9] The risk of pneumothorax seems to be limited to preterm infants receiving CPAP for treatment of respiratory distress syndrome (RDS) and is likely secondary to overdistention of some areas of the lung. It is rarely seen as a complication of CPAP for postextubation support.[20,21]

THE INCREASED USE OF NASAL HIGH FLOW

nHF use is widespread and increasing. Surveys have found that 77% of level II and III centers in the United Kingdom[22] and 89% of tertiary centers in Canada[23] used nHF in some capacity. Practice varies considerably between units. Only half of the 57 units surveyed in a UK study had a written guideline or policy regarding nHF use.[22] Unit approaches to choosing the nasal cannula size also varied, often contravening current recommendations. Manufacturers recommend a prong size approximately 50% of the diameter of the nares, which allows gas leak and avoids excessive pressure generation,[24–26] although this is difficult to achieve in very small infants.

PERCEIVED BENEFITS OF NASAL HIGH FLOW

The increased use of nHF has been prompted by several perceived advantages of this modality over CPAP. Parents and nursing staff report a preference for nHF over CPAP, particularly for older and more stable preterm infants.[13,27] Reported perceived benefits include increased parent-child interaction, improved comfort, easier skin-to-skin care, and improved oral feeding.[12,22]

The available evidence suggests that nHF causes less nasal trauma than CPAP. Most RCTs of nHF have reported nasal trauma as a secondary outcome. However, the trials differ in their classification system for nasal trauma, and also the underlying risk of the population, and are often unblinded. Nevertheless, a recent meta-analysis of seven studies found that nHF was associated with a significantly reduced rate of nasal injury compared with CPAP (risk ratio [RR], 0.46; 95% confidence interval [CI], 0.37–0.58; number needed to treat, 7).[10] nHF is often used for patients with nasal septal trauma who require ongoing respiratory support.

There are little empirical data to support several postulated benefits of nHF. Practice varies with regard to oral feeding on nHF and CPAP. Given the theoretic risk of aspiration, in some centers infants on CPAP are not offered oral feeds, whereas oral feeding with nHF is more common. In a retrospective observational study of patients with evolving BPD, Shetty and colleagues[28] reported quicker attainment of full oral feeds with the use of nHF from 34 weeks' postmenstrual age, compared with CPAP. However, the approach to oral feeding differed between the groups, with infants on CPAP not offered oral feeds. Only one RCT of 44 infants has specifically compared establishment of oral feeding in infants on nHF and CPAP,[29] and found no difference. Related outcomes, such as discharge weight, have not differed in the large RCTs of nHF as postextubation support.[21,30,31]

One small pediatric trial has reported improved patient comfort with the use of nHF, compared with face mask or low-flow oxygen.[32] Despite this, neonatal studies have not consistently shown a difference in validated pain scores. Whereas Klingenberg and colleagues[13] found no difference in pain scores in a single-center randomized crossover trial of nHF compared with CPAP, Osman and colleagues[11] reported lower pain scores and lower salivary cortisol concentrations with nHF. These conflicting findings may be caused by differences in the specific pain scales used, and difficulties in assessing comfort in neonates.

STATISTICAL NONINFERIORITY

RCTs are generally conducted as superiority trials. However, when a new treatment has some benefits over the current standard treatment, a noninferiority trial may be used.[33] When evaluating the primary outcome, if the efficacy of the new treatment falls within a margin of noninferiority, it is deemed to be no worse than the standard treatment. The perceived importance of the new treatment's benefits must justify this noninferiority. If a margin of noninferiority is too large, then this difference in efficacy may not be acceptable to the clinician. Conversely, a small margin requires a large sample size to demonstrate noninferiority.

With evolving evidence over recent years regarding the utility of nHF, its use in various settings has increased greatly. Evidence from RCTs suggests that, for certain indications, nHF is noninferior to CPAP. An assessment regarding the utility of nHF depends on the outcome measures that are deemed important by a particular clinician or neonatal unit. What difference in effectiveness is tolerable for the proposed benefits of nHF? Are these benefits sufficiently important that clinicians and caregivers would choose nHF over CPAP, accepting that the treatment failure rate may be higher?

WHICH OUTCOMES MATTER?
Death or Bronchopulmonary Dysplasia

Several trials have evaluated the incidence of death or BPD when nHF is used for primary respiratory support, compared with CPAP. A 2016 Cochrane Review pooled the available data regarding the effect of nHF use as primary respiratory support on death or BPD.[34] Four published and unpublished trials with a total of 439 preterm infants were included. There was no difference found in the primary outcomes of death (typical RR, 0.36; 95% CI, 0.01–8.73) or BPD (typical RR, 2.07; 95% CI, 0.64–6.64). Similarly, no difference was found in the incidence of death or BPD for infants managed with nHF versus CPAP following extubation.[34] Several of these trials permitted the use of rescue CPAP in the event of nHF failure; this may effectively reduce the power of the trials and pooled analyses to show a difference in these outcomes.

Several larger RCTs have been published since this time, which alter the evidence-based recommendations regarding nHF use as primary support of preterm RDS, but not the evidence regarding the impact on death or BPD. Few extremely preterm infants have been included in these RCTs, hence the impact of nHF use on BPD for those infants at highest risk is yet to be properly evaluated.

Treatment Failure: Primary Support

To date, seven RCTs have compared nHF with CPAP for initial treatment of preterm RDS (**Fig. 1**).[31,35–40] Data from Nair and colleagues (Comparison of the effects of Vapotherm and nasal CPAP in respiratory distress. Pediatric Academic Societies, Unpublished data, 2005), included in the 2016 Cochrane review,[34] were published only in abstract form and data from Ciuffini and colleagues[40] were included in a subsequent publication.[36] Hence both studies have been excluded from the current review. Four of the published RCTs have had a noninferiority design[36–39] and all were unblinded.

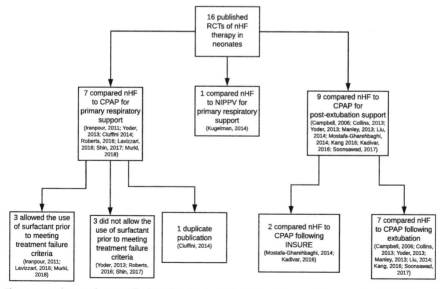

Fig. 1. Randomised controlled trials of nasal high flow therapy in neonates. NIPPV, nasal intermittent positive pressure ventilation.

There have been four noninferiority RCTs published since the 2016 Cochrane Review.[34] A single-center study by Lavizzari and colleagues[36] compared nHF with CPAP for primary respiratory support of mild-moderate RDS in 316 infants born 29 to 36 + 6 weeks' gestation. The primary outcome was the need for mechanical ventilation within 72 hours of randomization. Patients in the nHF group could not receive recue CPAP before intubation, whereas patients in the CPAP group could receive nasal intermittent positive pressure ventilation at clinician discretion. All infants were permitted to have surfactant administered by the INSURE (INtubation SURFactant Extubation) method if prespecified oxygenation criteria were met. Roberts and colleagues[38] conducted a multicenter trial in Australia and Norway, randomizing 564 infants born 28 to 36 + 6 weeks' gestation with RDS to nHF or CPAP within 24 hours of birth. The primary outcome was treatment failure, determined by objective criteria for hypoxia, respiratory acidosis, or apnea. Shin and colleagues,[39] in their trial of 85 patients, had a prespecified noninferiority margin of 20%, which was larger than in other trials. The primary outcome was the incidence of intubation and mechanical ventilation. Finally, in the most recent trial, Murki and colleagues[37] included 272 preterm infants greater than or equal to 28 weeks' gestation, randomizing them to nHF or CPAP on admission to the neonatal intensive care unit. The primary outcome was treatment failure. Patients could receive up to two doses of surfactant if fraction of inspired oxygen (F_{IO_2}) was greater than 0.3, without this being deemed treatment failure.

These trials of nHF for primary respiratory support have had different methodologic approaches to the use of rescue CPAP in the nHF arm, and also to surfactant provision. Three studies allowed the use of CPAP for patients in the nHF group, after treatment failure criteria were met, before mechanical ventilation.[37–39] In contrast, patients in the trial by Lavizzari and colleagues[36] underwent mechanical ventilation after predefined treatment failure criteria were reached. Use of rescue CPAP may avoid the need for intubation in a significant proportion of patients failing nHF therapy[38] and should be noted by units considering the use of nHF. The use of surfactant also differed in these trials: surfactant provision via the INSURE technique was permitted in some trials but not others. The efficacy of nHF likely differs in infants with atelectatic, surfactant-deplete lungs, compared with surfactant-replete lungs.

A secondary analysis of the trial by Roberts and colleagues[41] identified several factors associated with nHF treatment failure. This analysis examined clinical and demographic variables associated with nHF failure. Lower gestational age and higher prerandomization F_{IO_2} were associated with increased risk of nHF treatment failure. In all subgroups of this trial, CPAP was superior to nHF with respect to treatment failure. Therefore, for clinicians who still wish to use nHF as primary support for preterm RDS, careful choice of patient is important: more immature infants, and those with more severe RDS (as indicated by higher F_{IO_2}) are more likely to fail nHF treatment and require escalation of respiratory support.

Figs. 2 and 3 show the pooled analysis of trials comparing nHF with CPAP for primary respiratory support. Although nHF as first-line treatment of preterm RDS results in a significantly higher rate of treatment failure than CPAP, the rates of intubation are similar.

Treatment Failure: Postextubation Support

The use of nHF for respiratory support following extubation in preterm infants has been examined in nine trials. The 2016 Cochrane meta-analysis of nHF compared with CPAP to prevent extubation failure included six of these trials (934 infants) and found no difference in the rate of treatment failure (RR, 1.21; 95% CI, 0.95–1.55) or reintubation (typical RR, 0.91; 95% CI, 0.68–1.20) within 7 days.

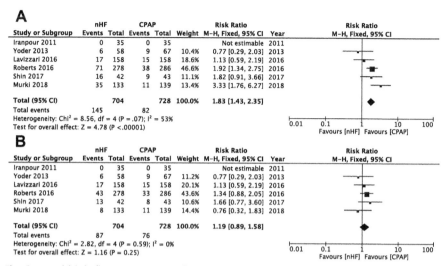

Fig. 2. Nasal high flow versus CPAP for primary respiratory support. Treatment failure (*A*) and reintubation (*B*) within 7 days.

Since publication of the Cochrane Review, three additional RCTs have examined the efficacy of nHF to prevent extubation failure. Kang and colleagues[42] randomized 161 preterm infants less than 32 weeks' gestation to nHF or CPAP postextubation. Overall, there was no significant difference in the rate of treatment failure or reintubation, but the authors did report a higher rate of nHF treatment failure in the most immature infants (26–28 weeks' gestation). Similarly, an RCT of 49 infants less than 32 weeks' gestation found no difference in the rate of reintubation with the use of nHF compared with CPAP.[43] Conversely, a single-center RCT of 54 patients using

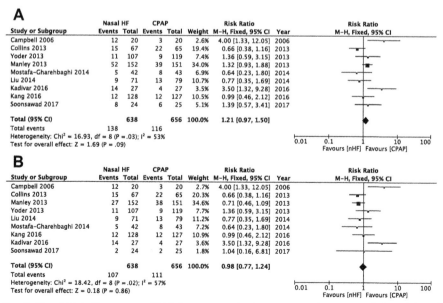

Fig. 3. Nasal high flow versus CPAP for postextubation support. Treatment failure (*A*) and reintubation (*B*) within 7 days.

nHF with gas flow less than 4 L/min by Kadivar and colleagues[44] found a higher rate of reintubation with nHF compared with CPAP.

Many of these trials permitted the use of rescue CPAP before reintubation in the event of nHF treatment failure. The largest study of nHF following extubation in preterm infants reported that 48% of infants who reached treatment failure with nHF were successfully treated with rescue CPAP, avoiding reintubation for at least 7 days.[21] The availability and application of rescue CPAP in the event of nHF failure is again an important consideration for neonatal units. If nHF is used as first-line therapy following extubation, CPAP should be available, to prevent mechanical ventilation in this subset of patients.

Only three RCTs have examined nHF for extremely preterm infants following extubation.[21,30,42] Collins and colleagues[30] reported no statistically significant difference in extubation failure between the nHF and CPAP groups for infants born less than 28 weeks' gestation (37% vs 52%; $P = .24$). Although there was no statistically significant difference between treatment groups, the study by Manley and colleagues,[21] which included the largest extremely preterm cohort, reported a high nHF treatment failure in infants born less than 26 weeks' gestation, and the authors advised caution using nHF for these infants. The third RCT similarly found a higher rate of treatment failure in infants 26 to 28 weeks' gestation.[42]

Duration of Respiratory Support

Several studies have found a longer duration of respiratory support or supplemental oxygen therapy in infants managed with nHF compared with CPAP.[21,31,38,45] However, there was no corresponding increase in the rate of BPD with nHF use. Several factors may have contributed to this finding. One study had a different weaning strategy for infants on nHF compared with those on CPAP[46] and two studies used lower nHF gas flows than suggested by current clinical practice recommendations.[45,46] Further research into weaning practices with the use of nHF in infants with evolving BPD is warranted.

Cost-Effectiveness

Cost-effectiveness is an important consideration when choosing between nHF and CPAP for noninvasive respiratory support. Cost-effectiveness analyses must consider clinician time, equipment purchase, consumables, and adverse events. An economic evaluation of nHF by the National Institute for Health Research in the United Kingdom found the higher capital equipment costs of CPAP were not outweighed by the higher consumable costs of nHF.[47] A recent economic evaluation[48] of the trial by Roberts and colleagues[49] demonstrated that as a sole primary support therapy, CPAP is likely to be more cost-effective than nHF. Although the cost of inpatient stay was lower with the use of nHF, the incidence of mechanical ventilation increased costs. nHF with rescue CPAP back up was the most cost-effective option overall.

Term Infants

Only one RCT of nHF therapy has included term infants,[31] with the results analyzed along with those of the preterm infants. Hence no conclusions can be drawn regarding nHF use in term neonates with respiratory distress.

Recommendations

Consensus practice recommendations regarding nHF use are difficult to reach, given differences in patient populations, resources, and availability of alternative respiratory support strategies between units. A recent survey of international experts sought to establish consensus guidelines for nHF in neonates.[50] The group reached agreement on the use of nHF following extubation of preterm infants greater than or equal to

28 weeks' gestation; however, agreement regarding nHF for primary respiratory support was not achieved. Two of the respondents supported the use of nHF for primary treatment of RDS in all populations, two did not support the use at all, and three recommended limiting use to babies greater than or equal to 30 weeks' gestation and with F_{IO_2} less than 0.3.

For all uses of nHF, practice should be consistent with that used in the published RCTs: appropriate choice of prong size to maintain a leak at the nares, gas flows up to 8 L/min, heated and humidified gas, regular review for the capacity of an infant to wean or stop therapy, and the use of rescue CPAP in the event of treatment failure. The current available evidence has guided the recommendations listed in **Box 1**.

Primary Support (Nasal High Flow for Initial Treatment of Preterm Respiratory Distress Syndrome)

CPAP is superior to nHF for the initial treatment of RDS in preterm infants. Depending on the perceived importance of the benefits of nHF, some clinicians may still wish to use nHF in this setting. Careful consideration of the infant's gestational age and F_{IO_2} requirement is essential, and caution is advised for those infants at high risk of treatment failure ($<$30 weeks' gestation or $F_{IO_2} \geq 0.3$).[41] If nHF is used, having CPAP available as a rescue therapy prevents the need for intubation and mechanical ventilation in some infants.

Postextubation Support (Nasal High Flow to Prevent Extubation Failure)

nHF is noninferior to CPAP for postextubation support of preterm infants greater than 28 weeks' gestation. It may therefore be considered an alternative to CPAP for this indication. Similar to primary support, the availability of rescue CPAP is important to prevent higher rates of intubation and mechanical ventilation in those infants in whom nHF treatment fails.

Extremely Preterm Infants

The available evidence surrounding the use of nHF in extremely preterm infants born less than 28 weeks' gestation is limited. To date, no published RCTs of nHF as primary respiratory support have included extremely preterm infants and only three trials of nHF for postextubation support have included this population. Limited data suggest that when using noninvasive support to prevent extubation failure in this high-risk group of infants, CPAP is likely to be superior to nHF.

Box 1
Best practices for use of noninvasive respiratory support in preterm infants

Recommendations for the use of noninvasive respiratory support in preterm infants
- Nasal CPAP is recommended for primary support in preterm infants with respiratory distress
- For clinicians and units who wish to use nasal high flow as primary respiratory support, it is recommended that use is limited to infants born $\geq$30 weeks' gestation and with supplemental oxygen requirement less than 30% on admission
- Nasal high flow is noninferior to CPAP for postextubation support of preterm infants and is considered in infants $\geq$28 weeks' gestation
- CPAP should be available for back up in units using nasal high flow, to avoid intubation in a subset of patients
- Nasal high flow should be considered for use in infants with nasal trauma, depending on clinical stability

WHAT IS NEXT FOR NASAL HIGH FLOW AND CONTINUOUS POSITIVE AIRWAY PRESSURE?

Several new applications of nHF and CPAP, and variations in the way they are used, show promise for improving noninvasive respiratory management of neonates. For CPAP, the use of neurally adjusted ventilatory assist (NAVA) and high-frequency nasal ventilation (HFNV) may broaden the applications of the modality. Future research questions for nHF include use during neonatal endotracheal intubation, for delivery room stabilization of preterm infants, using higher gas flows, and comparing commercially available devices.

Neurally Adjusted Ventilatory Assist

NAVA is a method of synchronization that is used as an adjunct to either invasive or noninvasive respiratory supports. NAVA detects diaphragmatic electrical activity via electrodes embedded in a nasogastric tube and uses this to control ventilator inflations. The inflation pressure delivered by the ventilator is proportional to the patient's respiratory effort.[51] Noninvasive NAVA improves synchrony[52] and lowers peak inspiratory pressure,[53] compared with conventional noninvasive ventilation. Although a promising new technology, no randomized studies have evaluated the safety and long-term outcomes of noninvasive NAVA and further research in this area is warranted.

High-Frequency Nasal Ventilation

Over recent years, HFNV has been increasingly used in neonates, despite limited evidence regarding efficacy and safety. HFNV applies an oscillatory waveform to the airways via a nasal interface. It has been postulated that this may increase improved gas exchange.[54] In a survey of five European countries, 17% of responding neonatal units used HFNV, most frequently in very low birth weight infants following CPAP failure.[55] Three RCTs have prospectively evaluated the use of HFNV. In an RCT of 39 patients born less than 1250 g, there was a lower rate of CPAP failure in infants randomized to HFNV compared with biphasic CPAP; however, this difference did not reach statistical significance.[56] Dumas De La Roque and colleagues[57] also reported decreased duration of respiratory distress in a cohort of term infants receiving HFNV. In a randomized crossover study of 40 stable preterm infants, Ruegger and colleagues[58] found a lower frequency of desaturation and bradycardia with the use of HFNV, but increase in overall oxygen requirement. Adequately powered RCTs are required to evaluate this therapy further.

Nasal High Flow to Support Endotracheal Intubation

Opportunities for junior staff to gain proficiency in neonatal endotracheal intubation are decreasing, and the procedure is technically challenging.[59] Furthermore, neonates are particularly vulnerable to acute deterioration during intubation. Applying nHF during apnea has been found to prolong the time to desaturation after induction of anesthesia in adults[60] and children,[61] a technique known as transnasal humidified rapid insufflation ventilatory exchange. It is postulated that because of a pressure differential between the airways and alveoli during apnea, gas exchange may still occur, prolonging the time to desaturation.[60] No studies have examined the use of nHF during endotracheal intubation of newborn infants. This technique may convey physiologic advantages compared with standard care and improve stability during neonatal endotracheal intubation.

Nasal High Flow for Delivery Room Stabilization of Preterm Infants

nHF may be of value as a method of stabilization for preterm infants in the delivery room. It is quick and easy to apply and may be used in place of CPAP and positive pressure ventilation. nHF use in the delivery room has only been reported in a single, small, observational study of infants born less than 30 weeks' gestation.[62] Most infants were successfully stabilized with nHF and overall intubation rates were lower than the unit average before the study. The provision of nHF for initial stabilization may enable extremely preterm infants to undergo transition with minimal intervention by the clinician, potentially reducing lung injury.

Higher Gas Flows with Nasal High Flow

Despite early concerns about possible lung overdistention with nHF, the available data suggest that the distending pressure is equivalent to, or slightly below, that provided by nasal CPAP.[63–65] Continuous distending pressure provided by nHF is determined by gas flow and leak; higher gas flow results in higher pharyngeal pressure.[64–66] Infant weight seems to be inversely associated with pressure,[63,65] with the smallest infants requiring less gas flow to generate the same distending pressure as in larger infants. No studies have investigated the use of gas flow rates greater than 8 L/min in preterm infants; this is to some extent limited by manufacturer recommendations, but it is possible that higher gas flows may be more efficacious, particularly in the smallest preterm infants.

Device Comparison

The two most widely used commercially available nHF devices are Optiflow Junior (Fisher & Paykel, Auckland, New Zealand) and Precision Flow (Vapotherm, Exeter, NH). Although both devices have been used in RCTs, only one single-center pilot study has compared the clinical efficacy of now superseded versions of the Vapotherm and Fisher & Paykel devices, in 40 preterm infants between 26 and 29 weeks' gestation.[67] There was no difference in the primary outcome of need for reintubation within 72 hours, nor any secondary outcomes. Because some clinicians express a preference for one device or the other, comparison of the two devices is warranted. The continual evolution of equipment confounds long-term recommendations regarding choice of device.

SUMMARY

Evidence evaluating the use of nHF in newborn infants and neonates has accumulated over recent years. nHF therapy is a reasonable alternative to CPAP for postextubation support of infants greater than 28 weeks' gestation. There is no difference in the rate of death and BPD, and nHF is noninferior to CPAP for preventing extubation failure, provided rescue CPAP is available. In contrast, CPAP is a superior therapy to nHF for primary support of RDS and for all indications in infants less than 28 weeks' gestation, although evidence is limited. However, nHF has some benefits over CPAP: ease of use, lower rates of nasal trauma, and parent and nursing staff preference. Clinicians and units who consider these benefits of great importance may choose to use nHF, acknowledging the lower rate of therapeutic success.

REFERENCES

1. March of Dimes, PMNCH, Save the Children, WHO. Born Too Soon: The Global Action Report on Preterm Birth. In: Howson CP, Kinney MV, Lawn JE, editors. Geneva: World Health Organization; 2012.

2. Kitchen WH, Campbell DG. Controlled trial of intensive care for very low birth weight infants. Pediatrics 1971;48:711–4.

3. Liggins GC, Howie RN. A controlled trial of antepartum glucocorticoid treatment for prevention of the respiratory distress syndrome in premature infants. Pediatrics 1972;50(4):515–25.

4. Horbar JD, Wright EC, Onstad L. Decreasing mortality associated with the introduction of surfactant therapy. Pediatrics 1993;92(2):191–6.

5. Walsh MC, Szefler S, Davis J, et al. Summary proceedings from the bronchopulmonary dysplasia group. Pediatrics 2006;117:S52–6.

6. Davidson LM, Berkelhamer SK. Bronchopulmonary dysplasia: chronic lung disease of infancy and long-term pulmonary outcomes. J Clin Med 2017;6(1) [pii:E4].

7. Dunn MS, Kaempf J, de Klerk A, et al. Randomized trial comparing 3 approaches to the initial respiratory management of preterm neonates. Pediatrics 2011; 128(5):e1069–76.

8. Finer NN, Carlo WA, Walsh MC, et al. Early CPAP versus surfactant in extremely preterm infants. N Engl J Med 2010;362(21):1970–9.

9. Morley CJ, Davis PG, Doyle LW, et al. Nasal CPAP or intubation at birth for very preterm infants. N Engl J Med 2008;358(7):700–8.

10. Imbulana DI, Manley BJ, Dawson JA, et al. Nasal injury in preterm infants receiving non-invasive respiratory support: a systematic review. Arch Dis Child Fetal Neonatal Ed 2018;103(1):F29–35.

11. Osman M, Elsharkawy A, Abdel-Hady H. Assessment of pain during application of CPAP and high flow in preterm infants. J Perinatol 2015;35(4):263–7.

12. Roberts CT, Manley BJ, Dawson JA, et al. Nursing perceptions of high-flow nasal cannulae treatment for very preterm infants. J Paediatr Child Health 2014;50(10): 806–10.

13. Klingenberg C, Pettersen M, Hansen EA, et al. Patient comfort during treatment with heated humidified high flow nasal cannulae versus nasal continuous positive airway pressure: a randomised cross-over trial. Arch Dis Child Fetal Neonatal Ed 2014;99(2):F134–7.

14. Schmolzer GM, Kumar M, Pichler G, et al. Non-invasive versus invasive respiratory support in preterm infants at birth: systematic review and meta-analysis. BMJ 2013;347:f5980.

15. Committee on Fetus and Newborn, American Academy of Pediatrics. Respiratory support in preterm infants at birth. Pediatrics 2014;133(1):171–4.

16. Shah V, Hodgson K, Seshia M, et al. Golden hour management practices for infants <32 weeks gestational age in Canada. Paediatr Child Health 2018;23(4):e70–6.

17. Al-Mandari H, Shalish W, Dempsey E, et al. International survey on periextubation practices in extremely preterm infants. Arch Dis Child Fetal Neonatal Ed 2015; 100(5):F428–31.

18. Buzzella B, Claure N, D'Ugard C, et al. A randomized controlled trial of two nasal continuous positive airway pressure levels after extubation in preterm infants. J Pediatr 2014;164(1):46–51.

19. Imbulana DI, Owen LS, Dawson JA, et al. A randomized controlled trial of a barrier dressing to reduce nasal injury in preterm infants receiving binasal noninvasive respiratory support. J Pediatr 2018;201:34–9.e3.

20. Davis PG, Henderson-Smart DJ. Nasal continuous positive airway pressure immediately after extubation for preventing morbidity in preterm infants. Cochrane Database Syst Rev 2003;(2):CD000143.

21. Manley BJ, Owen LS, Doyle LW, et al. High-flow nasal cannulae in very preterm infants after extubation. N Engl J Med 2013;369(15):1425–33.

22. Ojha S, Gridley E, Dorling J. Use of heated humidified high-flow nasal cannula oxygen in neonates: a UK wide survey. Acta Paediatr 2013;102(3):249–53.
23. Mukerji A, Shah PS, Shivananda S, et al. Survey of noninvasive respiratory support practices in Canadian neonatal intensive care units. Acta Paediatr 2017; 106(3):387–93.
24. Dysart K, Miller TL, Wolfson MR, et al. Research in high flow therapy: mechanisms of action. Respir Med 2009;103(10):1400–5.
25. Milesi C. High-flow nasal cannula. Ann Intensive Care 2014;4:29.
26. Sivieri EM, Gerdes JS, Abbasi S. Effect of HFNC flow rate, cannula size, and nares diameter on generated airway pressures: an in vitro study. Pediatr Pulmonol 2013;48(5):506–14.
27. Engesland H, Johannessen B. Nurses' experiences by using heated humidified high flow cannula to premature infants versus nasal continuous positive airway pressure. J Neonatal Nurs 2016;22(1):21–6.
28. Shetty S, Hunt K, Douthwaite A, et al. High-flow nasal cannula oxygen and CPAP and full oral feeding in infants with BPD. Arch Dis Child Fetal Neonatal Ed 2016; 101(5):F408–11.
29. Glackin SJ, O'Sullivan A, George S, et al. High flow nasal cannula versus NCPAP, duration to full oral feeds in preterm infants: a randomised controlled trial. Arch Dis Child Fetal Neonatal Ed 2017;102(4):F329–32.
30. Collins CL, Holberton JR, Barfield C, et al. A randomized controlled trial to compare heated humidified high-flow nasal cannulae with nasal continuous positive airway pressure postextubation in premature infants. J Pediatr 2013;162(5): 949–54.e1.
31. Yoder BA, Stoddard RA, Li M, et al. Heated, humidified high-flow nasal cannula versus nasal CPAP for respiratory support in neonates. Pediatrics 2013;131(5): e1482–90.
32. Spentzas T, Minarik M, Patters AB, et al. Children with respiratory distress treated with high-flow nasal cannula. J Intensive Care Med 2009;24:323–8.
33. Scott IA. Non-inferiority trials. Med J Aust 2009;190(6):326–30.
34. Wilkinson D, Andersen C, O'Donnell CP, et al. High flow nasal cannula for respiratory support in preterm infants. Cochrane Database Syst Rev 2016;(2):CD006405.
35. Iranpour R, Sadeghnia A, Hesaraki M. 393 high-flow nasal cannula versus nasal continuous positive airway pressure in the management of respiratory distress syndrome. Arch Dis Child 2012;97:A115–6.
36. Lavizzari A, Colnaghi M, Ciuffini F, et al. Heated, humidified high-flow nasal cannula vs nasal continuous positive airway pressure for respiratory distress syndrome of prematurity: a randomized clinical noninferiority trial. JAMA Pediatr 2016. [Epub ahead of print].
37. Murki S, Singh J, Khant C, et al. High-flow nasal cannula versus CPAP for primary respiratory support in preterm infants with respiratory distress: a randomized controlled trial. Neonatology 2018;113(3):235–41.
38. Roberts CT, Owen LS, Manley BJ, et al. Nasal high-flow therapy for primary respiratory support in preterm infants. N Engl J Med 2016;375(12):1142–51.
39. Shin J, Park K, Lee EH, et al. Humidified high flow nasal cannula versus CPAP as initial respiratory support in preterm infants. J Korean Med Sci 2017;32(4):650–5.
40. Ciuffini F, Pietrasanta C, Lavizzari A, et al. Comparison between two different modes of non-invasive ventilatory support in preterm newborn infants with respiratory distress syndrome mild to moderate: preliminary data. Pediatr Med Chir 2014;36(4):88.

41. Manley BJ, Roberts CT, Frøisland DH, et al. Refining the use of nasal high-flow therapy as primary respiratory support for preterm infants. J Pediatr 2018;196: 65–70 e61.

42. Kang WQ, Xu BL, Liu DP, et al. Efficacy of heated humidified high-flow nasal cannula in preterm infants aged less than 32 weeks after ventilator weaning. Zhongguo Dang Dai Er Ke Za Zhi 2016;18(6):488–91 [in Chinese].

43. Soonsawad S, Swatesutipun B, Limrungsikul A, et al. Heated humidified high-flow nasal cannula for prevention of extubation failure in preterm infants. Indian J Pediatr 2017;84(4):262–6.

44. Kadivar M, Mosayebi Z, Razi N, et al. High flow nasal cannulae versus nasal CPAP in neonates with respiratory distress syndrome managed with INSURE method: a randomized clinical trial. Iran J Med Sci 2016;41(6):494–500.

45. Kugelman A, Riskin A, Said W, et al. A randomized pilot study comparing heated humidified high-flow nasal cannulae with NIPPV for RDS. Pediatr Pulmonol 2015; 50(6):576–83.

46. Abdel-Hady H, Shouman B, Aly H. Early weaning from CPAP to high flow nasal cannula in preterm infants is associated with prolonged oxygen requirement. Early Hum Dev 2011;87(3):205–8.

47. Fleeman N, Mahon J, Bates V, et al. The clinical effectiveness and cost-effectiveness of heated humidified high-flow nasal cannula compared with usual care for preterm infants. Health Technol Assess 2016;20(30):1–68.

48. Huang L, Roberts CT, Manley BJ, et al. Cost-effectiveness analysis of nasal continuous positive airway pressure versus nasal high flow therapy as primary support for infants born preterm. J Pediatr 2018;196:58–64 e52.

49. Roberts CT, Owen LS, Manley BJ, et al. High-flow support in very preterm infants in Australia and New Zealand. Arch Dis Child Fetal Neonatal Ed 2016;101(5): F401–3.

50. Yoder BA, Manley B, Collins C, et al. Consensus approach to nasal high-flow therapy in neonates. J Perinatol 2017;37(7):809–13.

51. Rossor TE, Hunt KA, Shetty S, et al. Neurally adjusted ventilatory assist compared to other forms of triggered ventilation for neonatal respiratory support. Cochrane Database Syst Rev 2017;(10):CD012251.

52. Lee J, Kim HS, Sohn JA, et al. Randomized crossover study of neurally adjusted ventilatory assist in preterm infants. J Pediatr 2012;161(5):808–13.

53. Firestone KS, Fisher S, Reddy S, et al. Effect of changing NAVA levels on peak inspiratory pressures and electrical activity of the diaphragm in premature neonates. J Perinatol 2015;35(8):612–6.

54. Null DM, Alvord J, Leavitt W, et al. High-frequency nasal ventilation for 21 d maintains gas exchange with lower respiratory pressures and promotes alveolarization in preterm lambs. Pediatr Res 2014;75(4):507–16.

55. Fischer HS, Bohlin K, Bührer C, et al. Nasal high-frequency oscillation ventilation in neonates: a survey in five European countries. Eur J Pediatr 2015;174(4): 465–71.

56. Mukerji A, Sarmiento K, Lee B, et al. Non-invasive high-frequency ventilation versus bi-phasic continuous positive airway pressure (BP-CPAP) following CPAP failure in infants <1250 g: a pilot randomized controlled trial. J Perinatol 2017;37(1):49–53.

57. Dumas De La Roque E, Bertrand C, Tandonnet O, et al. Nasal high frequency percussive ventilation versus nasal continuous positive airway pressure in transient tachypnea of the newborn: a pilot randomized controlled trial. Pediatr Pulmonol 2011;46(3):218–23.

58. Ruegger CM, Lorenz L, Kamlin COF, et al. The effect of noninvasive high-frequency oscillatory ventilation on desaturations and bradycardia in very preterm infants: a randomized crossover trial. J Pediatr 2018;201:269–73.e2.
59. O'Shea JE, Thio M, Kamlin CO, et al. Videolaryngoscopy to teach neonatal intubation: a randomized trial. Pediatrics 2015;136(5):912–9.
60. Patel A, Nouraei SA. Transnasal humidified rapid-insufflation ventilatory exchange (THRIVE): a physiological method of increasing apnoea time in patients with difficult airways. Anaesthesia 2015;70(3):323–9.
61. Humphreys S, Lee-Archer P, Reyne G, et al. Transnasal humidified rapid-insufflation ventilatory exchange (THRIVE) in children: a randomized controlled trial. Br J Anaesth 2017;118(2):232–8.
62. Reynolds P, Leontiadi S, Lawson T, et al. Stabilisation of premature infants in the delivery room with nasal high flow. Arch Dis Child Fetal Neonatal Ed 2016;101(4): F284–7.
63. Kubicka ZJ, Limauro J, Darnall RA. Heated, humidified high-flow nasal cannula therapy: yet another way to deliver continuous positive airway pressure? Pediatrics 2008;121(1):82–8.
64. Lampland AL, Plumm B, Meyers PA, et al. Observational study of humidified high-flow nasal cannula compared with nasal continuous positive airway pressure. J Pediatr 2009;154(2):177–82.
65. Wilkinson DJ, Andersen CC, Smith K, et al. Pharyngeal pressure with high-flow nasal cannulae in premature infants. J Perinatol 2008;28(1):42–7.
66. Spence KL, Murphy D, Kilian C, et al. High-flow nasal cannula as a device to provide continuous positive airway pressure in infants. J Perinatol 2007;27(12): 772–5.
67. Miller SM, Dowd SA. High-flow nasal cannula and extubation success in the premature infant: a comparison of two modalities. J Perinatol 2010;30(12):805–8.

Intermittent Hypoxemia in Preterm Infants

Juliann M. Di Fiore, BS[a],*, Peter M. MacFarlane, PhD[b], Richard J. Martin, MD[b]

KEYWORDS

- Intermittent hypoxemia • Hypoxia • Pulse oximetry • Retinopathy of prematurity
- Neurodevelopmental impairment • Outcomes

KEY POINTS

- Intermittent hypoxemia (IH) events are common in preterm infants during early postnatal life.
- In neonates, IH events have been associated with multiple morbidities, including retinopathy of prematurity, sleep disordered breathing, neurodevelopmental impairment, and death.
- The relationship between IH and morbidity may depend on the pattern of the IH events, although this needs further investigation.

INTRODUCTION

Although maintaining adequate oxygenation is a fundamental aspect of newborn care, clinicians are only beginning to appreciate how even subtle alterations in oxygen levels can affect both short-term and long-term outcomes. Before the implementation of noninvasive technologies, oxygen assessment was limited to intermittent arterial sampling, which only gave a glimpse of the true instability of oxygen levels that can occur during early postnatal life. Current continuous recordings of oxygen saturation reveal a much higher frequency of intermittent hypoxemia (IH) events that were previously undocumented in medical charts and provide insight to high-risk patterns associated with both short-term and long-term morbidity. This article summarizes what is currently known about the technology used to assess oxygen levels, patterns of IH during early postnatal life, underlying mechanisms associated with IH, and high-risk IH patterns that may induce a pathologic cascade.

Disclosures: The authors have nothing to disclose.
[a] Division of Neonatology, Case Western Reserve University, Rainbow Babies & Children's Hospital, Suite RBC 3100, Cleveland, OH 44106-6010, USA; [b] Case Western Reserve University, Rainbow Babies & Children's Hospital, 11100 Euclid Avenue, Suite RBC 3100, Cleveland, OH 44106-6010, USA
* Corresponding author.
E-mail address: jmd3@case.edu

HISTORICAL PERSPECTIVE

Before the mid-1970s, intermittent arterial sampling formed the basis for assessing and managing supplemental oxygen administration. There was no clear evidence that arterial oxygen tension (PaO_2) or arterial oxygen saturation (SaO_2) showed frequent fluctuations in preterm infants even though apnea of prematurity was known to be a problem. This situation changed with the advent of transcutaneous PO_2 ($TcPO_2$) monitors, which were widely used during the 1980s. It was remarkable to observe how positional changes and associated procedures, such as spinal taps, could cause $TcPO_2$ to decrease.[1] This finding led to the widespread acceptance of gentle care for fragile preterm infants.

However, $TcPO_2$ electrodes (later combined with $TcPCO_2$ electrodes) were cumbersome, required frequent recalibration, and resulted in site erythema from heating to 43°C to 44°C. There was also the realization in the 1980s that $TcPO_2$ increasingly underestimated PaO_2 with advancing postnatal age; this was especially a problem with the increasing incidence of bronchopulmonary dysplasia (BPD).[2–4] These patients were a new population of extremely low birth weight infants who no longer had arterial access. A solution was found in pulse oximetry and this technology has dominated neonatology since approximately 1990. As a result, the available literature on IH episodes in preterm infants is almost exclusively based on pulse oximetry.

PULSE OXIMETRY

Because stabilization of oxygenation is one of the primary challenges in the neonatal intensive care unit (NICU), pulse oximetry plays an important role in patient care. Bedside discussions often include oximetry-based histogram data to note percentage time in any given oxygen saturation range and/or nursing notation of IH events. However, treatment decisions based on medical chart documentation may be problematic because they significantly underestimate the true incidence of even prolonged events.[5] Adding to the confusion is that there is currently no criteria for a clinically relevant IH event and, therefore, corresponding pulse oximeter alarm settings. Most research trials have defined an IH event as a decrease less than 85% or 80%, but in the clinical setting a low threshold alarm is determined by the individual NICU oxygen saturation target. There is also wide variation in practice pertaining to the clinical significance of the duration of an IH event. For example, health care workers in some NICUs use a long pulse oximeter alarm delay as a tool to minimize nuisance alarms caused by short self-resolving IH, whereas others consider that even short events require intervention. Correspondingly, alarm delay criteria can vary widely between NICUs depending on the manufacturer (ranging from 0 to 15 seconds) and staff perception of the duration needed for a clinically relevant desaturation event.

Pulse oximeters have the advantage of obtaining longitudinal documentation of oxygen levels in a noninvasive and rapidly responding manner, but there are limitations that may affect measurement accuracy. The most widely acknowledged disadvantage of pulse oximetry is in the inability to detect hyperoxemia at levels of SpO_2 (oxygen saturation via pulse oximetry) exceeding approximately 97%.[6] Additional factors, including probe position, motion and ambient light interference, low perfusion, skin pigmentation, and variations in hemoglobin level, may result in delayed waveform recognition and/or underestimation of oxygen saturation levels.[7,8] Most manufacturers report an overall error of ±2% to 3% of full scale but, even under ideal conditions, accuracy may diminish with decreasing SpO_2.[9] In a study of 1664 preterm infants, overall mean differences between SaO_2 and SpO_2 (Masimo) were −1.8% ± 2.9% but less than 40% of infants were within 3% of the corresponding SaO_2 when SpO_2 decreased less than 88%. During very low oxygen saturation levels of less than 70%, which are impractical or unethical to target in infants, newborn lamb models have shown even larger differences, ranging from 13% to 17%.[10] Therefore, although pulse oximetry is often used to identify periods of IH, treatment decisions based on the absolute Spo_2 value should be made with caution, especially at low levels of oxygen saturation, as can occur in cardiac patients.

INCIDENCE OF INTERMITTENT HYPOXEMIA EVENTS AND UNDERLYING MECHANISMS

There is considerable current interest in the postnatal time course of IH events in preterm infants. This interest is precipitated by the fact that persistent IH events frequently delay hospital discharge and may be perceived as increasing the vulnerability of these infants. Barrington and colleagues[11] documented more than 20 years ago that apneic events of longer than 12 seconds are common in very low birth weight preterm infants before discharge, many of which would, presumably, have been associated with IH. Data for infants of 24 to 28 weeks' gestation show a marked change in IH events over time, with few hypoxemic episodes occurring during the first week of postnatal life, a progressive increase in weeks 2 to 3, a plateau around weeks 4 to 6, and then a decrease in weeks 6 to 8[12] (**Fig. 1**). It has been proposed that this postnatal increase in IH events may be related to a documented postnatal increase in periodic breathing, which is frequently associated with episodic desaturation.[13] In a subsequent study, the incidence of IH events was significantly increased in a low (85%–89%) versus high (91%–95%) baseline Spo_2 target.[14] This finding is consistent with earlier data in preterm infants with BPD.[15] More recently IH events (comprising a >10% decrease in baseline Spo_2) were reported in most preterm infants during home recordings of Spo_2, but declined between 36 and 44 weeks of postmenstrual age.[16]

Immature respiratory control resulting in apnea and respiratory pauses, as well as ineffective and/or obstructed inspiratory efforts, are the major precipitants of IH events,[17] but several physiologic parameters likely contribute to the resultant desaturation. The most important of these is probably pulmonary oxygen stores, which may reflect lung volume. Preterm infants are at risk for a low basal functional residual

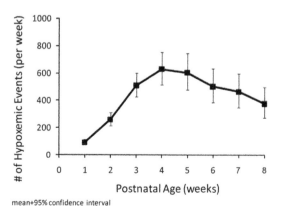

mean+95% confidence interval

Fig. 1. The progression of IH events during early postnatal life. Preterm infants have few IH events during the first week of life, followed by an increase during weeks 2 to 4, and a decrease thereafter. (*From* Di Fiore JM, Bloom JN, Orge F, et al. A higher incidence of intermittent hypoxemic episodes is associated with severe retinopathy of prematurity. *The Journal of pediatrics.* Jul 2010;157(1):69-73)

capacity because of both atelectasis and high chest wall compliance. Therapy with continuous positive airway pressure (CPAP) clearly benefits these infants by splinting the upper airway, stabilizing lung volume, and increasing baseline Spo_2, thereby minimizing the risk of desaturation. Other physiologic parameters, including blood oxygen capacity comprising blood volume and hemoglobin content,[18,19] may also be implicated in IH. Current neonatal practice attempts to minimize the use of mechanical ventilation via endotracheal intubation and favors the widespread use of CPAP or other noninvasive ventilation techniques. Synchronization methods during noninvasive ventilation to decrease IH events continue to be a challenge.[20] However, IH episodes are also common even in intubated, ventilated infants as a consequence of ineffective ventilator support and loss of the infant's lung volume.[21,22] Interestingly, intrauterine growth status also seems to be a factor. Small-for-gestational-age (SGA), versus appropriately grown, preterm infants are more vulnerable at a low baseline Spo_2 target, as manifested by higher mortality and increased incidence of IH events.[23] The mechanism of this increased vulnerability to IH is unclear, but pulmonary hypertension in SGA infants and resultant hypoxia-induced pulmonary vasoconstriction may contribute.

INTERMITTENT HYPOXEMIA AND OUTCOMES

Stabilizing the extreme fluctuations in oxygenation in preterm infants often requires a balance between the risks and benefits of oxygen supplementation and constant adjustments of fraction of inspired oxygen (Fio_2), which can be labor intensive. Therefore, with the current NICU focus on aggressive weaning protocols, knowledge of the association between IH and morbidity would be of great benefit in guiding clinical practice.

The evidence that suggests that IH may initiate a pathologic cascade is derived from animal models that show that intermittent hypoxia during adulthood increases extracellular superoxide concentration,[24] induces hypoxia-inducible factor (HIF) 1α expression,[25] degrades HIF-2α expression, and downregulates superoxide dismutase[26] leading to overall pro-oxidant signaling. In addition, exposure to IH during early postnatal life disrupts expression patterns of proteins involved with dopamine signaling[27] and causes a proinflammatory response, including increased levels of tumor necrosis factor alpha and interleukin-1β.[28] Thus, in infants, IH may induce a pathologic cascade via a pro-oxidant, proinflammatory, or neurotransmitter imbalance pathway (**Fig. 2**).

IH during early postnatal life has been associated with multiple poor outcomes, including retinopathy of prematurity (ROP), growth restriction, sleep disordered breathing, neurodevelopmental impairment, and mortality. Although it is well known that early postnatal hyperoxic exposure is the major risk factor for severe ROP, there is evidence that later IH causes rebound overexpression of growth factors (ie vascular endothelial growth factor, erythropoietin) associated with HIFs that may play a role in neovascularization.[29] Multiple animal models with various intermittent hypoxic paradigms have induced retinopathy[30] and have shown that the level of neovascularization may depend on the pattern of intermittent hypoxic exposure.[31] For example, rats exposed to cycles of IH in a clustered (10 minutes apart) versus equally dispersed (2 hours apart) pattern have more severe oxygen-induced retinopathy, including vascular tufts, leaky vessels, retinal hemorrhage, and vascular overgrowth in the clustered paradigm. Studies in preterm infants have shown similar findings with a higher number of IH events during early postnatal life in infants with severe ROP requiring laser therapy.[12] Closer examination of IH patterns revealed an association between ROP and IH of longer duration,[32,33] less severity, and a specific time interval between events of 1 to 20 minutes.[32] The time between IH events may play an important role in

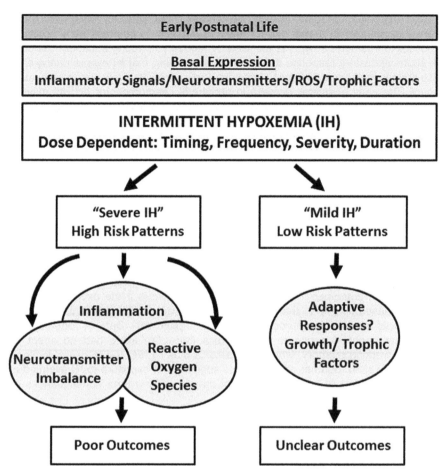

Fig. 2. The relationship between IH and outcomes may depend on the pattern of the hypoxemic events. IH has been associated with morbidity in preterm infants but not all IH has been shown to have deleterious effects. Therefore, these studies may represent severe IH in terms of frequency, severity, duration, and timing that induce inflammation, neurotransmitter imbalance, and reactive oxygen species (ROS) with a high risk of poor outcomes. In contrast, the effect of mild IH on outcomes is unclear.

initiating a pathophysiologic response, because rodent studies have revealed transient alterations in pro-oxidant signaling occurring during the resolution of the hypoxemic event.[24,25]

The relationship between IH events and growth restriction is currently limited to neonatal rodent models. For example, repetitive exposure to IH during the first week of life significantly reduced body weight by the third day, with subsequent growth restriction with every day of exposure.[34] After 21 days of recovery in room air, the rat pups showed catch-up growth, suggesting that IH events commonly seen in preterm infants during early postnatal life may play a role in weight gain, a common criterion for hospital discharge. However, to our knowledge, there are currently no available data for the potential effect of IH on growth restriction in human neonates.

IH events can have both short-term and long-term effects on respiratory stability and sleep disordered breathing. In rodents, early postnatal exposure to intermittent hypoxia enhanced the acute hypoxic chemoreflex immediately following intermittent hypoxia exposure[35] in males with no effect in females. In contrast, early postnatal exposure to intermittent hypoxia followed by recovery to young adulthood reduced the acute ventilatory response to hypoxia,[36] suggesting that IH events during early postnatal life may have divergent short-term versus long-term effects on respiratory control. The early postnatal increase in peripheral chemoreceptor activity may be one explanation why periodic breathing often develops within 2 to 4 weeks of life in preterm infants,[13] whereas the long-term reduction in peripheral chemoreceptor activity may be one component contributing to preterm birth being a risk factor for sleep disordered breathing at 8 to 11 years of age.[37]

Human trials in neonates have revealed associations between both delayed resolution[38,39] and increased frequency and/or severity of cardiorespiratory events[40,41] and neurodevelopmental impairment. The findings of these single-center studies have been confirmed by a recent retrospective analysis in the multicenter Canadian Oxygen Trial (COT).[33] Using continuous recordings of oxygen saturation in a large cohort of more than 1000 infants, the investigators found a correlation between time spent with hypoxemia during the first few months of life and adverse 18-month outcomes, including late death or disability, cognitive language delay, and motor impairment. Additional clinical trials have shown a relationship between BPD and poor cognitive outcomes,[42–45] which begs a question: is it the oxygen exposure or the increased IH events that can occur with chronic lung disease that may put these infants at risk for neurodevelopmental impairment? Data in rodents have shown that neonatal exposure to hyperoxia (65% O_2) alone had no effect on long-term working memory, whereas hyperoxia plus IH resulted in neurofunctional handicap.[46] Taken together, these studies suggest that exposure to IH events during a critical period of brain development may have long-term consequences on brain dysfunction.

In addition, patterns of oxygenation during the first few days of life have been associated with mortality. The Surfactant Positive Pressure and Oxygenation Trial (SUPPORT) randomized infants to a lower (85%–89%) versus higher (90%–95%) oxygen saturation target to reduce the incidence of severe ROP (SUPPORT[47]). One unexpected finding of the trial was a higher mortality in the lower target group that was limited to infants with intrauterine growth restriction.[48] Closer examination of achieved levels of oxygenation (as opposed to the randomized target) revealed an association between lower oxygen saturation ($\leq$92%) during the first 3 days of life and decreased 90-day survival in both appropriate gestational age (AGA) and SGA infants. However, SGA infants also had an enhanced mortality associated with an increased frequency of IH events that was not seen in the AGA infant cohort.[23]

Interestingly, not all patterns of IH may be deleterious and the effects of mild hypoxemia are not clear. For example, mild IH has been associated with later impaired sensorimotor performance in mice.[49] In contrast, various paradigms in both human and animal models have suggested that mild hypoxia/hypoxemia may be benign or even beneficial. In rodents, exposure to a single brief (5-minute) cycle of hypoxia during the first 24 hours after birth,[50] or longer (4 hours) and milder cycles of hypoxia during the first 3 to 4 weeks of life[51] enhanced long-term spatial learning,[51] memory,[50] and structural changes in both the hippocampus[50,51] and frontal cortex.[50] In neonates, short[33] or tightly clustered (<1 minute apart)[12] IH events were not associated with morbidity, but the risk associated with such patterns may be confounded by other factors, including intrauterine growth restriction.[23] In adults, various therapeutic mild IH paradigms are currently being examined for sleep apnea, systemic hypertension, depression, and neural inflammation.[52] These combined findings suggest that the compensatory versus maladaptive effects of IH may depend on the "dose" of IH. Because premature infants show a wide array of IH patterns with increasing postnatal age,[32] it is possible that early postnatal IH configurations contain both pathologic and beneficial components (see **Fig. 2**).

THERAPEUTIC OPTIONS

Management strategies for IH events focus primarily on their prevention. The aggressiveness of these approaches clearly depends on the likelihood of adverse effects of IH, and unanswered questions remain. Desaturation events are a consequence of immature respiratory control superimposed on an immature respiratory system and, in many cases, there is probably vulnerability to pulmonary hypertension. Two mainstays of management are, therefore, optimizing baseline oxygenation and enhancing respiratory control (**Fig. 3**).

1. Optimizing baseline oxygenation. There seems to be widespread consensus that baseline SpO_2 should be maintained in the 90% to 95% range, and that risks associated with restricting the upper limit to 89% outweigh the benefits.[53,54] As already noted, low baseline SpO_2 significantly increases the risk of desaturation, especially in SGA infants.[14,23] Over several decades, CPAP has proved an important means to stabilize oxygenation by supporting functional residual capacity and splinting the upper airway to prevent its closure during apnea. The role of red blood cell transfusions in decreasing apnea (and resultant desaturation) has been controversial. Most recent data show improvement in apnea and IH after red blood cell transfusion. Age-dependent improvement in frequency and severity of IH after transfusion have been documented beyond the first week of life when IH events begin to increase.[18] Another study documented a decrease in apnea associated with

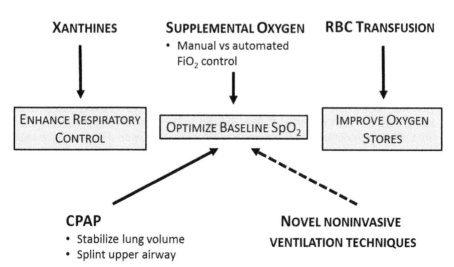

Fig. 3. Treatment strategies for IH include a multipronged approach; xanthines to enhance respiratory control, supplemental oxygen and pressure support to optimize baseline level of oxygenation, and red blood cell (RBC) transfusion to improve oxygen stores.

desaturation and bradycardia in the 12 hours after red cell transfusion.[55] It seems that the benefits of increasing red cell mass on IH outweigh the risk of transfusion in selected infants.

There is great interest in the rapid emergence of automated (vs manual) control of supplemental oxygen delivery in high-risk neonates, as addressed elsewhere in this issue. Initial automated systems focused on ventilated infants and had great success in reducing hyperoxic, but not hypoxic, episodes.[56] More recent studies by several European groups have had success in reducing IH events with automated versus manual Fio_2 control and further documented this benefit in infants on noninvasive as well as invasive ventilator support.[57,58] This technology is being used clinically in Europe and is undergoing further investigative trials in the United States. Although the available data are encouraging, it should be noted that the percentage of time that Spo_2 was in range (91%–95%) only increased from 58% to 62%,[58] emphasizing the major challenge in keeping preterm infants in any given target even with rapidly responding computer controlled feedback.

The application of near-infrared spectroscopy as a tool for assessing the relationship between Spo_2 and cerebral tissue oxygen saturation is still the subject of ongoing research. Although interpretation of absolute values of cerebral tissue oxygenation have yet to be determined, recent data have shown a greater adverse impact from IH than bradycardic events.[59] It remains to be seen whether this noninvasive technique can be used as a prognostic marker.[60] In addition, other novel new approaches are being explored. Two investigative groups are exploring afferent stimulation at the body surface to decrease apnea and resultant IH. Smith and colleagues[61] are using stochastic resonance stimulation via gentle mattress vibrations, whereas Kesavan and colleagues are using extremity vibration devices to enhance limb proprioceptive afferents.[61,62] Although both approaches show promise in decreasing IH events, it is unclear whether stabilization of oxygenation is a contributing mechanism.

2. Role of caffeine therapy. Xanthine therapy, notably caffeine, has become a mainstay of neonatal care and improves not only respiratory but also neurodevelopmental outcomes.[63] Although its mechanisms of benefit may be multifactorial, enhanced neonatal respiratory control with caffeine is well accepted.[64] Earlier data questioned whether caffeine improved hypoxemic episodes in preterm infants,[65] but recent data clearly show a reduction in IH.[66] This is not surprising, given that caffeine reduces the incidence of apnea of prematurity. There are still interesting issues regarding optimal caffeine administration for preterm infants. The first issue is when this therapy should begin. Available data support early (even prophylactic) dosing in high-risk neonates; however, these data are largely based on retrospective reviews and associations rather than randomized trials.[67] The second issue is when this therapy should stop. Rhein and colleagues[66] showed a reduction in IH events with prolonged therapy until approximately 36 weeks of postmenstrual age and even beyond. This finding is under further study but runs the potential risk of either prolonging hospitalization or increasing home monitor use. The third and most challenging issue is whether doses higher than those traditionally used should be used in either a loading or maintenance mode. Available data comparing high versus standard dosing are limited by low-quality outcome measures, small sample sizes, and diverse caffeine dosing regimens.[68] Benefit versus safety of such an approach must be carefully studied because adenosine receptor subtype inhibition (the presumed main mechanism of action for xanthines) is variable and dose dependent, raising potential safety concerns.[69,70] The challenge is to weigh the potential consequences of IH episodes against the pros and cons of any therapeutic intervention.

SUMMARY

Intermittent hypoxemic events are ubiquitous in preterm infants and are a major challenge in clinical care. Early arterial blood gas sampling limited the ability to monitor oxygen levels over small windows of time, whereas implementation of pulse oximetry has increased knowledge of the transient progression of IH during early postnatal life. Current treatment modalities used in the clinical setting have only been partially successful in reducing the incidence of apnea and accompanying IH but the risks and benefits of more aggressive interventions must include knowledge of the relationship between IH and morbidity. Future clinical challenges that may assist in mitigating IH and possible sequelae include identification of optimum oxygen saturation targets, recognition of high-risk (and possibly beneficial) IH patterns, and implementation of Fio_2 automated controllers and other novel therapies to avoid periods of both hyperoxemia and hypoxemia.

ACKNOWLEDGMENTS

HL 056470, HL 138402 and Gerber Foundation Reference # 1082-4005.

Best Practices

What is the current practice for IH?

Best practice/guideline/care path objectives
- Continuous oxygen saturation monitoring at the bedside
- Identify periods of hypoxemia
- Interventions include
  - Caffeine
  - CPAP or nasal cannula support
  - Cautious use of supplemental oxygen

What changes in current practice are likely to improve outcomes?

- Identification of optimal oxygen saturation targets

- Implementation of automated oxygen control systems to minimize fluctuations in oxygenation and improve time in target

- Optimization of caffeine therapy dosing and duration

Major recommendations/rating for the strength of the evidence

- The current recommended oxygen saturation target is 90% to 95%, although strength of evidence remains modest

- Maintenance of adequate ventilation and lung volume to support oxygenation can be provided by CPAP, nasal cannula or noninvasive ventilation

- Caffeine may be administered prophylactically to reduce intermittent hypoxemic events and minimize ventilatory support

Bibliographic sources: Refs.[53,57,66]

REFERENCES

1. Gleason CA, Martin RJ, Anderson JV, et al. Optimal position for a spinal tap in preterm infants. Pediatrics 1983;71(1):31–5.
2. Rome ES, Stork EK, Carlo WA, et al. Limitations of transcutaneous PO2 and PCO2 monitoring in infants with bronchopulmonary dysplasia. Pediatrics 1984;74(2): 217–20.

3. Solimano AJ, Smyth JA, Mann TK, et al. Pulse oximetry advantages in infants with bronchopulmonary dysplasia. Pediatrics 1986;78(5):844–9.

4. Ramanathan R, Durand M, Larrazabal C. Pulse oximetry in very low birth weight infants with acute and chronic lung disease. Pediatrics 1987;79(4):612–7.

5. Brockmann PE, Wiechers C, Pantalitschka T, et al. Under-recognition of alarms in a neonatal intensive care unit. Arch Dis Child Fetal Neonatal Ed 2013;98(6): F524–7.

6. Poets CF, Wilken M, Seidenberg J, et al. Reliability of a pulse oximeter in the detection of hyperoxemia. J Pediatr 1993;122(1):87–90.

7. Poets CF, Southall DP. Noninvasive monitoring of oxygenation in infants and children: practical considerations and areas of concern. Pediatrics 1994;93(5): 737–46.

8. Trivedi NS, Ghouri AF, Shah NK, et al. Effects of motion, ambient light, and hypoperfusion on pulse oximeter function. J Clin Anesth 1997;9(3):179–83.

9. Rosychuk RJ, Hudson-Mason A, Eklund D, et al. Discrepancies between arterial oxygen saturation and functional oxygen saturation measured with pulse oximetry in very preterm infants. Neonatology 2012;101(1):14–9.

10. Dawson JA, Bastrenta P, Cavigioli F, et al. The precision and accuracy of Nellcor and Masimo oximeters at low oxygen saturations (70%) in newborn lambs. Arch Dis Child Fetal Neonatal Ed 2014;99(4):F278–81.

11. Barrington KJ, Finer N, Li D. Predischarge respiratory recordings in very low birth weight newborn infants. J Pediatr 1996;129(6):934–40.

12. Di Fiore JM, Bloom JN, Orge F, et al. A higher incidence of intermittent hypoxemic episodes is associated with severe retinopathy of prematurity. J Pediatr 2010; 157(1):69–73.

13. Patel M, Mohr M, Lake D, et al. Clinical associations with immature breathing in preterm infants: part 2-periodic breathing. Pediatr Res 2016;80(1):28–34.

14. Di Fiore JM, Walsh M, Wrage L, et al. Low oxygen saturation target range is associated with increased incidence of intermittent hypoxemia. J Pediatr 2012;161(6): 1047–52.

15. McEvoy C, Durand M, Hewlett V. Episodes of spontaneous desaturations in infants with chronic lung disease at two different levels of oxygenation. Pediatr Pulmonol 1993;15(3):140–4.

16. Hunt CE, Corwin MJ, Weese-Mayer DE, et al. Longitudinal assessment of hemoglobin oxygen saturation in preterm and term infants in the first six months of life. J Pediatr 2011;159(3):377–83.e1.

17. Di Fiore JM, Arko MK, Miller MJ, et al. Cardiorespiratory events in preterm infants referred for apnea monitoring studies. Pediatrics 2001;108(6):1304–8.

18. Abu Jawdeh EG, Martin RJ, Dick TE, et al. The effect of red blood cell transfusion on intermittent hypoxemia in ELBW infants. J Perinatol 2014;34(12):921–5.

19. Sands SA, Edwards BA, Kelly VJ, et al. Mechanism underlying accelerated arterial oxygen desaturation during recurrent apnea. Am J Respir Crit Care Med 2010;182(7):961–9.

20. de Waal CG, van Leuteren RW, de Jongh FH, et al. Patient-ventilator asynchrony in preterm infants on nasal intermittent positive pressure ventilation. Arch Dis Child Fetal Neonatal Ed 2018;104(3):F280–4.

21. Dimaguila MA, Di Fiore JM, Martin RJ, et al. Characteristics of hypoxemic episodes in very low birth weight infants on ventilatory support. J Pediatr 1997; 130(4):577–83.

22. Esquer C, Claure N, D'Ugard C, et al. Role of abdominal muscles activity on duration and severity of hypoxemia episodes in mechanically ventilated preterm infants. Neonatology 2007;92(3):182–6.

23. Di Fiore JM, Martin RJ, Li H, et al. Patterns of oxygenation, mortality, and growth status in the surfactant positive pressure and oxygen trial cohort. J Pediatr 2017; 186:49–56.e1.

24. Fabian RH, Perez-Polo JR, Kent TA. Extracellular superoxide concentration increases following cerebral hypoxia but does not affect cerebral blood flow. Int J Dev Neurosci 2004;22(4):225–30.

25. Yuan G, Nanduri J, Khan S, et al. Induction of HIF-1alpha expression by intermittent hypoxia: involvement of NADPH oxidase, Ca2+ signaling, prolyl hydroxylases, and mTOR. J Cell Physiol 2008;217(3):674–85.

26. Nanduri J, Wang N, Yuan G, et al. Intermittent hypoxia degrades HIF-2alpha via calpains resulting in oxidative stress: implications for recurrent apnea-induced morbidities. Proc Natl Acad Sci U S A 2009;106(4):1199–204.

27. Decker MJ, Rye DB. Neonatal intermittent hypoxia impairs dopamine signaling and executive functioning. Sleep Breath 2002;6(4):205–10.

28. Del Rio R, Moya EA, Iturriaga R. Differential expression of pro-inflammatory cytokines, endothelin-1 and nitric oxide synthases in the rat carotid body exposed to intermittent hypoxia. Brain Res 2011;1395:74–85.

29. Chow LC, Wright KW, Sola A. Can changes in clinical practice decrease the incidence of severe retinopathy of prematurity in very low birth weight infants? Pediatrics 2003;111(2):339–45.

30. Penn JS, Henry MM, Wall PT, et al. The range of PaO2 variation determines the severity of oxygen-induced retinopathy in newborn rats. Invest Ophthalmol Vis Sci 1995;36(10):2063–70.

31. Coleman RJ, Beharry KD, Brock RS, et al. Effects of brief, clustered versus dispersed hypoxic episodes on systemic and ocular growth factors in a rat model of oxygen-induced retinopathy. Pediatr Res 2008;64(1):50–5.

32. Di Fiore JM, Kaffashi F, Loparo K, et al. The relationship between patterns of intermittent hypoxia and retinopathy of prematurity in preterm infants. Pediatr Res 2012;72(6):606–12.

33. Poets CF, Roberts RS, Schmidt B, et al. Association between intermittent hypoxemia or bradycardia and late death or disability in extremely preterm infants. JAMA 2015;314(6):595–603.

34. Pozo ME, Cave A, Koroglu OA, et al. Effect of postnatal intermittent hypoxia on growth and cardiovascular regulation of rat pups. Neonatology 2012;102(2): 107–13.

35. Julien C, Bairam A, Joseph V. Chronic intermittent hypoxia reduces ventilatory long-term facilitation and enhances apnea frequency in newborn rats. Am J Physiol Regul Integr Comp Physiol 2008;294(4):R1356–66.

36. Reeves SR, Mitchell GS, Gozal D. Early postnatal chronic intermittent hypoxia modifies hypoxic respiratory responses and long-term phrenic facilitation in adult rats. Am J Physiol Regul Integr Comp Physiol 2006;290(6):R1664–71.

37. Rosen CL, Larkin EK, Kirchner HL, et al. Prevalence and risk factors for sleep-disordered breathing in 8- to 11-year-old children: association with race and prematurity. J Pediatr 2003;142(4):383–9.

38. Janvier A, Khairy M, Kokkotis A, et al. Apnea is associated with neurodevelopmental impairment in very low birth weight infants. J Perinatol 2004;24(12):763–8.

39. Pillekamp F, Hermann C, Keller T, et al. Factors influencing apnea and brady-cardia of prematurity - implications for neurodevelopment. Neonatology 2007; 91(3):155–61.

40. Taylor HG, Klein N, Schatschneider C, et al. Predictors of early school age out-comes in very low birth weight children. J Dev Behav Pediatr 1998;19(4):235–43.

41. Greene MM, Patra K, Khan S, et al. Cardiorespiratory events in extremely low birth weight infants: neurodevelopmental outcome at 1 and 2 years. J Perinatol 2014;34(7):562–5.

42. Short EJ, Klein NK, Lewis BA, et al. Cognitive and academic consequences of bronchopulmonary dysplasia and very low birth weight: 8-year-old outcomes. Pe-diatrics 2003;112(5):e359.

43. Gray PH, O'Callaghan MJ, Rogers YM. Psychoeducational outcome at school age of preterm infants with bronchopulmonary dysplasia. J Paediatr Child Health 2004;40(3):114–20.

44. Anderson PJ, Doyle LW. Neurodevelopmental outcome of bronchopulmonary dysplasia. Semin Perinatol 2006;30(4):227–32.

45. Twilhaar ES, Wade RM, de Kieviet JF, et al. Cognitive outcomes of children born extremely or very preterm since the 1990s and associated risk factors: a meta-analysis and meta-regression. JAMA Pediatr 2018;172(4):361–7.

46. Ratner V, Kishkurno SV, Slinko SK, et al. The contribution of intermittent hypox-emia to late neurological handicap in mice with hyperoxia-induced lung injury. Neonatology 2007;92(1):50–8.

47. Carlo WA, Finer NN, Walsh MC, et al. Target ranges of oxygen saturation in extremely preterm infants. N Engl J Med 2010;362(21):1959–69.

48. Walsh MC, Di Fiore JM, Martin RJ, et al. Association of oxygen target and growth status with increased mortality in small for gestational age infants: further analysis of the surfactant, positive pressure and pulse oximetry randomized trial. JAMA Pediatr 2016;170(3):292–4.

49. Juliano C, Sosunov S, Niatsetskaya Z, et al. Mild intermittent hypoxemia in neonatal mice causes permanent neurofunctional deficit and white matter hypo-myelination. Exp Neurol 2015;264:33–42.

50. Martin N, Pourie G, Bossenmeyer-Pourie C, et al. Conditioning-like brief neonatal hypoxia improves cognitive function and brain tissue properties with marked gender dimorphism in adult rats. Semin Perinatol 2010;34(3):193–200.

51. Zhang JX, Chen XQ, Du JZ, et al. Neonatal exposure to intermittent hypoxia en-hances mice performance in water maze and 8-arm radial maze tasks. J Neurobiol 2005;65(1):72–84.

52. Navarrete-Opazo A, Mitchell GS. Therapeutic potential of intermittent hypoxia: a matter of dose. Am J Physiol Regul Integr Comp Physiol 2014;307(10):R1181–97.

53. Manja V, Saugstad OD, Lakshminrusimha S. Oxygen saturation targets in preterm infants and outcomes at 18-24 Months: a systematic review. Pediatrics 2017; 139(1) [pii:e20161609].

54. Stenson BJ. Oxygen saturation targets for extremely preterm infants after the NeOProM trials. Neonatology 2016;109(4):352–8.

55. Zagol K, Lake DE, Vergales B, et al. Anemia, apnea of prematurity, and blood transfusions. J Pediatr 2012;161(3):417–421 e411.

56. Claure N, Bancalari E, D'Ugard C, et al. Multicenter crossover study of automated control of inspired oxygen in ventilated preterm infants. Pediatrics 2011;127(1): e76–83.

57. Waitz M, Schmid MB, Fuchs H, et al. Effects of automated adjustment of the inspired oxygen on fluctuations of arterial and regional cerebral tissue

oxygenation in preterm infants with frequent desaturations. J Pediatr 2015;166(2): 240–244 e1.

58. van Kaam AH, Hummler HD, Wilinska M, et al. Automated versus manual oxygen control with different saturation targets and modes of respiratory support in preterm infants. J Pediatr 2015;167(3):545–50.e1-2.

59. Schmid MB, Hopfner RJ, Lenhof S, et al. Cerebral oxygenation during intermittent hypoxemia and bradycardia in preterm infants. Neonatology 2015;107(2): 137–46.

60. Korcek P, Stranak Z, Sirc J, et al. The role of near-infrared spectroscopy monitoring in preterm infants. J Perinatol 2017;37(10):1070–7.

61. Smith VC, Kelty-Stephen D, Qureshi Ahmad M, et al. Stochastic resonance effects on apnea, bradycardia, and oxygenation: a randomized controlled trial. Pediatrics 2015;136(6):e1561–8.

62. Kesavan K, Frank P, Cordero DM, et al. Neuromodulation of limb proprioceptive afferents decreases apnea of prematurity and accompanying intermittent hypoxia and bradycardia. PLoS One 2016;11(6):e0157349.

63. Schmidt B, Roberts RS, Anderson PJ, et al. Academic performance, motor function, and behavior 11 Years after neonatal caffeine citrate therapy for apnea of prematurity: an 11-year follow-up of the CAP randomized clinical trial. JAMA Pediatr 2017;171(6):564–72.

64. Abu-Shaweesh JM, Martin RJ. Caffeine use in the neonatal intensive care unit. Semin Fetal Neonatal Med 2017;22(5):342–7.

65. Bucher HU, Duc G. Does caffeine prevent hypoxaemic episodes in premature infants? A randomized controlled trial. Eur J Pediatr 1988;147(3):288–91.

66. Rhein LM, Dobson NR, Darnall RA, et al. Effects of caffeine on intermittent hypoxia in infants born prematurely: a randomized clinical trial. JAMA Pediatr 2014;168(3):250–7.

67. Lodha A, Seshia M, McMillan DD, et al. Association of early caffeine administration and neonatal outcomes in very preterm neonates. JAMA Pediatr 2015; 169(1):33–8.

68. Vliegenthart R, Miedema M, Hutten GJ, et al. High versus standard dose caffeine for apnoea: a systematic review. Arch Dis Child Fetal Neonatal Ed 2018;103(6): F523–9.

69. Chavez Valdez R, Ahlawat R, Wills-Karp M, et al. Correlation between serum caffeine levels and changes in cytokine profile in a cohort of preterm infants. J Pediatr 2011;158(1):57–64, 64 e51.

70. McPherson C, Neil JJ, Tjoeng TH, et al. A pilot randomized trial of high-dose caffeine therapy in preterm infants. Pediatr Res 2015;78(2):198–204.

Targeting Arterial Oxygen Saturation by Closed-Loop Control of Inspired Oxygen in Preterm Infants

Nelson Claure, MSc, PhD*, Eduardo Bancalari, MD

KEYWORDS

- Premature infant • Oxygenation • Automatic • Supplemental oxygen
- Oxygen therapy

KEY POINTS

- In premature infants the severity and duration of spontaneous episodes of intermittent hypoxemia can be influenced by the caregiver's response. In contrast, episodes of hyperoxemia are induced by excessive fraction of inspired oxygen.
- Maintenance of the target range of SpO_2 is limited by staff availability and tolerance of high SpO_2 is common.
- In clinical studies, closed loop Fio_2 control has been shown to improve SpO_2 targeting while reducing exposure to hyperoxemia, high-inspired oxygen, and prolonged and severe episodes of hypoxemia.
- The selection of the target range of SpO_2 during closed loop Fio_2 control should be done cautiously, as beneficial or detrimental effects may become apparent because of the tighter maintenance of the selected range.
- Clinical trials are needed to determine the impact of closed loop FiO_2 control on ophthalmic, respiratory, and neurodevelopmental outcomes.

Most extreme premature infants require oxygen supplementation to maintain adequate arterial oxygen levels, and the need for supplemental oxygen can extend for several weeks after birth. Although essential for avoiding the deleterious effects of hypoxia,[1–3] excessive arterial oxygen levels have been associated with eye, lung,

Conflict of Interest Statement: One of the systems for closed loop inspired oxygen discussed here was developed and patented by Drs N. Claure and E. Bancalari, who are Faculty of the University of Miami. The University of Miami, the assignee for this patent, has a licensing agreement with Vyaire Medical. Vyaire Medical provided support to some of the studies with this system.

Division of Neonatology, Department of Pediatrics, University of Miami Miller School of Medicine, PO Box 016960 R-131, Miami, FL 33101, USA
* Corresponding author.
E-mail address: NClaure@miami.edu

and central nervous system (CNS) damage.[4–9] More recently, clinical trials have shown increased mortality with exposure to lower saturation ranges[10,11] and detrimental pulmonary and hemodynamic effects associated with insufficient oxygenation.[12–16] Of greater concern is the reported association between exposure to prolonged episodes of intermittent hypoxemia (IH) and neurodevelopmental impairment.[17] Hence, maintenance of adequate oxygenation with the least exposure to hyperoxemia and episodes of hypoxemia seem essential for improving the outcome of extreme premature infants, and effective targeting of arterial oxygen saturation (SpO_2) in the neonatal intensive care unit (NICU) is key for achieving these goals.

SpO_2 TARGETING IN PREMATURE INFANTS

Targeting a prescribed range of SpO_2 in premature infants is primarily done by adjusting the fraction of inspired oxygen (FiO_2) while steps are taken to maintain sufficient respiratory support for adequate gas exchange. In doing this, FiO_2 is continually titrated by the clinical staff to keep SpO_2 within the target range and to avoid exposure to the high and low SpO_2 levels (**Fig. 1**). This, however, is not achieved consistently, and premature infants on supplemental oxygen usually spend less than half of the time within the target range.[18,19] As reported, these infants spend more than one-third of the time with SpO_2 above the targeted range,[18] which can exceed 50% of the time in more chronic infants.[20,21] This prolonged exposure to hyperoxemia in extreme premature infants is always induced by administration of excessive O_2.

Extreme premature infants also spend considerable time with SpO_2 less than the targeted range.[18] This is the result of spontaneous episodes of IH.[21–27] The duration and severity of these episodes can be influenced by the caregiver's response. However, frequently episodes of IH also lead to exposure to hyperoxemia if the caregiver provides an excessive FiO_2 in response to an episode of IH.[28] The occurrence of IH episodes can be influenced by the basal or target range of SpO_2 with a higher frequency when the basal SpO_2 is near or less than 90%.[22,29,30] In order to prevent episodes of IH, many caregivers tend to maintain a high basal SpO_2, which often exceeds the target range.[20,27] This was confirmed in large clinical trials where the actual SpO_2 levels consistently exceeded the target ranges.[10,31–33] Also in these trials,

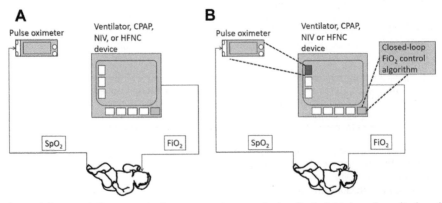

Fig. 1. (*A*) Manual FiO_2 control where a caregiver conducts adjustments based on displayed values of SpO_2. (*B*) A closed loop FiO_2 control system where adjustments by the automated algorithm are based on direct readings from an external or a built-in pulse oximeter.

the time spent with extremely low SpO_2 values was considerably longer among the infants assigned to the lower target range, whereas infants assigned to the higher target range spent considerable more time with excessive SpO_2 values.[32]

HUMAN FACTORS AFFECTING SpO_2 TARGETING

Limited staff and lack of expertise can reduce the efficacy of SpO_2 targeting by manual Fio_2 titration. SpO_2 targeting is compromised with lower nurse:infant ratios.[19,20] Unfortunately, this comes at the cost of an increased time in hyperoxemia, which is even more evident in convalescent premature infants. Commonly there are also inconsistencies between center's policies and actual clinical practice. In a survey in the United States, less than half of the nurses could identify their centers policies on SpO_2 targeting.[34] It is also common that although low SpO_2 alarms levels are kept as intended, the high SpO_2 alarms are increased above the intended level.[18] Caregiver training seems to be the most effective means to improve SpO_2 targeting.[35] This was particularly effective in reducing the exposure to hyperoxemia but it was accompanied by an increased time with SpO_2 less than target range.

RATIONALE FOR AUTOMATIC CONTROL OF Fio_2

In spite of the efforts to avoid hyperoxemia and IH, SpO_2 targeting is not consistently achieved. More importantly, there is considerable tolerance of SpO_2 values that exceed the target range in the NICU. This is particularly common in preterm infants who present with frequent episodes of IH. Under ideal circumstances where staff availability is not limited, manual titration of Fio_2 should keep SpO_2 within the prescribed target range for most of the time. However, this is a very demanding task that cannot be reasonably achieved under routine clinical conditions. Hence, the use of automatic closed loop Fio_2 control has been proposed to address the limitations in SpO_2 targeting resulting from the intrinsic respiratory instability of the patient population and the factors affecting the caregiver's response. The general objective of automatic Fio_2 control is to maintain SpO_2 within the range selected by the clinicians, thereby reducing exposure to extreme high/low SpO_2 values, while minimizing exposure to high inspired oxygen.

SYSTEMS FOR CLOSED LOOP Fio_2 CONTROL

Systems for closed loop Fio_2 control include a SpO_2 monitoring device, gas delivery system (eg, ventilator), and the algorithm determining the Fio_2 adjustments (**Fig. 1**B). Although the algorithms used in these systems may vary, they all increase or decrease Fio_2 in proportion to the decline or increase in SpO_2 outside the target range, respectively, as well as any upward or downward trend. These algorithms also attempt to provide a commensurate response so that an episode of IH or hyperoxemia does not result in under- or overshooting.

IMPACT ON SpO_2 TARGETING

In multiple clinical studies, closed loop Fio_2 control systems have been shown to be consistently more effective in maintaining SpO_2 within the target range than manual titration by the clinical staff and similar or better than a fully dedicated caregiver at the bedside (**Table 1**).[36–50] Although all studies showed improved SpO_2 targeting by closed loop Fio_2 control, there was considerable variability on the achieved percentage of time in range as well as on the difference to the manual Fio_2 control mode. This variability is likely related to the entry criteria that determined the population of

Table 1
SpO$_2$ targeting during closed loop and manual Fio$_2$ control

	Target Range of SpO$_2$	% Time in Target		P	Type of Manual Fio$_2$ Control
		Closed-Loop	Manual		
Bhutani et al,[36] 1992	94%–96%	81	54	<.01	Routine
			69		Dedicated
Morozoff,[53] 1993	90%–95%	50	39	.04	Routine
Claure et al,[38] 2001	88%–96%	75	66	<.05	Dedicated
Urschitz et al,[39] 2004	87%–96%	91	82	.004	Routine
			91	.002	Dedicated
Claure et al,[40] 2009	88%–95%	58	42	<.001	Routine
Morozoff and Smyth,[41] 2009	90%–96%	73	57	n/a	Routine
Claure et al,[42] 2011	87%–93%	47	39	<.001	Routine
Hallenberger et al,[43] 2014	All 4 centers	72	61	<.001	Routine
	90%–95%	71	63		
	80%–92%	69	64		
	83%–93%	66	43		
	85%–94%	84	65		
Zapata et al,[44] 2014	85%–93%	58	34	<.01	Routine
Waitz et al,[47] 2015	88%–96%	76	69	<.01	Routine
Lal et al,[46] 2015	90%–95%	69	60	.031	Routine
van Kaam et al,[45] 2015	89%–93%[a]	62	54	<.001	Routine
	91%–95%[a]	62	58	<.05	
Plottier et al,[48] 2017	91%–95%[a]	81	56	.0001	Routine
van Zanten et al,[49] 2017	90%–95%[a]	62	48	<.01	Routine
Gajdos et al,[50] 2018	88%–96%	78	69	.0012	Routine

Abbreviation: n/a, not available.
[a] Includes time with SpO$_2$ > target range while Fio$_2$ = 0.21.

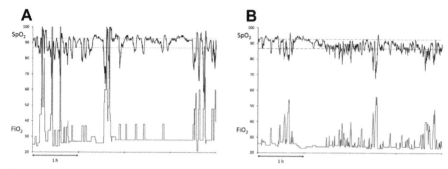

Fig. 2. (*A*) SpO$_2$ and Fio$_2$ recordings from a premature infant undergoing conventional manual Fio$_2$ control by the caregiver. Frequent manual changes are required to assist during episodes of intermittent hypoxemia. (*B*) SpO$_2$ and Fio$_2$ recordings from the same patient while on closed loop Fio$_2$ control. Automatic adjustments to Fio$_2$ are proportional to the severity and duration of the episodes of hypoxemia with a rapid return to the basal level when the episode resolves.

premature infants enrolled in each of these studies. In some of these studies, entry criteria included infants with a minimum frequency of episodes of IH, a selected population that represents the most challenging for both manual and closed loop Fio$_2$ control. An example of the adjustments made by a caregiver and a system of closed loop Fio$_2$ control is shown in **Fig. 2**. These studies also varied in regard to the postnatal age and the forms of invasive or noninvasive respiratory support the enrolled infants were receiving at the time of the study. These differences between studies combined with the consistent improvement in SpO$_2$ targeting provide proof of principle to the use of closed-loop Fio$_2$ control for this population.

IMPACT ON HYPEROXEMIA

Clinical studies showed closed loop Fio$_2$ control systems were effective in reducing the time with SpO$_2$ in hyperoxemia (**Table 2**). As expected, greater reductions were noted in studies where manual Fio$_2$ control was suboptimal. It is also possible that in some of these studies awareness of the study may have increased the attentiveness of the staff to avoid hyperoxemia. The study by van Zanten and colleagues[49] documented the actual impact of introducing closed loop Fio$_2$ control in the NICU.

IMPACT ON EPISODES OF INTERMITTENT HYPOXEMIA

Data from clinical studies showed the systems of closed loop Fio$_2$ control did not consistently influence the frequency of episodes with SpO$_2$ decreasing to less than the target range (**Table 3**). This is not an unexpected finding because these automatic systems were not designed to prevent the occurrence or produce an immediate resolution of the episodes of IH but instead to attenuate their severity or shorten their duration. In some clinical studies there were more episodes with SpO$_2$ less than the target range during closed loop than during manual Fio$_2$ control. In those studies, tolerance of SpO$_2$ values that exceeded the target range was common and was likely in an attempt to attenuate the occurrence of IH. A consistent finding in clinical studies was the reduction in episodes of more severe or prolonged hypoxemia, in particular those episodes where SpO$_2$ declined to less than 80%, which lasted for at least

Table 2
Hyperoxemia during closed loop and manual Fio_2 control

| | SpO$_2$ Range | % Time in Range | | | Type of Manual Fio$_2$ Control |
		Closed-Loop	Manual	P	
Morozoff,[53] 1993	>95%	23	39	.008	Routine
Claure et al,[38] 2001	>96%	10	15	ns	Dedicated
Urschitz et al,[39] 2004	>96%	1.3[b]	4.9[b]	n/a	Routine
			1.8[b]	n/a	Dedicated
Claure et al,[40] 2009	>95%	9	31	<.001	Routine
	>97%	3	16	<.001	
Claure et al,[42] 2011	>93%[a]	21	37	<.001	Routine
	>98%[a]	0.7	5.6	.003	
Hallenberger et al,[43] 2014	4 centers (>95%, >92%, >93% or >94%)	16	16	.108	Routine
Zapata et al,[44] 2014	>95%	27	55	<.01	Routine
Waitz et al,[47] 2015	>96%	6.6	10	.02	Routine
Lal et al,[46] 2015	>95%	4.8	10	.026	Routine
	>97%	0.08	1.7	.001	
van Kaam et al,[45] 2015	Target 89%–93%:				Routine
	>93%[a]	21	25	<.001	
	>98%[a]	0.2	0.7	<.001	
	Target 91%–95%:				
	>95%[a]	22	19	ns	
	>98%[a]	0.7	1.7	<.01	
Plottier et al,[48] 2017	>95%[a]	5.1	25	.0003	Routine
	>98%[a]	0	0.5	.001	
van Zanten et al,[49] 2017	>95%	19	42	<.001	Routine
	>98%	2	10	<.0005	
Gajdos et al,[50] 2018	>96%	4	6	.189	Routine

Abbreviations: n/a, not available; ns, nonsignificant.
[a] Excludes time with $Fio_2 = 0.21$.
[b] Estimated.

1 minute. Reassuringly, studies report minimal rates of overshoot into hyperoxemia following an automatic increase in Fio_2 during an episode of hypoxemia.

In these studies the proportion of time spent less than the target range was largely unaffected by closed loop Fio_2 control, whereas the time spent less than lower thresholds of SpO$_2$ (eg, 80%) was reduced compared with manual Fio_2 control (data not shown).

These data suggest that the timely and more consistent response of closed loop Fio_2 control systems can indeed attenuate the severity of IH episodes. Conceivably, this could ameliorate the damaging effects of IH episodes on the developing eye and CNS.[17,23,51]

IMPACT ON WORKLOAD AND INTERACTION WITH THE CAREGIVER

As expected, clinical studies reported striking reductions in the number of manual adjustments to Fio_2 by the clinical team during closed loop Fio_2 compared with routine care.[37–45,48] This reduction was even more striking when compared with the number of adjustments done by a nurse at bedside who was fully dedicated to Fio_2 titration.

Table 3
Episodes of intermittent hypoxemia during closed loop and manual Fio_2 control

	SpO₂ Range of Hypoxemia and Episode Duration	# Of Episodes per 24 h			Type of Manual Fio_2 Control
		Closed-Loop	Manual	P	
Claure et al,[38] 2001	<88%, >5s	386	360[a]	ns	Dedicated
	<85%, >5s	257	257[a]	ns	
	<75%, >5s	31	31[a]	ns	
Urschitz et al,[39] 2004	<87%, >5s	223	305[a]	ns	Routine
			209[a]	ns	Dedicated
Claure et al,[40] 2009	<88%, ≥10s	552	360[a]	.001	Routine
	<85%, >120s	15	33[a]	.022	
	<75%, >60s	12	23[a]	.022	
Claure et al,[42] 2011	<87%, ≥10s	456	264	<.001	Routine
	<85%, >120s	22	35	<.001	
	<75%, >60s	3	10	.001	
Waitz et al,[47] 2015	<88%, ≥10s	586	588	.07	Routine
	<85%, >120s	54	115	<.01	
	<75%, >60s	2	13	<.01	
van Kaam et al,[45] 2015	Target 89%–93%:				Routine
	<80%, >60s	4	15	<.001	
	Target 91%–95%:				
	<80%, >60s	4	13	<.001	
Plottier,[48] 2017	<85%, >60s	0	11[a]	.0001	Routine
	<80%, >60s	0	3.1[a]	.001	
Gajdos et al,[50] 2018	<88%, >10s	526	597	.14	Routine
	<88%, >60s	35	91	<.001	
	<80%, >10s	405	457	.13	
	<80%, >60s	43	75	<.001	

Abbreviation: ns, nonsignificant.
[a] Extrapolated to 24 hours.

These numbers, however, do not provide a full indication of the reduction in the actual time spent by an attentive caregiver who cannot predict when the next episode of IH will occur or when it occurs, how soon the episode will resolve. An example of the manual Fio_2 adjustments conducted by a caregiver to maintain SpO₂ within the target range is shown in **Fig. 2**B.

Closed loop Fio_2 control systems could in theory lead to an unwanted reduction in caregiver attentiveness. Although this has not been evidenced in the clinical studies conducted to date, this could occur if caregivers rely on the automatic system to keep adequate oxygenation and do not monitor the basal Fio_2 requirement, the adequacy of ventilation, and the infant's general respiratory status. An automatic increase in basal Fio_2 could potentially mask a respiratory deterioration that would otherwise lead to persistent hypoxemia alarms. In order to mitigate this risk, closed loop Fio_2 control systems need to include additional warnings that alert the caregiver when a higher basal Fio_2 is required to keep SpO₂ within range.

The selection of the prescribed target range of SpO₂ by the clinician is a very important aspect during the use of closed loop Fio_2 control systems in premature infants. Different than what occurs during routine manual control, the prescribed target range will be consistently maintained during closed loop Fio_2 control. The tighter maintenance of a given SpO₂ range could uncover important physiologic effects on respiratory and oxygenation stability as well as the effects related to oxygen availability to different organ systems. For this reason, the selection of the target range for clinical or research purposes has to be done with caution, as the impact on the infant's outcome may be related not only to the use of closed loop systems but also to the selected range.

SUMMARY

Exposure to hyperoxemia from excessive inspired oxygen and episodes of IH have been associated with deleterious effects affecting the developing eye, lung, and CNS in premature infants. The infant's inherent respiratory instability combined with resource limitations during routine care in the NICU often can lead to poor maintenance of the SpO_2 target range and exposure to extreme high and low SpO_2 ranges. Data from clinical studies have provided proof of principle and documented the efficacy of systems using closed loop Fio_2 control in improving SpO_2 targeting. Robust randomized clinical trials are needed to determine the true impact of this strategy on the long-term clinical outcomes of these infants.[52] The timing of these trials is crucial before this novel technology becomes widely adopted in the NICU without sufficient evidence of benefit or safety as it has happened with many other therapies.

Best Practices

What is the current practice for maintaining arterial oxygen saturation targets in extreme premature infants in the NICU?

Best Practice/Guideline/Care Path Objective

- Neonatal centers determine their target range of arterial oxygen saturation (SpO_2) with focus on reducing exposure to low and high SpO_2.

- Clinical staff in neonatal centers aim at maintaining SpO_2 within the target range by manual titration of the fraction of inspired oxygen (Fio_2).

What changes in current practice are likely to improve outcomes?

- Better maintenance of SpO_2 within the center's target range.

- Reducing exposure to extreme high and low SpO_2 levels.

- Reducing exposure to high Fio_2.

- Neonatal centers have developed algorithms and quality improvement initiatives to improve maintenance SpO_2 within target range. Some of these algorithms are published in the literature.

- Although clinical algorithms can improve SpO_2 targeting, their use is limited by staff availability and the high-time demands of this task.

Major recommendations

- In short-term clinical studies closed loop Fio_2 control has consistently shown to be more effective than manual titration in SpO_2 targeting. These studies showed reduction in the more severe and prolonged episodes of hypoxemia and hyperoxemia.

- Randomized clinical trials with longer-term use of automated Fio_2 control are required to determine the impact of these systems on short- and long-term clinical outcomes. Some of these trials are underway.

- Definition of the optimal SpO_2 target when using automated Fio_2 control systems must be carefully evaluated.

ACKNOWLEDGMENTS

We are grateful to the University of Miami Project NewBorn for their continued support.

REFERENCES

1. Cross KW. Cost of preventing retrolental fibroplasia? Lancet 1973;2(7835):954–6.
2. Avery ME. Recent increase in mortality from hyaline membrane disease. J Pediatr 1960;57:553–9.
3. Bolton DP, Cross KW. Further observations on cost of preventing retrolental fibroplasia. Lancet 1974;1(7855):445–8.
4. Flynn JT, Bancalari E, Snyder ES, et al. A cohort study of transcutaneous oxygen tension and the incidence and severity of retinopathy of prematurity. The New England Journal of Medicine 1992;326(16):1050–4.
5. Collins MP, Lorenz JM, Jetton JR, et al. Hypocapnia and other ventilation-related risk factors for cerebral palsy in low birth weight infants. Pediatr Res 2001;50(6):712–9.
6. Back SA, Luo NL, Mallinson RA, et al. Selective vulnerability of preterm white matter to oxidative damage defined by F2-isoprostanes. Ann Neurol 2005;58(1):108–20.
7. Haynes RL, Folkerth RD, Keefe RJ, et al. Nitrosative and oxidative injury to premyelinating oligodendrocytes in periventricular leukomalacia. J Neuropathol Exp Neurol 2003;62(5):441–50.
8. Supplemental therapeutic oxygen for prethreshold retinopathy of prematurity (STOP-ROP), a randomized, controlled trial. I: primary outcomes. Pediatrics 2000;105(2):295–310.
9. Askie LM, Henderson-Smart DJ, Irwig L, et al. Oxygen-saturation targets and outcomes in extremely preterm infants. N Engl J Med 2003;349(10):959–67.
10. Carlo WA, Finer NN, Walsh MC, et al. Target ranges of oxygen saturation in extremely preterm infants. N Engl J Med 2010;362(21):1959–69.
11. Stenson B, Brocklehurst P, Tarnow-Mordi W. Increased 36-week survival with high oxygen saturation target in extremely preterm infants. N Engl J Med 2011;364(17):1680–2.
12. Tay-Uyboco JS, Kwiatkowski K, Cates DB, et al. Hypoxic airway constriction in infants of very low birth weight recovering from moderate to severe bronchopulmonary dysplasia. J Pediatr 1989;115(3):456–9.
13. Abman SH, Wolfe RR, Accurso FJ, et al. Pulmonary vascular response to oxygen in infants with severe bronchopulmonary dysplasia. Pediatrics 1985;75(1):80–4.
14. Skinner JR, Hunter S, Poets CF, et al. Haemodynamic effects of altering arterial oxygen saturation in preterm infants with respiratory failure. Arch Dis Child Fetal Neonatal Ed 1999;80(2):F81–7.
15. Noori S, Patel D, Friedlich P, et al. Effects of low oxygen saturation limits on the ductus arteriosus in extremely low birth weight infants. J Perinatol 2009;29(8):553–7.
16. Halliday HL, Dumpit FM, Brady JP. Effects of inspired oxygen on echocardiographic assessment of pulmonary vascular resistance and myocardial contractility in bronchopulmonary dysplasia. Pediatrics 1980;65(3):536–40.
17. Poets CF, Roberts RS, Schmidt B, et al. Association between intermittent hypoxemia or bradycardia and late death or disability in extremely preterm infants. JAMA 2015;314(6):595–603.

18. Hagadorn JI, Furey AM, Nghiem TH, et al. Achieved versus intended pulse oximeter saturation in infants born less than 28 weeks' gestation: the AVIOx study. Pediatrics 2006;118(4):1574–82.

19. Lim K, Wheeler KI, Gale TJ, et al. Oxygen saturation targeting in preterm infants receiving continuous positive airway pressure. J Pediatr 2014;164(4):730–6.e1.

20. Sink DW, Hope SA, Hagadorn JI. Nurse:patient ratio and achievement of oxygen saturation goals in premature infants. Arch Dis Child Fetal Neonatal Ed 2011; 96(2):F93–8.

21. Durand M, McEvoy C, MacDonald K. Spontaneous desaturations in intubated very low birth weight infants with acute and chronic lung disease. Pediatr Pulmonol 1992;13(3):136–42.

22. Di Fiore JM, Walsh M, Wrage L, et al. Low oxygen saturation target range is associated with increased incidence of intermittent hypoxemia. J Pediatr 2012;161(6): 1047–52.

23. Di Fiore JM, Kaffashi F, Loparo K, et al. The relationship between patterns of intermittent hypoxia and retinopathy of prematurity in preterm infants. Pediatr Res 2012;72(6):606–12.

24. Bolivar JM, Gerhardt T, Gonzalez A, et al. Mechanisms for episodes of hypoxemia in preterm infants undergoing mechanical ventilation. J Pediatr 1995;127(5):767–73.

25. Esquer C, Claure N, D'Ugard C, et al. Mechanisms of hypoxemia episodes in spontaneously breathing preterm infants after mechanical ventilation. Neonatology 2008;94(2):100–4.

26. Esquer C, Claure N, D'Ugard C, et al. Role of abdominal muscles activity on duration and severity of hypoxemia episodes in mechanically ventilated preterm infants. Neonatology 2007;92(3):182–6.

27. Jain D, D'Ugard C, Bello J, et al. Hypoxemia episodes during day and night and their impact on oxygen saturation targeting in mechanically ventilated preterm infants. Neonatology 2018;113(1):69–74.

28. van Zanten HA, Tan RN, Thio M, et al. The risk for hyperoxaemia after apnoea, bradycardia and hypoxaemia in preterm infants. Arch Dis Child Fetal Neonatal Ed 2014;99(4):F269–73.

29. McEvoy C, Durand M, Hewlett V. Episodes of spontaneous desaturations in infants with chronic lung disease at two different levels of oxygenation. Pediatr Pulmonol 1993;15(3):140–4.

30. Laptook AR, Salhab W, Allen J, et al. Pulse oximetry in very low birth weight infants: can oxygen saturation be maintained in the desired range? J Perinatol 2006;26(6):337–41.

31. Stenson BJ, Tarnow-Mordi WO, Darlow BA, et al. Oxygen saturation and outcomes in preterm infants. N Engl J Med 2013;368(22):2094–104.

32. Schmidt B, Roberts RS, Whyte RK, et al. Impact of study oximeter masking algorithm on titration of oxygen therapy in the Canadian oxygen trial. J Pediatr 2014; 165(4):666–71.e2.

33. Schmidt B, Whyte RK, Asztalos EV, et al. Effects of targeting higher vs lower arterial oxygen saturations on death or disability in extremely preterm infants: a randomized clinical trial. JAMA 2013;309(20):2111–20.

34. Nghiem TH, Hagadorn JI, Terrin N, et al. Nurse opinions and pulse oximeter saturation target limits for preterm infants. Pediatrics 2008;121(5):e1039–46.

35. Ford SP, Leick-Rude MK, Meinert KA, et al. Overcoming barriers to oxygen saturation targeting. Pediatrics 2006;118(Suppl 2):S177–86.

36. Bhutani VK, Taube JC, Antunes MJ, et al. Adaptive control of inspired oxygen delivery to the neonate. Pediatr Pulmonol 1992;14(2):110–7.

37. Morozoff PE, Evans RW. Closed-loop control of SaO2 in the neonate. Biomed Instrum Technol 1992;26(2):117–23.

38. Claure N, Gerhardt T, Everett R, et al. Closed-loop controlled inspired oxygen concentration for mechanically ventilated very low birth weight infants with frequent episodes of hypoxemia. Pediatrics 2001;107(5):1120–4.

39. Urschitz MS, Horn W, Seyfang A, et al. Automatic control of the inspired oxygen fraction in preterm infants: a randomized crossover trial. Am J Respir Crit Care Med 2004;170(10):1095–100.

40. Claure N, D'Ugard C, Bancalari E. Automated adjustment of inspired oxygen in preterm infants with frequent fluctuations in oxygenation: a pilot clinical trial. J Pediatr 2009;155(5):640–5, e1-2.

41. Morozoff EP, Smyth JA. Evaluation of three automatic oxygen therapy control algorithms on ventilated low birth weight neonates. Conf Proc IEEE Eng Med Biol Soc 2009;2009:3079–82.

42. Claure N, Bancalari E, D'Ugard C, et al. Multicenter crossover study of automated control of inspired oxygen in ventilated preterm infants. Pediatrics 2011;127(1):e76–83.

43. Hallenberger A, Poets CF, Horn W, et al. Closed-loop automatic oxygen control (CLAC) in preterm infants: a randomized controlled trial. Pediatrics 2014;133(2):e379–85.

44. Zapata J, Gomez JJ, Araque Campo R, et al. A randomised controlled trial of an automated oxygen delivery algorithm for preterm neonates receiving supplemental oxygen without mechanical ventilation. Acta Paediatr 2014;103(9):928–33.

45. van Kaam AH, Hummler HD, Wilinska M, et al. Automated versus manual oxygen control with different saturation targets and modes of respiratory support in preterm infants. J Pediatr 2015;167(3):545–50, e1-2.

46. Lal M, Tin W, Sinha S. Automated control of inspired oxygen in ventilated preterm infants: crossover physiological study. Acta Paediatr 2015;104(11):1084–9.

47. Waitz M, Schmid MB, Fuchs H, et al. Effects of automated adjustment of the inspired oxygen on fluctuations of arterial and regional cerebral tissue oxygenation in preterm infants with frequent desaturations. J Pediatr 2015;166(2):240–4.e1.

48. Plottier GK, Wheeler KI, Ali SK, et al. Clinical evaluation of a novel adaptive algorithm for automated control of oxygen therapy in preterm infants on non-invasive respiratory support. Arch Dis Child Fetal Neonatal Ed 2017;102(1):F37–43.

49. Van Zanten HA, Kuypers KL, Stenson BJ, et al. The effect of implementing an automated oxygen control on oxygen saturation in preterm infants. Arch Dis Child Fetal Neonatal Ed 2017;102(5):F395–9.

50. Gajdos M, Waitz M, Mendler MR, et al. Effects of a new device for automated closed loop control of inspired oxygen concentration on fluctuations of arterial and different regional organ tissue oxygen saturations in preterm infants. Archives of disease in childhood fetal and neonatal edition 2018.

51. Di Fiore JM, Bloom JN, Orge F, et al. A higher incidence of intermittent hypoxemic episodes is associated with severe retinopathy of prematurity. J Pediatr 2010;157(1):69–73.

52. Poets CF, Franz AR. Automated FiO2 control: nice to have, or an essential addition to neonatal intensive care? Arch Dis Child Fetal Neonatal Ed 2017;102(1):F5–6.

53. Morozoff PE, Evans RW, Smyth JA. Automatic-control of blood-oxygen saturation in premature-infants. Second Ieee Conference on Control Applications 1993;1-2:415–20.

Meta-analysis of Oxygenation Saturation Targeting Trials

Do Infant Subgroups Matter?

Lisa Maree Askie, PhD, MPH, BN, FHEA

KEYWORDS

- Oxygen saturation targeting • Prospective meta-analysis • Subgroup analysis
- Extremely preterm infants

KEY POINTS

- Infants born extremely preterm (less than 28 weeks' gestation) should have their oxygen saturation levels targeted between 91% and 95%.
- No particular subgroup of infants benefits more or less from this target range, so this practice can be implemented for all infants less than 28 weeks from birth or soon thereafter.
- There are potential benefits from the higher target range (decreased mortality and necrotizing enterocolitis) but also potential harms (increased retinopathy of prematurity treatment and bronchopulmonary dysplasia), which should be considered in decision-making.

INTRODUCTION

Oxygen therapy has been used in the treatment of small and sick newborns since the 1940s. Despite being one of the most commonly used drugs in neonatal care, there have been few randomized trials that have objectively assessed what is the best range to target a preterm infant's oxygen saturation as measured by pulse oximetry. Before his death in 2004, Silverman wrote how the use of supplemental oxygen in the care of preterm infants was "a cautionary tale" and "the albatross of neonatal medicine" given the failure to properly assess the effects of oxygen therapy. At that time Silverman

Disclosure Statement: Professor L.M. Askie is the coordinator of the neonatal oxygen prospective meta-analysis (NeOProM) Collaboration and a co-convenor of the Cochrane Prospective Meta-analysis Methods Group. She has no other commercial or financial conflicts of interest to disclose. The NeOProM data analysis was supported by grant R03HD 079867 from the Eunice Kennedy Shriver National Institute of Child Health and Human Development, National Institutes of Health, Department of Health and Human Services, Washington DC, USA.
NHMRC Clinical Trials Centre, University of Sydney, Medical Foundation Building, 92-94 Parramatta Road, Camperdown, New South Wales, 2050, Australia
E-mail address: lisa.askie@ctc.usyd.edu.au

asserted that "there has never been a shred of convincing evidence to guide limits for the rational use of supplemental oxygen in the care of extremely premature infants. For decades, the optimum range of oxygenation (to balance four competing risks: mortality, ROP-blindness, chronic lung disease, and brain damage) was, and remains to this day, unknown."[1]

A few very small randomized trials in the 1950s[2,3] and 2 slightly larger trials in the early 2000s,[4,5] which assessed preterm infants still oxygen dependent many weeks after birth, and numerous observational studies[6-8] added to the evidence base but were unable to reliably assess the 4 competing risks that Silverman referred to with sufficient certainty to ensure that any expected benefits from a lower target range, such as reduced retinopathy of prematurity (ROP) and bronchopulmonary dysplasia (BPD), would not come at the expense of small but important increases in death or major disability. To resolve this situation investigators from 5 countries (United States, Canada, United Kingdom, New Zealand, and Australia) formed a collaboration in 2003[9] in which 5 randomized trials with similar protocols were conducted separately but all agreed prospectively, before the results of any of the trials were known, to combine their individual participant data (IPD) once completed in a prospective meta-analysis.[10] This group was known as the Neonatal Oxygenation Prospective Meta-analysis (NeOProM) Collaboration. The main NeOProM results were published in *JAMA* in 2018[11] and included a full list of all prespecified subgroup analyses results in the online supplement the article.

The main NeOProM study findings concluded that a higher target range of oxygen saturation as measured by pulse oximetry (Spo_2), 91% to 95%, compared with a lower range of Spo_2, 85% to 89%, decreases the risk of death and NEC, increases the risk of ROP treatment and BPD, and has no effect on major disability. Because application of these findings in practice requires trade-offs between benefits and harms, there is interest in whether particular subgroups of infants could benefit more or less from the different target ranges. Hence, clinicians ask themselves, do infant subgroups matter?

DO INFANT SUBGROUPS MATTER?

The 2016 American Academy of Pediatrics clinical report guidelines[12] state that "the ideal physiologic target range for oxygen saturation for infants of [extremely low birth weight] is likely patient specific and dynamic and depends on various factors, including gestational age, chronologic age, underlying disease, and transfusion status." These guidelines also conclude that a target oxygen saturation "range of 90% to 95% may be safer than 85% to 89% at least for some infants" but that more definitive evidence is forthcoming from the NeOProM Collaboration findings.

A major strength of the NeOProM Collaboration was the ability to synthesize (meta-analyze) the line-by-line IPD for all outcomes from all infants randomized in the 5 participating trials. By doing so, NeOProM was able to explore whether findings from 1 particular trial also were found consistently across other trials and whether different definitions of particular subgroup variables across trials (for example, small-for-gestational-age [SGA infants]) changed the results. The meta-analysis also provided increased statistical power to reliably detect any important subgroup differences that would not be possible within individual trials. The plans for these subgroup analyses were prespecified prior to the results of any of the trials being known (a core feature of the prospective meta-analysis method), were published in a protocol,[10] and were not driven or influenced by the trials' results data or post hoc analyses.

The primary outcome of the NeOProM meta-analysis was death or major disability at 18 months to 24 months corrected age. There was no statistically significant difference in this outcome for the higher (Spo_2 91%–95%) compared with the lower (Spo_2 85%–89%) oxygen saturation target group (relative risk [RR] 1.04; 95% CI, 0.98–1.09; $P = .21$). The prespecified subgroup variables examined in NeOProM were gestational age (<26 weeks vs ≥26 weeks), outborn, use of any antenatal corticosteroids, gender, SGA infants, multiple pregnancy, type of delivery (vaginal vs cesarean), time intervention started (<6 hours age vs ≥6 hours age), and oximeter software type (original vs revised). There were no statistically significant differences in the composite outcome of death or major disability or for major disability alone within any of these prespecified subgroups.

Outcomes Favoring Higher Targets

The NeOProM meta-analysis revealed, however, that there were 2 important neonatal outcomes for which the higher oxygen target range showed reduced risks: death and necrotizing enterocolitis (NEC).

When the full NeOProM meta-analysis data set was used to explore any potential differences in death rates by different types (subgroups) of infants, none were found—including for those infants born SGA infants (RR 1.36; 95% CI, 1.04–1.78) compared with non-SGA infants (RR 1.14; 95% CI, 1.00–1.30) (interaction $P = .287$), when using the definitions from each individual trial (**Table 1**). This contradicted previously published findings,[13] which found that SGA infants within the surfactant, positive pressure, and oxygenation randomized (SUPPORT) trial had a higher death rate (38.5%) compared with non-SGA infants (16.4%) ($P<.01$). The NeOProM analysis confirmed the differences in death rates for SGA infants (RR 1.99; 95% CI, 1.22–3.24; $P = .006$) compared with non-SGA infants (RR 1.16; 95% CI, 0.91–1.48; $P = .27$) reported by Walsh and colleagues[13] but this observation was not found in the other 4 trials as no other trial found a statistically significant difference in death between the higher and lower target groups for SGA infants (see **Table 1**). Having access to the IPD from all 5 trials allowed further investigation of this finding to see if it was robust to changes in the definition of SGA infants. The NeOProM meta-analysis found that when a common definition of SGA[14] was applied across all trials, the statistically significant difference in death in Walsh and colleagues' study[13] disappeared (RR 1.11; 95% CI, 0.74–1.68) (**Table 2**) and when the SUPPORT definition of SGA[15] was used across all NeOProM trials, there again was no significant difference in the risk of death in SGA infants versus non-SGA infants (interaction $P = .203$) (**Table 3**). Thus, there does not seem to be any particular types or subgroups of SGA infants for whom the risk of death is any better or worse, so targeting the higher range (Spo_2 91%–95%) can be recommended for all infants born less than 28 weeks' gestation.

There was 1 other characteristic for which there was a significant difference in the risk of death: the type of oximeter software. Whilst 3 of the NeOProM trials (Canadian oxygen trial, benefits of oxygen saturation targeting (BOOST) II UK, and BOOST II Australia) were still recruiting, an artifact in the Masimo oximeter algorithm was identified[16] and the software was revised accordingly. Subsequently, the data safety monitoring committees of the United Kingdom and Australian BOOST trials requested a pooled interim analysis of mortality data stratified by oximeter software type. The results showed a significantly larger treatment effect for mortality in the revised software oximeters.[17] As a result, both these trials were terminated early, when 81% and 95% of their recruitment targets, respectively, had been enrolled. This finding was confirmed in the full NeOProM subgroup analysis by oximeter type, which showed a statistically significant difference in the risk of death when targeting the lower Spo_2 range for infants using

Table 1
Death by small-for-gestational-age using trialists' definition

Subgroup: Small-for-Gestational-Age (Trialist Defined)		Lower Oxygen Saturation		Higher Oxygen Saturation		Adjusted Relative Risk	Adjusted Relative Risk (95% CI)	Interaction
Outcome: Death	Trial	n (%)	N	n (%)	N	Adjusted Relative Risk	Treatment effect P Value	P Value
No	SUPPORT	116 (19.6)	592	102 (17.2)	593	1.16 (0.91–1.48)	.237	.287
	COT	83 (15.6)	531	74 (14.1)	526	1.11 (0.83–1.47)	.481	
	BOOST II NZ	24 (15.7)	153	23 (14.6)	157	1.06 (0.63–1.77)	.834	
	BOOST II UK	100 (24.6)	407	79 (19.4)	408	1.26 (0.97–1.64)	.077	
	BOOST II AUS	75 (15.6)	481	73 (15.1)	485	1.04 (0.77–1.40)	.810	
	NeOProM	398 (18.4)	2164	351 (16.2)	2169	1.14 (1.00–1.30)	.047	
Yes	SUPPORT	24 (58.5)	41	16 (29.1)	55	1.99 (1.22–3.24)	.006	
	COT	14 (25.9)	54	14 (27.5)	51	0.95 (0.51–1.74)	.856	
	BOOST II NZ	1 (5.9)	17	4 (30.8)	13	0.18 (0.02–1.44)	.106	
	BOOST II UK	21 (28.0)	75	17 (23.6)	72	1.74 (0.98–3.09)	.345	
	BOOST II AUS	25 (31.6)	79	14 (18.2)	77	1.24 (0.53–2.87)	.618	
	NeOProM	85 (32.0)	266	65 (24.3)	268	1.36 (1.04–1.78)	.033	

Abbreviations: AUS, Australia; NZ, New Zealand; tx, treatment; UK, United Kingdom.
Data from: Askie LM, Darlow BA, Finer N, et al. *JAMA.* 2018;319(21):2190–2201. Supplement 3, eTable 15.

Table 2
Death by small-for-gestational-age using NeOProM definition

Subgroup: Small-for-Gestational-Age (Neonatal Oxygenation Prospective Meta-analysis Defined)		Lower Oxygen Saturation		Higher Oxygen Saturation			Adjusted Relative Risk (95% CI)		Interaction
Outcome: Death	Trial	n (%)	N	n (%)	N	Adjusted Relative Risk	Treatment Effect P Value	P Value
No	SUPPORT	110 (20.3)	541	84 (15.8)	533	1.31 (1.01–1.70)	.043	.674
	COT	83 (15.6)	531	74 (14.1)	526	1.11 (0.83–1.47)	.481	
	BOOST II NZ	24 (15.7)	153	23 (14.6)	157	1.06 (0.63–1.77)	.834	
	BOOST II UK	105 (24.6)	427	81 (19.0)	427	1.29 (0.99–1.67)	.055	
	BOOST II AUS	75 (15.6)	481	73 (15.1)	485	1.04 (0.77–1.40)	.810	
	NeOProM	397 (18.6)	2133	335 (15.7)	2128	1.18 (1.04–1.35)	.012	
Yes	SUPPORT	30 (32.6)	92	34 (29.6)	115	1.11 (0.74–1.68)	.605	
	COT	14 (25.9)	54	14 (27.5)	51	0.95 (0.51–1.74)	.856	
	BOOST II NZ	1 (5.9)	17	4 (30.8)	13	0.18 (0.02–1.44)	.106	
	BOOST II UK	17 (29.8)	57	17 (30.4)	56	0.93 (0.51–1.68)	.799	
	BOOST II AUS	25 (31.6)	79	14 (18.2)	77	1.24 (0.53–2.87)	.618	
	NeOProM	87 (29.1)	299	83 (26.6)	312	1.08 (0.83–1.40)	.572	

Data from: Askie LM, Darlow BA, Finer N, et al. *JAMA.* 2018;319(21):2190-2201. Supplement 3, eTable 15.

Table 3
Death by small-for-gestational-age using SUPPORT definition

Subgroup: Small-for-Gestational-Age (SUPPORT Defined)		Lower Oxygen Saturation		Higher Oxygen Saturation		Adjusted Relative Risk (95% CI)		
Outcome: Death	Trial	n (%)	N	n (%)	N	Adjusted Relative Risk	Treatment Effect P Value	Interaction P Value
No	SUPPORT	116 (19.6)	592	102 (17.2)	593	1.16 (0.91–1.48)	.237	.203
	COT	85 (15.6)	545	77 (14.2)	543	1.10 (0.83–1.45)	.509	
	BOOST II NZ	24 (15.1)	159	24 (14.7)	163	1.00 (0.60–1.65)	.989	
	BOOST II UK	109 (24.7)	442	87 (19.6)	443	1.25 (0.97–1.60)	.082	
	BOOST II AUS	83 (16.4)	505	79 (15.6)	508	1.06 (0.80–1.40)	.697	
	NeOProM	417 (18.6)	2243	369 (16.4)	2250	1.14 (1.00–1.29)	.047	
Yes	SUPPORT	24 (58.5)	41	16 (29.1)	55	1.99 (1.22–3.24)	.006	
	COT	12 (30.0)	40	11 (32.4)	34	0.93 (0.47–1.83)	.827	
	BOOST II NZ	1 (9.1)	11	3 (42.9)	7	0.21 (0.03–1.66)	.139	
	BOOST II UK	13 (31.0)	42	11 (27.5)	40	1.13 (0.57–2.21)	.752	
	BOOST II AUS	17 (30.9)	55	8 (14.8)	54	2.09 (0.98–4.42)	.625	
	NeOProM	67 (35.4)	189	49 (25.8)	190	1.42 (1.05–1.92)	.020	

Abbreviation: SUPPORT, surfactant, positive pressure, and oxygenation randomized trial.
Data from: Askie LM, Darlow BA, Finer N, et al. *JAMA.* 2018;319(21):2190–2201. Supplement 3, eTable 33.

revised oximeters (RR 1.38; 95% CI, 1.14–1.68) compared with infants using the original oximeters (RR 1.06; 95% CI, 0.91–1.23), interaction P = .03 (see Fig. 5 in Askie and colleagues[11]). The revised software is now used routinely in Masimo oximeters worldwide. There has been much debate, both within the NeOProM group and beyond, as to why such a large change in mortality risk was found when the oximeter software changed.[17–22] As with any subgroup analysis, this result may be a spurious finding (particularly because the SUPPORT trial had found similar results but with the original algorithm), or it may be that the 17% relative increase in the risk of death with lower targeting found in the main NeOProM analysis (RR 1.17; 95% CI, 1.04–1.31) is an underestimate of the true treatment effect that would be seen in real-world practice with the use of current Masimo oximeters, which would be akin to a 38% relative increase in death.

The other outcome for which there was a significantly increased risk with lower oxygen targeting was NEC. The risk of NEC was higher when targeting the lower Spo_2 range for all infants (P value = .003), inborn infants (interaction P = .015), and singletons (interaction P = .034) (see eTable 26 in Supplement 3 in Askie and colleagues[11]). The subgroup findings may have occurred due to low power (for example, the number of outborn NeOProM infants is small: n = 322) or may have occurred by chance due to multiple testing, so the implications of these results are unclear.

Outcomes Favoring Lower Targets

There were 2 important neonatal outcomes in the NeOProM meta-analysis for which the lower oxygen target range showed reduced risks: retinopathy of prematurity (ROP) requiring treatment and supplemental oxygen at 36 weeks' postmenstrual age (BPD).

The combined NeOProM meta-analysis showed that targeting the lower Spo_2 range (85%–89%) significantly reduced the risk of ROP requiring treatment (RR 0.74; 95% CI, 0.63–0.86; $P<.001$) (see Fig. 3 in Askie and colleagues[11]). This finding had substantial heterogeneity (I^2 = 80%), however, because SUPPORT was the only trial within NeOProM to find a significant reduction in the need for ROP treatment (**Tables 4** and **5**). If the 4% absolute difference (11% in the lower target group vs 15% in the higher target group) in the rate of ROP treatment in NeOProM is true, each trial would alone have needed a sample size of 2050 infants to detect a risk difference of this size. None of the NeOProM trials alone had a sample size this large, so any failure to detect a difference of this magnitude may be due to insufficient power within the individual trials. The unusually large effect on treated ROP seen in the SUPPORT trial (7% in the lower target group vs 18% in the higher target group), however, raises some questions about whether SUPPORT was different from the other NeOProM trials in other ways that may have influenced this outcome. SUPPORT required antenatal consent so the investigators were able to enroll all-comers because they could not exclude the sickest babies prior to birth, and all infants were inborn. The other 4 trials obtained informed consent after delivery and commenced the targeting intervention within the first 24 hours of life. Consequently, infants in SUPPORT started their targeting intervention much earlier compared with those in the other trials.

The earlier enrollment in the SUPPORT trial can been seen in the subgroup analysis of the NeOProM trials by time of intervention start. As shown in **Table 4**, there was a significant difference in the effect of lower targeting between infants who commenced before 6 hours of age compared with those who commenced at 6 hours or later (interaction P = .0006). The large treatment effect seen in the infants who started their targeting intervention before 6 hours, however, was predominantly due to the effect seen within SUPPORT because there were few infants from the other trials who commenced the intervention before 6 hours of age. In the trials where most infants commenced the

Table 4
Retinopathy of prematurity treatment by trial

Outcome: Retinopathy of Prematurity Treatment	Lower Oxygen Saturation		Higher Oxygen Saturation		Adjusted Relative Risk (95% CI)		
Trial	n (%)	N	n (%)	N	Adjusted Relative Risk	Treatment Effect P Value	Heterogeneity
SUPPORT	36 (7.5)	482	93 (18.1)	514	0.41 (0.28–0.60)	<.001	
COT	64 (12.8)	500	66 (13.1)	503	0.90 (0.66–1.21)	.485	
BOOST II NZ	14 (8.9)	158	13 (8.7)	150	0.88 (0.45–1.73)	.715	
BOOST II UK	69 (17.6)	393	88 (21.9)	401	0.82 (0.62–1.08)	.153	
BOOST II AUS	37 (7.6)	487	48 (9.7)	497	0.79 (0.52–1.19)	.259	
NeOProM	220 (10.9)	2020	308 (14.9)	2065	0.74 (0.63–0.86)	<.001	$I^2 = 80\%$

Data from: Askie LM, Darlow BA, Finer N, et al. *JAMA.* 2018;319(21):2190–2201. Row 6 from Figure 3. Rows 1–5: previously unpublished.

Table 5
Retinopathy of prematurity treatment by intervention start time

Subgroup: Intervention Start Time	Trial	Lower Oxygen Saturation		Higher Oxygen Saturation		Adjusted Relative Risk (95% CI)		
		n (%)	N	n (%)	N	Adjusted Relative Risk	Treatment Effect P Value	Interaction P Value
Outcome: Retinopathy of Prematurity Treatment								
Start <6 h	SUPPORT	36 (7.5)	478	93 (18.2)	510	0.41 (0.28–0.59)	<.001	.0006
	COT	3 (12.5)	24	2 (8.7)	23	1.45 (0.27–7.72)	.665	
	BOOST II NZ	3 (11.5)	26	2 (7.4)	27	1.00 (0.99–1.01)	.545	
	BOOST II UK					Not available		
	BOOST II AUS	1 (2.0)	49	6 (10.7)	56	0.19 (0.02–1.53)	.119	
	NeOProM	42 (7.3)	572	101 (16.5)	611	0.44 (0.31–0.62)	<.001	
≥6 h	SUPPORT	0	4	0	4	Not estimable		
	COT	61 (12.8)	476	64 (13.3)	480	0.88 (0.65–1.20)	.417	
	BOOST II NZ	11 (8.3)	132	11 (8.9)	123	0.88 (0.41–1.88)	.738	
	BOOST II UK					Not available		
	BOOST II AUS	36 (8.3)	436	42 (9.5)	441	0.87 (0.57–1.34)	.529	
	NeOProM	108 (10.3)	1048	117 (11.2)	1048	0.93 (0.72–1.18)	.53	

Data from: Askie LM, Darlow BA, Finer N, et al. *JAMA.* 2018;319(21):2190–2201. Supplement 3, eTable 27.

study intervention at or beyond 6 hours of age, there was no significant difference between the 2 target ranges in the rates of ROP treatment. It is likely that in actual clinical practice, where written informed consent is not required, that oxygen saturation targeting would commence before 6 hours of age. Although the large treatment effect of lower targeting seen in SUPPORT may be more akin to a real-world scenario, this cannot be formally tested within the NeOProM data because too few infants from the other trials commenced the intervention early and thus any differences seen may be due to differences in other features of SUPPORT (eg, ROP was a coprimary outcome so ascertainment of this outcome may have been better in SUPPORT than the other trials) rather than the earlier timing of intervention commencement itself. It is possible, however, that the 26% RR reduction (RR 0.74; 95% CI, 0.63–0.86) in ROP treatment seen with lower targeting in the full NeOProM meta-analysis is an underestimate of the true treatment effect, which could be as large as a 59% RR reduction (RR 0.41; 95% CI, 0.28–0.60) if real-world conditions are more akin to the SUPPORT protocol scenario.

Continued use of supplemental oxygen at 36 weeks' postmenstrual age also was significantly reduced in infants targeting the lower range in the NeOProM meta-analysis (RR 0.81; 95% CI, 0.74–0.90; $P<.001$) (see Fig. 3 in Askie and colleagues[11]). The effect of this finding was larger among SGA infants (interaction $P = .005$) (see eTable 30 in Supplement 3 in Askie and colleagues[11]). The relevance of this finding is unclear because Stenson and Saugstad[23] noted that in the 2 trials that used an oxygen reduction test to assess oxygen need at 36 weeks there was no difference in the rates of BPD between the higher and lower target groups. An oxygen reduction test definition of physiologic BPD was not a prespecified NeOProM outcome, so there are no subgroup analyses available using this more objective definition. The SUPPORT trial, however, required the oxygen reduction test definition of BPD and revealed no difference in physiologic BPD.

DISCUSSION

From the combined meta-analysis of approximately 5000 extremely preterm infants in the NeOProM Collaboration, there is no clear group of infants who benefit more or less from targeting a higher oxygen saturation range compared with a lower oxygen saturation range. Thus, the current AAP guidelines[12] should be revised to remove caveats referring to the ideal range to target preterm infant oxygen saturation as patient specific because the meta-analysis data do not support this statement: infant subgroups do not matter for this clinical question.

In the NeOProM subgroup analyses, there were some statistically significant findings for some outcomes in some subgroups. The number of subgroup analyses undertaken, however, was large (more than 300) and approximately 5% were nominally significant, which is what would have been expected by chance. In addition, no formal statistical adjustment was made for multiple testing. To reduce the risk of spurious findings due to multiple testing, subgroup analyses often are restricted to just the primary outcome (and its components if a composite outcome).[24]

As always, when undertaking the large number of analyses that the availability of IPD permits, results should be interpreted using the pattern and totality of the evidence, not by just selecting isolated statistically significant findings within a particular subgroup analysis. Thus, the test for interaction between subgroups is the most relevant finding rather than whether individual subgroups themselves cross or do not cross the line of unity. Other issues to consider when interpreting subgroup analyses findings include the general lack of power to detect statistically significant differences within a subset of the overall evidence base (as demonstrated in the SUPPORT SGA infants analysis, referred to previously), which increases the risk of spurious findings and problems regarding bias and interpretation if the subgroup analyses are not pre-specified but rather are data-driven post hoc analyses. For these reasons, subgroup analyses usually are considered hypothesis generating rather than hypothesis testing, and their findings should be interpreted with the due caution that this distinction brings.

BEST PRACTICES

The best available evidence regarding what oxygen saturation range should be targeted for extremely preterm infants from birth or soon thereafter comes from the NeO-ProM prospective meta-analysis using harmonized IPD from 5 randomized trials and approximately 5000 infants. The NeOProM data suggest that targeting a higher Spo_2 range (91%–95%), compared with a lower Spo_2 range (85%–89%), has both benefits (reduced mortality and NEC) and harms (increased ROP treatment and BPD but not physiologic BPD). Subgroup analyses have not identified any specific subgroups of infants who seem to benefit more or less from the higher target range, so the higher target range can be recommended for all infants born at less than 28 weeks' gestation.

The finding of reduced mortality with higher targets may be an underestimate of the true treatment effect when using the revised oximeter software in current clinical practice. Conversely, the finding of increased ROP treatment with higher targets also may be an underestimate of the true treatment effect if the targeting intervention is applied in practice more in line with the SUPPORT protocol, that is, is commenced very soon after birth, is given to all comers, and is in a setting where most babies are inborn.

Clinicians need to assess this balance between benefits and harms within their own settings and should ensure that any policy change regarding oxygen saturation targets to a higher range is accompanied by stringent adherence to policies that maximize the prevention and early treatment of ROP and BPD.

Best Practices

What is the current practice?

The range at which to target oxygen saturation for extremely preterm infants varies across centers from 85% to 95%.

Five randomized trials and their meta-analyzed data aimed at assessing whether targeting the lower (85%–89%) or higher (90%–95%) end of this spectrum was best. The meta-analysis also assessed whether some infants benefited more or less from either target range.

What changes in current practice are likely to improve outcomes?

Targeting the higher range (Spo_2 90%–95%) resulted in less death and NEC but more ROP requiring treatment and supplemental oxygen at 36 weeks' postmenstrual age.

All infants born before 28 weeks' gestation should target an Spo_2 range of 90% to 95% from birth or soon thereafter.

Moving to a higher target range should be accompanied by stringent surveillance for the prevention and early treatment of ROP.

Strength of the evidence: strong recommendation for implementation[2,11]

Summary statement

There are no specific subgroups of infants who benefit more or less from the higher oxygen saturation target range, so all extremely preterm infants should be managed using this protocol.

REFERENCES

1. Silverman WA. A cautionary tale about supplemental oxygen: the albatross of neonatal medicine. Pediatrics 2004;113(2):394–6.
2. Askie LM, Darlow BA, Davis PG, et al. Effects of targeting lower versus higher arterial oxygen saturations on death or disability in preterm infants. Cochrane Database Syst Rev 2017;(4):CD011190.
3. Askie LM, Henderson-Smart DJ, Ko H. Restricted versus liberal oxygen exposure for preventing morbidity and mortality in preterm or low birth weight infants. Cochrane Database Syst Rev 2009;(1):CD001077.
4. STOP-ROP Investigators. Supplemental therapeutic oxygen for Prethreshold retinopathy of prematurity (STOP-ROP), a randomized, controlled trial. I: primary outcomes. Pediatrics 2000;105(2):295–310.
5. Askie LM, Henderson-Smart DJ, Irwig L, et al. Oxygen-saturation targets and outcomes in extremely preterm infants. N Engl J Med 2003;349(10):959–67.
6. Tin W, Milligan DW, Pennefather P, et al. Pulse oximetry, severe retinopathy, and outcome at one year in babies of less than 28 weeks gestation. Arch Dis Child Fetal Neonatal Ed 2001;84(2):F106–10.
7. Chow LC, Wright KW, Sola S, CSMC Oxygen Administration Study Group. Can changes in clinical practice decrease the incidence of severe retinopathy in very low birth weight infants? Pediatrics 2003;111(2):339–45.
8. Anderson CG, Benitz WE, Madan A. Retinopathy of prematurity and pulse oximetry: a national survey of recent practices. J Perinatol 2004;24(3):164–8.
9. Cole CH, Wright KW, Tarnow-Mordi W, et al. Pulse oximetry saturation trial for prevention of retinopathy of prematurity planning study group. Resolving our uncertainty about oxygen therapy. Pediatrics 2003;112(6 Pt 1):1415–9.
10. Askie LM, Brocklehurst P, Darlow BA, et al. NeOProM: neonatal oxygenation prospective meta-analysis collaboration study protocol. BMC Pediatr 2011;11:6.
11. Askie LM, Darlow BA, Finer N, et al. Association between oxygen saturation targeting and death or disability in extremely preterm infants in the neonatal oxygenation prospective meta-analysis collaboration. JAMA 2018;319(21):2190–201.
12. AAP Committee on Fetus and Newborn, ACOG Committee on Obstetric Practice. In: Kilpatrick SJ, Papile L, Macones GA, editors. Guidelines for perinatal care. 8th edition; 2017.
13. Walsh MC, Di Fiore JM, Martin RJ, et al. Association of oxygen target and growth status with increased mortality in small for gestational age infants: further analysis of the Surfactant, Positive Pressure and Pulse Oximetry Randomized Trial. JAMA Pediatr 2016;170(3):292–4.
14. Kramer MS, Platt RW, Wen SW, et al. A new and improved population-based Canadian reference for birth weight for gestational age. Pediatrics 2001;108(2):E35.
15. Alexander GR, Himes JH, Kaufman RB, et al. A United States national reference for fetal growth. Obstet Gynecol 1996;87(2):163–8.
16. Johnston ED, Boyle B, Juszczak E, et al. Oxygen targeting in preterm infants using the Masimo SET Radical pulse oximeter. Arch Dis Child Fetal Neonatal Ed 2011;96(6):F429–33.
17. Stenson B, Brocklehurst P, Tarnow-Mordi W. Increased 36-week survival with high oxygen saturation target in extremely preterm infants. N Engl J Med 2011;364(17):1680–2.
18. Stenson BJ. Oxygen targets for preterm infants. Neonatology 2013;103(4):341–5.

19. Schmidt B, Roberts RS, Whyte RK, et al. Impact of study oximeter masking algorithm on titration of oxygen therapy in the Canadian Oxygen Trial. J Pediatr 2014; 165(4):666–71.e2.
20. Cummings JJ. Oxygen-saturation targets in preterm infants. N Engl J Med 2016; 375(2):186–8.
21. Whyte RK, Nelson H, Roberts RS, et al. Benefits of oxygen saturation targeting trials: oximeter calibration software revision and infant saturations. J Pediatr 2017;182:382–4.
22. Stenson BJ, Donoghoe M, Brocklehurst P, et al. Pulse oximeter saturation targeting and oximeter changes in the benefits of oxygen saturation targeting (BOOST)-II Australia and BOOST-II UK oxygen trials. J Pediatr 2019;204: 301–4.e2.
23. Stenson B, Saugstad OD. Oxygen treatment for immature infants beyond the delivery room: lessons from randomized studies. J Pediatr 2018;200:12–8.
24. Sun X, Briel M, Walter SD, et al. Is a subgroup effect believable? Updating criteria to evaluate the credibility of subgroup analyses. BMJ 2010;340:c117.

Oxygen Saturation and Retinopathy of Prematurity

Rosemary D. Higgins, MD

KEYWORDS

- Oxygen • Retinopathy of prematurity • Prematurity

KEY POINTS

- Retinopathy of prematurity (ROP) affects the infants at lower gestational ages and birth weight.
- Oxygen exposure in preterm infants is associated with ROP.
- Recent oxygen saturation targeting trials show increased mortality with lower target ranges; target ranges above 90% saturation are current suggested for premature infants.
- Prevention, early intervention and treatment regimens are needed to improve ROP outcomes.

BRIEF HISTORY OF RETINOPATHY OF PREMATURITY

Retinopathy of prematurity (ROP) is a serious vasoproliferative disorder affecting premature infants. It was first described as "retrolental fibroplasia" because of the white appearance of the pupil in infants who survived but were blind.[1] The white appearance was due to retinal detachment. Early treatment for premature infants involved administration of oxygen into incubators. Oxygen use was curtailed following the Kinsey Study,[2] which assigned infants administered oxygen of more than 50% or less than 40% to 50%. The results showed that the infants in the restrictive group had less retinopathy and oxygen use was subsequently restricted resulting in less retinopathy. For infants less than 1000 g birthweight, the estimate of absolute numbers of infants affected with ROP was anticipated to increase secondarily to increased survival.[3]

RETINOPATHY OF PREMATURITY EPIDEMIOLOGY AND PATHOLOGY

ROP occurs more commonly with lower gestational age (GA), and is associated with duration of oxygen exposure. Black infants are less likely to develop severe ROP.[4] Small for GA infants are at higher risk of development of ROP.[5]

Disclosure Statement: The author has no relationship with a commercial company that has a direct financial interest in subject matter or materials discussed in article or with a company making a competing product.

College of Health and Human Services, George Mason University, 4400 University Drive, 2G7, Peterson Family Health Science Hall, Room 5415, Fairfax, VA 22030, USA

E-mail address: rhiggin@gmu.edu

Premature birth results in a relative hyperoxia compared with in utero. Further, the retinal vessels are not fully mature and the relative hyperoxia initially inhibits vessel growth. In the meantime, the retina grows in thickness. Over time, a gradual retinal hypoxia develops, and growth factors, including vascular endothelial growth factor, are released, resulting in excessive blood vessel growth. The result is ROP.

RETINOPATHY OF PREMATURITY CLASSIFICATION AND TREATMENT STUDIES

With the advent of modern neonatal care, including neonatal intensive care units (NICUs) and mechanical ventilation, and additional technologies, smaller preterm infants were surviving and ROP increased in the 1970s.[3] During the 1980s, the International Classification of ROP was developed; this was the first attempt at standardizing the grading system for ROP[6] and this has been recently updated.[7] This classification was used in the Cryotherapy for Retinopathy of Prematurity (CRYO-ROP) trial conducted in the mid-1980s.[8] The results of the CRYO-ROP trial now availed treatment for advanced ROP when previously none existed.

Laser therapy was then developed for ROP. Several smaller trials were conducted, and the ET-ROP (Early Treatment for Retinopathy of Prematurity) trial[9] showed reduced unfavorable visual acuity with earlier treatment from 19.5% to 14.5% ($P = .01$). Type 1 ROP was defined as follows: zone I, any stage ROP with plus disease; zone I, stage 3 ROP with or without plus disease; zone II, stage 2 or 3 ROP with plus disease.[9] Plus disease was defined as 2 or more quadrants (6 clock hours) of dilation or tortuosity of the peripheral retinal vessels.[9] Thus, the laser treatment occurred earlier than treatment occurred in the CRYO-ROP study. Further comparison between the ET-ROP and CRYO-ROP studies showed more zone I disease in the ET-ROP study.[10] There were more infants in the ET-ROP study with lower birth weights and lower GA, likely accounting for the increase in zone I disease.

ADVENT OF OXYGEN SATURATION TARGETING TRIALS: SMALLER REPORTS THAT SPURRED LARGE TRIALS

A retrospective review of outcomes for infants admitted to NICUs in England showed that infants managed with lower oxygen saturation ranges (70%–90%) compared with higher ranges (88%–98%) in the first 8 weeks of life had lower rates of cryotherapy.[11] The infants in the lower saturation range did not have an increased risk of mortality or neurodevelopmental impairment.[11] Use of transcutaneous oxygen monitoring showed a decrease in ROP in a subgroup of infants $\geq$1100 g.[12] Chow and colleagues[13] showed that implementation of an oxygen policy to avoid higher oxygen saturations (93%–95%) and to prevent large swings in oxygen saturations for 2 to 8 weeks of age in infants 500 to 1500 g birth weight, resulted in a significant decrease in the rate of severe ROP and an improvement in survival over time.

The relationship of oxygen and ROP continued to be explored in the 1990s. The Supplemental Therapy with Oxygen to Prevent Retinopathy of Prematurity (STOP-ROP) trial[14] and the Benefits of Oxygen Saturation Targeting Study (BOOST)[15] were conducted to test the role of supplemental oxygen for ROP. The STOP-ROP trial[14] enrolled premature infants with prethreshold ROP in at least 1 eye to target oxygen saturations of 96% to 99% versus 89% to 94% saturation to test the hypothesis that a higher level would reduce the rate of progression of ROP to threshold disease. The trial enrolled 649 infants with an average GA at birth of 25.4 weeks and an average postmenstrual age of 35.4 ± 2.5 weeks. The progression of ROP from prethreshold to threshold disease was not reduced in the higher saturation group. Infants who did not have plus disease, defined as posterior pole dilation and/or tortuosity, at the time of enrollment had less progression to threshold with supplemental oxygen. However, the supplemental oxygen group (96%–99%) had higher rates of pulmonary adverse events.[14]

The BOOST Study[15] was designed to look at 2 saturation targets; 91% to 95% or 95% to 98% begun at 32 weeks postmenstrual age with outcomes of improving growth and development at 1 year of age. There were 358 infants enrolled with no differences observed in growth or major developmental outcomes. The investigators concluded that optimal oxygen saturation range for preterm infants soon after birth should be determined with a large trial.[15]

SATURATION TRIALS OF THE 2000S

Based on the conclusions from the BOOST trial, several large oxygen saturation–targeting trials were developed and executed. The investigators from these trials agreed to pool data and perform a prospective individual patient meta-analysis.[16] The meta-analysis[17] showed that death occurred in 484 (19.9%) of 2433 infants in the lower SpO2 target group and 418 (17.1%) of 2440 infants in the higher SpO2 target group (risk difference 2.8%; 95% confidence interval [CI] 0.6%–5.0%; relative risk (RR) 1.17; 95% CI 1.04–1.31; $P = .01$). Treatment for ROP was administered to 220 (10.9%) of 2020 infants in the lower SpO2 target group and 308 (14.9%) of 2065 infants in the higher SpO2 target group (risk difference −4.0%; 95% CI −6.1% to −2.0%; RR 0.74; 95% CI 0.63–0.86; $P<.001$).[17] These trials would not have been conducted if a mortality difference had been anticipated in advance of the studies. Nevertheless, they have provided valuable clinical evidence to guide practice with respect to oxygen therapy. The individual trial results are described as follows.

The Surfactant, Positive Pressure, and Pulse Oximetry Randomized Trial (SUPPORT)[18] was conducted from 2005 to 2009 in the National Institute of Child Health and Human Development (NICHD) Neonatal Research Network. Primary outcome showed no difference in the primary outcome of death or ROP between a higher oxygen target saturation (91%–95%) and a lower oxygen target saturation (85%–89%). However, secondary outcome of ROP was lower in the lower saturation group compared with the higher saturation group. The death rate was higher in the lower saturation group, which was an unexpected finding. At follow-up at 18 to 22 months,[19] death or neurodevelopmental impairment was in 30.2% of the infants in the lower oxygen saturation group (185 of 612), versus 27.5% of those in the higher oxygen saturation group (171 of 622) (relative risk 1.12; 95% CI 0.94–1.32; $P = .21$).

The Canadian Oxygen Trial (COT)[20] was conducted from 2006 to 2012. There was no difference in the rate of retinopathy or death in the higher versus lower target saturation groups. Infants who were assigned to the lower target range, 298 (51.6%) died or survived with disability compared with 283 (49.7%) of the 569 infants assigned to the higher target range (odds ratio adjusted for center 1.08; 95% CI 0.85–1.37; $P = .52$).[20] The rates of death were 16.6% for those in the 85% to 89% group and 15.3% for those in the 91% to 95% group (adjusted odds ratio 1.11; 95% CI 0.80–1.54; $P = .54$).[20] Differences between baseline characteristics of patients in COT and SUPPORT may account for the different study results.

The Benefits of Oxygen Saturation Targeting (BOOST II) in New Zealand[21] was conducted from 2006 to 2012, in the United Kingdom from 2007 to 2014, and in Australia from 2006 to 2013.[22] Targeting an oxygen saturation below 90% in extremely preterm infants was associated with an increased risk of death in infants whose treatment used the revised oximeter-calibration algorithm. The rate of death was significantly higher in the lower-target group than in the higher-target group (23.1% vs 15.9%; relative risk in the lower-target group 1.45; 95% CI 1.15–1.84; P = .002). Those in the lower-target group for oxygen saturation had a reduced rate of ROP (10.6% vs 13.5%; relative risk 0.79; 95% CI 0.63–1.00; P = .045). For the Australia and UK studies,[23] an interim analysis showed increased mortality at a corrected GA of 36 weeks. Enrollment was stopped after 1135 infants in Australia and 973 infants in the United Kingdom had been enrolled in the trial. The mortality rate in the lower oxygen saturation arm was 21.2% compared with 17.7% in the higher oxygen saturation arm (RR 1.20; 95% CI 1.01–1.43). No difference was shown in severe vision loss between the higher and lower saturation arms of the trial (0.4% vs 0.7%).

CURRENT OXYGEN TARGET SATURATION PARAMETERS

The guidelines of the American Academy of Pediatrics (AAP)[24] as of 2007 stated, "The optimal range for oxygen saturation and Pao_2 that balances tissue metabolism, growth and development, and toxicity has not been elucidated fully for preterm infants receiving supplemental oxygen. Oxygen saturation values between 85% and 95% and Pao_2 values between 50 mm Hg and 80 mm Hg are examples of ranges pragmatically determined by some clinicians to guide oxygen therapy in preterm infants. Additional research is needed to determine the 'optimal' oxygen saturation and Pao_2 needed. Of note, even with careful monitoring, oxygen saturation and Pao_2 may fluctuate outside specified ranges, particularly in neonates with cardiopulmonary disease." This recommendation was published in 2007,[24] while the vast majority of oxygen saturation targeting studies were occurring around the world.

In 2012, shortly after the publication of the SUPPORT trial, the AAP recommendations[25] were updated to state, "Data from cohort studies initially suggested that lower saturation ranges may decrease ROP. However, 3 RCTs demonstrated that although a target saturation range of 85% to 89% was associated with a decrease in severe ROP, it was also associated with an increase in mortality, compared with a target saturation range of 91% to 95%. These findings resulted in early study closure of 2 of these 3 studies, and a recommendation to target a saturation range higher than 85% to 89%. Of note, even with careful monitoring, oxygen saturation and Pao_2 may fluctuate outside specified ranges, particularly in neonates with cardiopulmonary disease."[25]

A recent survey to assess variations in oxygen saturation targets in 2015 and 2016 was conducted across the networks of the International Network for Evaluating Outcomes in Neonates (iNeo).[26] The upper SpO2 target limit was 94% or 95% (range 90%–98%) in 68% of the NICUs. The lower SpO2 limit was 90%; however, there was considerable variation in saturation targets was found in this survey.

GAPS IN KNOWLEDGE

Despite the rigorous oxygen saturation trials, there are still many areas in need of study for oxygen saturation for preterm infants to optimize outcomes. An NICHD workshop in 2006[27] identified several areas for study. The oxygen saturation trials did provide evidence for a saturation target that may cause harm. In the NEO-PROM meta-analysis, infants assigned to 85% to 89% target saturation had a higher mortality.[17] Other questions that persist include the following: What is the therapeutic range of inspired oxygen? What is the toxic range of inspired oxygen? What explains the variability in toxicity? How do specific disease processes affect toxicity?[27] Titrating a sweet spot that allows for maximal survival and minimal ROP based on age of the infant, GA at birth, and other factors still eludes physicians.

Minimization of saturation variability persists as a gap in knowledge. Preterm infants can have labile cardiorespiratory status. Development of automatic feedback systems are needed to maintain saturation at stable targets. Technology such as feedback devices to keep oxygenation constant, closed-loop oxygen controllers, or oxygen delivery systems with pulse oximetry regulation have the potential to advance care for preterm and sick infants. Defining the optimal saturation target for various populations of infants is needed. Further, investigation of target saturation at various developmental periods and GA are needed to better inform clinical practice.

FUTURE OF OXYGEN AND RETINOPATHY OF PREMATURITY

Although lower GA and birthweight are strong predictors of the development of ROP, oxygen remains in the causal pathway. Additional prevention, early intervention, and treatment strategies are needed to relieve the burden of ROP.

Best Practices

What is the current practice for oxygen management and ROP?

Best Practice/Guideline/Care Path Objective(s)
- Avoid preterm birth
- AAP recommendation to target a saturation range higher than 85% to 89%
- Emerging evidence-based consensus to target the 91% to 95% saturation range
- Vigilance with oxygen saturation monitoring
- Screening for ROP in conjunction with ophthalmology
- Follow-up eye examinations at established intervals
- Intervention with laser treatment if Type I ROP develops

What changes in current practice are likely to improve outcomes?

- Prevention of preterm birth
- Further research to include the following:
  - Balance between adequate inspired oxygen versus toxicity at various developmental periods
  - Automated feedback systems to maintain saturation targets
  - Saturation target variability
  - Prevention and early intervention therapies

Major Recommendations
- AAP recommendation to target a saturation range higher than 85% to 89% but evidence-based emerging consensus to target the 91% to 95% saturation range
- ROP screening performed as per guidelines
- Treatment if Type 1 ROP occurs
- Appropriate follow-up

Rating for the Strength of the Evidence

Saturation targeting

Saturation targeting in the range of 91% to 95% is supported by an individual participant meta-analysis, which is the highest level of evidence.

Bibliographic Source(s)[17,25]

REFERENCES

1. Terry TL. Retrolentral fibroplasia. J Pediatr 1946;29(6):770–3.
2. Kinsey VE. Retrolental fibroplasia; cooperative study of retrolental fibroplasia and the use of oxygen. AMA Arch Ophthalmol 1956;56(4):481–543.
3. Phelps DL. Retinopathy of prematurity: an estimate of vision loss in the United States–1979. Pediatrics 1981;67(6):924–5.
4. Saunders RA, Donahue ML, Christmann LM, et al. Racial variation in retinopathy of prematurity. The cryotherapy for retinopathy of prematurity cooperative group. Arch Ophthalmol 1997;115(5):604–8.
5. Ahn YJ, Hong KE, Yum HR, et al. Characteristic clinical features associated with aggressive posterior retinopathy of prematurity. Eye (Lond) 2017;31(6):924–30.
6. The Committee for the Classification of Retinopathy of Prematurity. An international classification of retinopathy of prematurity. Arch Ophthalmol 1984;102:1130–4.
7. International Committee for the Classification of Retinopathy of Prematurity. The international classification of retinopathy of prematurity revisited. Arch Ophthalmol 2005;123(7):991–9.
8. Multicenter trial of cryotherapy for retinopathy of prematurity. Preliminary results. Cryotherapy for Retinopathy of Prematurity Cooperative Group. Arch Ophthalmol 1988;106(4):471–9.
9. Early Treatment for Retinopathy of Prematurity Cooperative Group. Revised indications for the treatment of retinopathy of prematurity: results of the early treatment for retinopathy of prematurity randomized trial. Arch Ophthalmol 2003;121(12):1684–94.
10. Good WV, Hardy RJ, Dobson V, et al, Early Treatment for Retinopathy of Prematurity Cooperative Group. The incidence and course of retinopathy of prematurity: findings from the early treatment for retinopathy of prematurity study. Pediatrics 2005;116(1):15–23.
11. Tin W, Milligan DW, Pennefather P, et al. Pulse oximetry, severe retinopathy, and outcome at one year in babies of less than 28 weeks gestation. Arch Dis Child Fetal Neonatal Ed 2001;84(2):F106–10.
12. Bancalari E, Flynn J, Goldberg RN, et al. Influence of transcutaneous oxygen monitoring on the incidence of retinopathy of prematurity. Pediatrics 1987;79:663–9.
13. Chow LC, Wright KW, Sola A. Can changes in clinical practice decrease the incidence of severe retinopathy of prematurity in very low birth weight infants? Pediatrics 2003;111(2):339–45.
14. Phelps DL, Lindblad A, Bradford JD, et al. Supplemental therapeutic oxygen for prethreshold retinopathy of prematurity (STOP-ROP), a randomized, controlled trial. I: primary outcomes. Pediatrics 2000;105(2):295–310.
15. Askie LM, Henderson-Smart DJ, Irwig L, et al. Oxygen-saturation targets and outcomes in extremely preterm infants. N Engl J Med 2003;349(10):953–61.
16. Askie LM, Brocklehurst P, Darlow BA, et al, NeOProM Collaborative Group. NeOProM: neonatal oxygenation prospective meta-analysis collaboration study protocol. BMC Pediatr 2011;11:6.
17. Askie LM, Darlow BA, Finer N, et al, Neonatal Oxygenation Prospective Meta-Analysis (NeOProM) Collaboration. Association between oxygen saturation targeting and death or disability in extremely preterm infants in the neonatal oxygenation prospective meta-analysis collaboration. JAMA 2018;319(21):2190–201.

18. Carlo WA, Finer NN, Walsh MC, et al. SUPPORT study group of the Eunice Kennedy Shriver NICHD neonatal research network. Target ranges of oxygen saturation in extremely preterm infants. N Engl J Med 2010;362(21):1959-69.
19. Vaucher YE, Peralta-Carcelen M, Finer NN, et al. SUPPORT study group of the Eunice Kennedy Shriver NICHD neonatal research network. Neurodevelopmental outcomes in the early CPAP and pulse oximetry trial. N Engl J Med 2012; 367(26):2495-504.
20. Schmidt B, Whyte RK, Asztalos EV, et al, Canadian Oxygen Trial (COT) Group. Effects of targeting higher vs lower arterial oxygen saturations on death or disability in extremely preterm infants: a randomized clinical trial. JAMA 2013; 309(20):2111-20.
21. Darlow BA, Marschner SL, Donoghoe M, et al, Benefits of Oxygen Saturation Targeting-New Zealand (BOOST-NZ) Collaborative Group. Randomized controlled trial of oxygen saturation targets in very preterm infants: two year outcomes. J Pediatr 2014;165(1):30-5.
22. Stenson BJ, Tarnow-Mordi WO, Darlow BA, et al, BOOST II United Kingdom Collaborative Group, BOOST II Australia Collaborative Group, BOOST II New Zealand Collaborative group. Oxygen saturation and outcomes in preterm infants. N Engl J Med 2013;368(22):2094-104.
23. Tarnow-Mordi W, Stenson B, Kirby A, et al, BOOST-II Australia and United Kingdom Collaborative Groups. Outcomes of two trials of oxygen-saturation targets in preterm infants. N Engl J Med 2016;374(8):749-60.
24. American Academy of Pediatrics and the American College of Obstetricians and Gynecologists. Guidelines for perinatal care. In: Lockwood CJ, Lemons JA, editors. Clinical considerations in the use of oxygen. 6th edition. Elk Grove, (IL): AAP; 2007. p. 259–63. ACOG; Washington, DC.
25. American Academy of Pediatrics and the American College of obstetricians and Gynecologists. Guidelines for perinatal care. In: Riley LE, Stark AR, editors. Respiratory complications: oxygen. 7th edition. Elk Grove, (IL): AAP; 2012. p. 343–5. ACOG; Washington, DC.
26. Darlow BA, Vento M, Beltempo M, et al. Variations in oxygen saturation targeting, and retinopathy of prematurity screening and treatment criteria in neonatal intensive care units: an international survey. Neonatology 2018;114:323–31.
27. Higgins RD, Bancalari E, Willinger M, et al. Executive summary of the workshop on oxygen in neonatal therapies: controversies and opportunities for research. Pediatrics 2007;119(4):790–6.

Achieved Oxygenation Saturations and Outcome in Extremely Preterm Infants

Benjamin J. Stenson, MD

KEYWORDS

- Oxygen • Oxygenation • Oximetry • Infant mortality • Necrotizing enterocolitis
- Retinopathy of prematurity • Infant • Extremely premature

KEY POINTS

- In the Neonatal Oxygenation Prospective Meta-analysis (NeOProM) trials, differences in outcomes between groups are likely to be related to differences in achieved peripheral capillary oxygen saturation (SpO_2).
- Mortality and necrotizing enterocolitis were increased in infants randomized to the low SpO_2 target range groups (85%–89%), but low-target group infants who experienced these outcomes had SpO_2 distributions centered around 90% to 92%.
- Achieved SpO_2 patterns were not different between infants randomized to higher SpO_2 targets (91%–95%) who did or did not require treatment of retinopathy of prematurity (ROP).
- Trials of slightly higher SpO_2 targets than 91% to 95% may help determine whether there is further survival advantage obtainable. These will be associated with increased risk of the need for ROP treatment.

INTRODUCTION

The Neonatal Oxygenation Prospective Meta-analysis (NeOProM) trials have shown that small differences in target ranges for peripheral capillary oxygen saturation (SpO_2) in extremely preterm infants influence the risk of mortality and morbidity.[1] In older patient age groups too, the clinical community is waking up to the reality that oxygen must be administered carefully based on evidence rather than according to habit.[2]

The intervention in the NeOProM trials was to target SpO_2 to the ranges 85% to 89% or 91% to 95%. This was delivered by nursing staff manually adjusting fraction of inspired oxygen (Fio_2) with the aim of maintaining SpO_2 within a desired range. The NeOProM trials were masked by the use of specially adjusted oximeters so that infants enrolled in both randomization groups were targeted to the same displayed SpO_2 range

Disclosure Statement: The author has nothing to disclose.
Neonatal Unit, Royal Infirmary of Edinburgh, 46 Little France Crescent, Edinburgh EH16 4SA, UK
E-mail address: Ben.stenson@luht.scot.nhs.uk

and caregivers were unaware of their group allocation. This design was pioneered in the first Benefits of Oxygen Saturation Targeting (BOOST) trial.[3] This method should have minimized the risk that caregiver biases could influence the treatment of the infants in other ways that were unbalanced between randomization groups and makes it reasonable to conclude that differences in outcomes between groups were determined by the trial intervention and its effect on achieved SpO_2. This is further supported by the little heterogeneity between the NeOProM trials for the key outcomes despite the trials being conducted independently in different settings and parts of the world.

Although there was not a statistically significant difference between groups in the NeOProM trials in the primary composite outcome of death or severe neurodevelopmental disability, infants targeted to the lower SpO_2 range had a significantly increased risk of death and of severe necrotizing enterocolitis (NEC), defined as requiring surgery or causing death. There was no difference between groups in the risk of severe neurodevelopmental disability. Infants randomized to the higher target groups had an increased risk of requiring treatment of retinopathy of prematurity (ROP), but there was not a significant difference between groups in the number of infants with severe visual impairment. In fact, this was numerically higher in the infants randomized to the lower SpO_2 target.

It is vital to understand the achieved SpO_2 patterns that were obtained in association with these outcomes in the trials because, unlike in retrospective observational studies of achieved or targeted SpO_2 in which multiple confounders may explain differences in outcomes, in these trials there can be much greater confidence that outcomes were related at least in part to differences in achieved SpO_2.

SpO_2 varies widely in unwell preterm infants and there is great difficulty in keeping it within a target range.[4] Whatever target range is used, infants spend varying proportions of time inside or outside that intended range. Success in targeting SpO_2 is influenced by the target range selected.[5–7] There are probably multiple contributors to this observation. It is suggested that caregivers may prefer higher SpO_2.[4] It is also the case that SpO_2 readings below 90% are on the steep part of the hemoglobin-oxygen dissociation curve, where small changes in alveolar oxygen tension will result in much larger fluctuations in SpO_2 than they would at higher SpO_2 readings.[8] In the BOOST-II UK and BOOST-II Australia trials, with a masked intervention and both groups targeted to the same displayed SpO_2, infants allocated to the lower target range spent less time in their intended range than infants allocated to the higher target range.[5] The advantages of automated oxygen adjustment in terms of time spent within intended target range seem smaller in comparison with manual adjustment when higher SpO_2 targets are used.[7] These observations are important because the lower target range group infants in the NeOProM trials had higher than intended achieved SpO_2. The differences in outcomes between groups that were observed may underestimate the differences that would have been observed if the lower target groups had been targeted more effectively and spent more time in their intended target range.

It would be a mistake to consider that all the infants in each randomization group achieved SpO_2 distributions similar to those of the group as a whole. As well as considering the overall achieved SpO_2 patterns of the randomization groups, there is value in considering the patterns of achieved SpO_2 in the infants within the randomization groups who developed the adverse outcomes of interest.

The individual trials in the NeOProM collaboration have reported their achieved SpO_2 in different ways and in varying detail. Post hoc analyses of the associations between achieved SpO_2 patterns from the trials and clinical outcomes should be considered hypothesis-generating rather than high-level evidence. If observations are replicable between trials that may increase their information value.

MEDIAN PERIPHERAL CAPILLARY OXYGEN SATURATION

So far, the only information published from the trials relating achieved SpO_2 to outcome has come from the Surfactant, Positive Pressure, and Pulse Oximetry Randomized Trial (SUPPORT)[9,10] and relates the risk of mortality to achieved median SpO_2 and intermittent hypoxia. The subject of intermittent hypoxia is excluded from this discussion. (See Juliann M. Di Fiore and colleagues' article, "Intermittent Hypoxemia in Preterm Infants," in this issue.) In the SUPPORT,[9] SpO_2 data were continuously sampled every 10 seconds (Masimo, Radical, Yorba, CA, USA). Each infant's median SpO_2 was determined and histograms were presented in the trial report for the distribution of these medians. Values were not provided for the median of these values in each group in the trial report but it was stated that the actual median levels of oxygen saturation were slightly higher than targeted levels in both groups. This implies that the median SpO_2 in the low-target group over the whole duration of the intervention was greater than 89% and the median SpO_2 in the high-target group was greater than 95%. In other words, the low-target group in this trial had a higher risk of mortality despite achieving a median SpO_2 of at least 90%.

In a post hoc analysis of SpO_2 data from the first 3 days of life from the SUPPORT,[10] the median SpO_2 of infants in the low SpO_2 target group (target range 85%–89%) with birthweight appropriate for gestational age was 93%. Low-target group infants who were small for gestational age in the SUPPORT had a median SpO_2 in the first 3 days of 90%.

Median oxygen saturation for all infants was divided into quartiles. The lowest quartile for oxygen saturation was less than or equal to 92%. Appropriately grown infants with a median oxygen saturation during the first 3 days after birth greater than 92% had the highest 90-day survival rate at 90.8%. In comparison with these infants, there was a lower 90-day survival in both infants who were appropriately grown (83.2%, $P = .0013$) and those who were small for gestational age (54.3%, $P<.0001$), with median SpO_2 in the first 3 days less than or equal to 92% (**Fig. 1**).

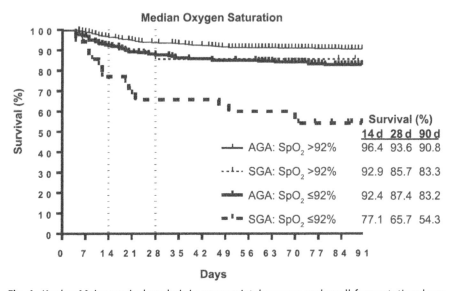

Fig. 1. Kaplan Meier survival analysis in appropriately grown and small for gestational age infants in the SUPPORT according to median achieved SpO_2 during the first 3 days of life. AGA, appropriate for gestational age; SGA, small for gestational age. (*From* Di Fiore JM, Martin RJ, Li H, et al. Patterns of oxygenation, mortality and growth status in the surfactant, positive pressure and oxygen trial cohort. J Pediatr 2017;186:49–56.e1; with permission.)

OVERALL PERIPHERAL CAPILLARY OXYGEN SATURATION DISTRIBUTION

In the 3 BOOST-II trials,[5] SpO_2 readings were also recorded every 10 seconds throughout the duration of monitoring. For each trial, SpO_2 readings were pooled from all infants and the percentage of time that the infants in each randomization group spent at each SpO_2 was calculated. This was plotted by randomization group in the form of frequency histograms indicating the percentage of time spent at each SpO_2 (**Fig. 2**) and was also tabulated in the supplementary data. Separate results were given for each trial. During the trials, there was a change in the study oximeters to correct an artifact that had been identified in their calibration,[11] and separate plots and tables were provided for the different oximeter types. Differences between randomization groups in achieved SpO_2 and in clinical outcomes were clearer after the revision of the trial oximeters.[5,12,13]

As in the SUPPORT, infants in the low-target groups in the BOOST-II trials had higher than intended SpO_2. Infants in the high-target groups had SpO_2 distributions that were centered in their intended SpO_2 target range. Increased mortality was observed in infants targeted to lower SpO_2 (85%–89%) in the BOOST-II UK and BOOST-II Australia trials[12] even though the median SpO_2 of infants in the low-target groups in these trials (89%–90%) was at the upper limit of the intended low-target range of 85% to 89%.

To explore the achieved SpO_2 distributions in relation to clinical outcome in the BOOST-II UK trial, there has been a further post hoc analysis to produce plots of achieved SpO_2 distributions, separating the infants by randomization groups and also according to whether they died or developed severe NEC or ROP requiring treatment (**Figs. 3–5**). Most infants in the UK trial were treated with oximeters that had revised software and the plots are restricted to data from these infants.

For the outcomes mortality and NEC that were increased in the infants randomized to lower SpO_2 targets in the NeOProM trials, all time on the oximeter was analyzed. This is because lower SpO_2 readings were the focus and these were allowed by protocol in lower target group infants whether or not they were breathing supplemental oxygen. Low SpO_2 readings would be modifiable whether the infant was breathing air or supplemental oxygen. For ROP, the analysis was for time that the infants were breathing supplemental oxygen because high SpO_2 readings were the focus. High SpO_2 readings in infants breathing air were not considered to be modifiable and to be unlikely to be associated with underlying hyperoxia, whereas high readings in infants on supplemental oxygen may indicate hyperoxia and were amenable to modification.

Fig. 3 shows data for mortality. In both randomization groups, the distribution of achieved SpO_2 was lower in infants who died than in infants who survived. In both randomization groups, these differences were apparent at higher but not at lower SpO_2 in which the curves overlaid each another. Consistent with the significantly increased risk of mortality observed in infants randomized to lower SpO_2 in the NeOProM trials overall, the difference in SpO_2 distribution between infants who lived and died in the BOOST-II UK trial was greater in low-target group infants than in high-target group infants. Low-target group infants who survived had a distribution of SpO_2 similar to that of high-target group infants. In comparison, the SpO_2 distribution of low-target group infants who died was shifted markedly to the left but was still higher than their intended target range, with a peak at 90%. The difference in achieved SpO_2 between low-target group of infants who lived and died was greatest at SpO_2

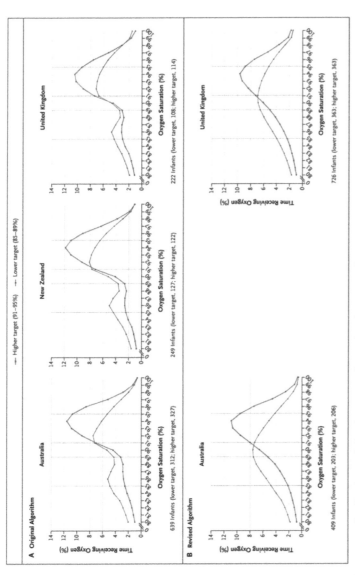

Fig. 2. Average frequency distributions of the time spent by each infant at each oxygen saturation level from 80% to 100% while receiving supplemental oxygen. For trials in the United Kingdom and Australia, separate distributions are provided for infants managed using the original oximeter-calibration algorithm (A) and those managed using the revised algorithm (B), according to whether they were assigned to receive a higher target of oxygen saturation (91%–95%) or a lower target (85%–89%). Revised oximeters were not used in the New Zealand trial. Vertical dotted lines indicate the intended target SpO$_2$ ranges of the randomization groups. (*From* The BOOST II United Kingdom, Australia, and New Zealand Collaborative Groups, Oxygen Saturation and Outcomes in Preterm Infants. Volume 368 N Engl J Med. 2013 May 30;368(22):2094–104. https://doi.org/10.1056/NEJMoa1302298. Epub 2013 May 5. Copyright © (2013) Massachusetts Medical Society. Reprinted with permission.)

Proportion of time at each saturation for all time on the oximeter

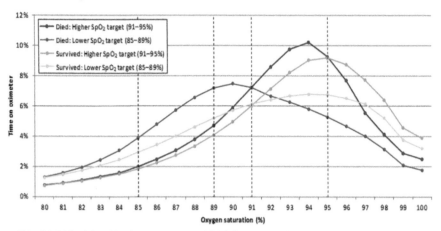

Died 160 babies (95 lower target, 65 higher target)
Survived 577 babies (276 lower target, 301 higher target)

Fig. 3. Achieved SpO$_2$ distributions from the BOOST-II UK trial, with randomization groups plotted separately according to whether the infants survived or died. Data are for all time on the oximeter. Vertical dotted lines indicate the intended target SpO$_2$ ranges of the randomization groups.

Proportion of time at each saturation for all time on the oximeter

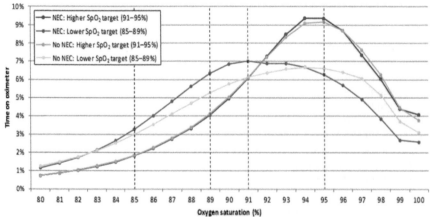

NEC 95 babies (54 lower target, 41 higher target)
No NEC 639 babies (317 lower target, 322 higher target)

Fig. 4. Achieved SpO$_2$ distributions from the BOOST-II UK trial, with randomization groups plotted separately according to whether or not the infant developed severe NEC. Data are for all time on the oximeter. Vertical dotted lines indicate the intended target SpO$_2$ ranges of the randomization groups.

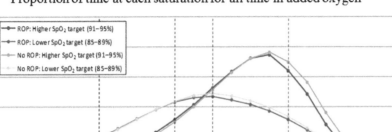

Proportion of time at each saturation for all time in added oxygen

ROP 108 babies (49 lower target, 59 higher target)
No ROP 493 babies (244 lower target, 249 higher target)

Fig. 5. Achieved SpO_2 distributions from the BOOST-II UK trial, with randomization groups plotted separately according to whether or not the infant developed ROP requiring treatment. Data are for times when the infants were breathing supplemental oxygen. Vertical dotted lines indicate the intended target SpO_2 ranges of the randomization groups.

readings within and above the intended low-target SpO_2 range and not at lower SpO_2 readings.

Fig. 4 shows data for severe NEC. Severe NEC was increased in low-target group infants in the NeOProM trials. Infants in the high-target group of the BOOST-II UK trial who got severe NEC had an SpO_2 distribution that was not different from unaffected infants in the same group. In contrast, infants in the low-target group who developed severe NEC differed quite clearly from unaffected infants in their SpO_2 distribution. As was observed with mortality, low-target group infants who did not develop severe NEC had SpO_2 distribution similar to that of high-target group infants. Low-target group infants who developed severe NEC had a SpO_2 distribution that was shifted to the left. The peak of this distribution, at 92% to 93%, was 3 to 4 points higher than the intended target range for the low-target group. There was not a difference in exposure to very low SpO_2 between infants who did or did not develop severe NEC in the low-target group.

Fig. 5 shows data for ROP requiring treatment. In both randomization groups, the achieved SpO_2 distribution of infants who developed ROP requiring treatment was indistinguishable from that of infants in the same randomization group who did not.

DISCUSSION

These analyses were not prespecified at the time that the trials were planned and consequently must be considered hypothesis-generating rather than fully explanatory. However, they are surprising and thought-provoking, and there would be value in seeing whether they are replicated in the other trials.

The data show that the risks of mortality and severe NEC, which were increased in infants randomized to the low SpO_2 target range, were not associated with greater exposure than other infants to very low SpO_2 readings. The difference in achieved SpO_2 observed with these adverse outcomes was mainly increased time spent in the intended low-target SpO_2 range and even slightly above it. The data suggest that there may be value in studying the risks and benefits of a slightly higher SpO_2 target range than 91% to 95% to see if further reductions in risk of mortality and NEC are achievable.

In the NeOProM trials there was more ROP requiring treatment in infants targeted to 91% to 95%. In the BOOST-II UK trial, the achieved SpO_2 patterns of the infants in this high-target group who got ROP were not different from those who did not, suggesting that their ROP was not simply a reflection of less effective targeting in some infants than others. The implication may be that it will be hard to avoid further increases in ROP requiring treatment if higher ranges are studied, even with meticulous targeting.

The intended target ranges in the NeOProM trials of 85% to 89% and 91% to 95% were the same in all 5 NeOProM trials. Consequently, although the trial data suggest that, of these 2 ranges, the higher range should be preferred, the optimal target range remains unknown because other ranges have not been studied. Some may consider that an intermediate range between the 2 is worthy of study. It has been speculated that the optimal SpO_2 target range may be dynamic, changing with advancing post-natal age.[14] The use of servocontrol systems might enable more successful targeting, lowering the associated ROP risk of higher SpO_2 targets. If these achieved SpO_2 data are considered alongside these hypotheses, they suggest that these speculations are approaches that should not be used outside randomized controlled trials. The adverse outcomes, death, NEC, and ROP, move in opposite directions with different SpO_2 target ranges and their causation overlaps in timing, so it is likely to be challenging to minimize all of them simultaneously. Careful measurement of these competing risks is required.

If an intermediate range of 88% to 92% was targeted, then the infants targeted most successfully would have a distribution of achieved SpO_2 centered around 90%, similar to that described in the low-target group infants in BOOST-II UK trial who died. They would have median SpO_2 values less than 92%, which was associated with a greater risk of mortality in the SUPPORT.[10] If, like the infants in the NeOProM trials, infants targeted to this intermediate range had a distribution of SpO_2 that was a few points higher than intended, then it may still be similar to that described in infants who developed severe NEC in the BOOST-II UK trial.

Most cases of NEC and some cases of mortality occur in the early weeks after birth. The increase in these outcomes observed in the low-target group infants in the NeOProM trials should caution against uncontrolled use of lower SpO_2 targets in the early weeks after birth. The achieved SpO_2 distributions from the SUPPORT and BOOST-II UK trial add further to this caution. The BOOST-II UK trial achieved SpO_2 histograms that do not support a hypothesis that the risk of death was associated with time spent with deep hypoxia that might be avoided by more careful targeting of the lower SpO_2 range than was achieved in the trial. Both the SUPPORT and the BOOST-II UK trial achieved SpO_2 data that suggest that mortality was increased in low-target group infants despite their having achieved SpO_2 higher than the intended low-target range. Targeting this lower range has already been tested and shown to worsen outcome.

A variety of automated oxygen adjustment systems has been evaluated and the technology is becoming available for clinical use both for ventilated infants and infants receiving noninvasive support.[15–18] These devices are effective and it is clear that achieved SpO_2 distributions in infants on automated adjustment systems differ from those of infants treated using manual adjustment. Therefore, it is likely that introduction of automated oxygen adjustment systems into clinical practice will influence the risks of ROP, NEC, and death. Clinicians considering using these devices have little to guide them in terms of device settings. The best evidence presently available is that mortality risk will be lower in infants with achieved SpO_2 distributions, such as those achieved in the high-target group survivors in the NeOProM trials. Setting automated control devices to achieve a value centered around the middle of the range 91% to 95% would probably achieve a lower SpO_2 distribution than was seen in the trials and could conceivably increase the risk of mortality or NEC. Trials are required to determine the optimum target for automated adjustment systems.

SUMMARY

Data relating achieved SpO_2 to clinical outcome from the SUPPORT and BOOST-II UK trial facilitate their interpretation and add caution regarding variation in practice in this area outside the context of further clinical trials. The best current evidence for clinical safety is to target the SpO_2 range 91% to 95% by manual oxygen adjustment. This should be the baseline comparator for further studies of different SpO_2 target ranges and targeting technologies. Increased risks of mortality and NEC were observed in association with SpO_2 distributions centered around 90% to 93%, suggesting value in testing whether or not a higher SpO_2 target range, such as 92% to 97%, could be associated with further survival advantage. It is unlikely that a higher range could be studied without an increased risk of the need for ROP treatment; however, with advances in the treatment of this condition, the need for ROP treatment is not as important an adverse outcome as death or severe NEC, and may be a price worth paying.

ACKNOWLEDGMENTS

The author is grateful to Mr Andy King, BOOST-II UK Trial Statistician, for providing the analyses and histograms of achieved SpO_2 readings from the BOOST-II UK trial. The BOOST-II UK Trial was supported by the Medical Research Council (Grant number 73460).

REFERENCES

1. Askie LM, Darlow BA, Finer N, et al, Neonatal Oxygenation Prospective Meta-analysis (NeOProM) Collaboration. Association between oxygen saturation targeting and death or disability in extremely preterm infants in the Neonatal Oxygenation Prospective Meta-Analysis collaboration. JAMA 2018;319(21): 2190–201.
2. Chu DK, Kim LH, Young PJ, et al. Mortality and morbidity in acutely ill adults treated with liberal versus conservative oxygen therapy (IOTA): a systematic review and meta-analysis. Lancet 2018;391(10131):1693–705.
3. Askie LM, Henderson-Smart DJ, Irwig L, et al. Oxygen-saturation targets and outcomes in extremely preterm infants. N Engl J Med 2003;349(10):959–67.
4. Hagadorn JI, Furey AM, Nghiem TH, et al, AVIOx Study Group. Achieved versus intended pulse oximeter saturation in infants born less than 28 weeks' gestation: the AVIOx study. Pediatrics 2006;118:1574–82.
5. BOOST-II United Kingdom Collaborative Group, BOOST II Australia Collaborative Group, BOOST II New Zealand Collaborative Group, Stenson BJ, Tarnow-Mordi WO, Darlow BA, et al. Oxygen saturation and outcomes in preterm infants. New Engl J Med 2013;368:2094–104.

6. van Zanten HA, Pauws SC, Stenson BJ, et al. Effect of a smaller target range on the compliance in targeting and distribution of oxygen saturation in preterm infants. Arch Dis Child Fetal Neonatal Ed 2018;103(5):F430–5.

7. van Kaam AH, Hummler HD, Wilinska M, et al. Automated versus manual oxygen control with different saturation targets and modes of respiratory support in preterm infants. J Pediatr 2015;167:545–50.e1–2.

8. Jones JG, Lockwood GG, Fung N, et al. Influence of pulmonary factors on pulse oximeter saturation in preterm infants. Arch Dis Child Fetal Neonatal Ed 2016; 101(4):F319–22.

9. Carlo WA, Finer NN, Walsh MC, et al, SUPPORT Study Group of the Eunice Kennedy Shriver NICHD Neonatal Research Network. Target ranges of oxygen saturation in extremely preterm infants. New Engl J Med 2010;362:1959–69.

10. Di Fiore JM, Martin RJ, Li H, et al, SUPPORT Study Group of the Eunice Kennedy Shriver National Institute of Child Health, and Human Development Neonatal Research Network. Patterns of oxygenation, mortality, and growth status in the surfactant positive pressure and oxygen trial cohort. J Pediatr 2017;186: 49–56.e1.

11. Johnston ED, Boyle B, Juszczak E, et al. Oxygen targeting in preterm infants using the Masimo SET Radical pulse oximeter. Arch Dis Child Fetal Neonatal Ed 2011;96:F429–33.

12. BOOST-II Australia and United Kingdom Collaborative Groups, Tarnow-Mordi W, Stenson B, Kirby A, et al. Outcomes of two trials of oxygen-saturation targets in preterm infants. N Engl J Med 2016;374:749–60.

13. Stenson BJ, Donoghoe M, Brocklehurst P, et al. Pulse oximeter saturation targeting and oximeter changes in the Benefits of Oxygen Saturation Targeting (BOOST)-II Australia and BOOST-II UK oxygen trials. J Pediatr 2019;204: 301–4.e2.

14. Cummings JJ, Polin RA, Committee on Fetus and Newborn. Oxygen targeting in extremely low birth weight infants. Pediatrics 2016;138 [pii:e20161576].

15. Claure N, Bancalari E. Closed-loop control of inspired oxygen in premature infants. Semin Fetal Neonatal Med 2015;20(3):198–204.

16. Dargaville PA, Sadeghi Fathabadi O, Plottier GK, et al. Development and preclinical testing of an adaptive algorithm for automated control of inspired oxygen in the preterm infant. Arch Dis Child Fetal Neonatal Ed 2017;102(1):F31–6.

17. Poets CF, Franz AR. Automated FiO_2 control: nice to have, or an essential addition to neonatal intensive care? Arch Dis Child Fetal Neonatal Ed 2017;102(1):F5–6.

18. Reynolds PR, Miller TL, Volakis LI, et al. Randomised cross-over study of automated oxygen control for preterm infants receiving nasal high flow. Arch Dis Child Fetal Neonatal Ed 2018. https://doi.org/10.1136/archdischild-2018-315342.

Oxygen Therapy and Pulmonary Hypertension in Preterm Infants

Samuel J. Gentle, MD[a],*, Steven H. Abman, MD[b],
Namasivayam Ambalavanan, MD[a]

KEYWORDS

- Oxygen • Bronchopulmonary dysplasia
- Bronchopulmonary-associated pulmonary hypertension • Infant mortality • Infant
- Extremely premature

KEY POINTS

- Hypoxemia induces pulmonary hypertension in animal studies and within multiple patient populations.
- The randomized controlled trials on oxygen saturation targeting in extremely preterm infants did not systematically identify pulmonary hypertension as a potential complication.
- Based on experiments in animals and analyses of data from neonatal human studies, it is possible that borderline low oxygen saturations lead to acquired pulmonary hypertension in preterm infants.

INTRODUCTION

Elevated pulmonary vascular pressures normally occur during fetal life and decrease partially in response to an increase in oxygen tension at birth. Whereas persistent pulmonary hypertension characterizes the failure of this extrauterine transition in term infants, extremely preterm infants typically present with pulmonary hypertension at birth in association with respiratory distress syndrome.[1,2] The pathophysiology and risk factors for late pulmonary hypertension overlap with those for bronchopulmonary dysplasia (BPD). Pulmonary hypertension may result from underdevelopment in the setting of pulmonary hypoplasia[3] or growth restriction,[4] maldevelopment as a result of damaging postnatal exposures (eg, mechanical ventilation[5]) or genetic predisposition (eg, single nucleotide polymorphisms associated with decreased nitric oxide

Disclosure Statement: The authors have nothing to disclose.
[a] The University of Alabama at Birmingham, 176F Suite 9390F, Women and Infants Center, 619 South 20th St., Birmingham, AL 35233, USA; [b] University of Colorado, Children's Hospital Colorado, 13123 E 16th Ave B395, Aurora, CO 80045, USA
* Corresponding author.
E-mail address: sjgentle@uabmc.edu

production[6]), or as a result of maladaptation to other inflammatory or infectious insults, but these are also risks for BPD.[3,7] More recently, late-onset pulmonary hypertension in association with the development of moderate or severe BPD has been described.[4] Around 20% of infants with BPD will also develop pulmonary hypertension.[8,9] The optimal oxygen saturation targeting strategy to prevent and/or support extremely preterm infants with pulmonary hypertension remains unclear. In this article, the authors review the influence of hypoxemia on development of pulmonary hypertension and the limited evidence from the NeOProM trials about the risks for pulmonary hypertension. They also review the evidence for use of oxygen therapy in established pulmonary hypertension.

EPIDEMIOLOGY OF BRONCHOPULMONARY DYSPLASIA–ASSOCIATED PULMONARY HYPERTENSION

Whereas descriptions of early pulmonary hypertension in extremely preterm infants predate the trials included in NeOProM,[2] the overall incidence and impact of late pulmonary vascular disease within a more recent prospective cohort were later described.[4] One of the first large prospective studies in extremely preterm infants performed echocardiography starting at 4 weeks after birth in 145 infants with a median gestational age of 26 weeks. Of these infants 6% had evidence of pulmonary hypertension on initial ultrasound, and 12% were later diagnosed with pulmonary hypertension on a subsequent echocardiogram, emphasizing the importance of serial echocardiograms.[4] In another large prospective cohort study of 277 infants between 500 to 1250 g at birth receiving a 7 day and 36 weeks postmenstrual age (PMA) echocardiogram, 42% of infants had early and 14% had late pulmonary hypertension.[10] Other retrospective studies are limited by selection bias and only report rates of pulmonary hypertension in those infants receiving echocardiography. The true incidence of BPD-associated pulmonary hypertension is unknown, as cardiac catheterization, the most sensitive modality for diagnosing pulmonary hypertension,[11] is not routinely performed in infants with BPD. Echocardiography, the more common modality used to screen for pulmonary hypertension, estimates pulmonary arterial pressure from the tricuspid regurgitation jet velocity and/or other findings including right ventricular hypertrophy, septal flattening, and right atrial or ventricular dilatation. The American Heart Association and American Thoracic Society now recommend early screening in infants with severe respiratory distress syndrome or in those infants with established BPD.[11]

HYPOXEMIA AND RISK FOR PULMONARY HYPERTENSION

Defining a "normal" arterial oxygen tension in extremely preterm infants remains a challenge. By extension, defining hypoxemia or "below normal" arterial oxygen tensions is also a challenge. Although sometimes used synonymously, hypoxia refers to an imbalance in oxygen delivery and consumption sufficient to preclude metabolism by only aerobic means. In utero, infants' arterial oxygen tension in the umbilical vein is ∼30 mm Hg. At birth and if only exposed to ambient oxygen, the Pao_2 in preterm infants increases to around 65 mm Hg.[12] Whether oxygen saturation targeting in the extremely preterm infant should approximate lower targets to mirror in utero conditions or higher targets considered physiologically normal in term infants prompted the conception of the NeOProM trials to better determine oxygen saturation targets in the extremely preterm infant.

Inferences from data from other patient populations and animal data may suggest that targeting lower oxygen saturations presents a hypoxemic exposure that can increase extremely preterm infants' risk for developing pulmonary hypertension. Humans living at high altitudes provide a simple and straightforward example of pulmonary vascular remodeling from hypoxemia having increased pulmonary arterial pressures reversible on oxygen administration and pulmonary arteriole thickening, a known attribute of pulmonary hypertension.[13] Literature in human adults suggests that pulmonary hypertension can develop at oxygen saturations between 88% and 90%.[14] Histologic features of hypoxia-induced pulmonary hypertension in animal models include an increase in smooth muscle cells and extracellular matrix proteins in the pulmonary vasculature[15] as well as a reduction in the number of small blood vessels, thereby reducing the cross-sectional area available for gas exchange.[16] Lakshminrusimha and colleagues[17] evaluated the relationship between arterial Po_2 and pulmonary vascular resistance in a lamb model for persistent pulmonary hypertension in which fetal ductal ligation had been performed. Pulmonary vascular resistance increased at a Po_2 less than or equal to 52 mm Hg in control lambs (corresponding to a SpO_2 of ~86%) and at a Pao_2 less than or equal to 60 mm Hg (corresponding to a SpO_2 of ~90%) in lambs with persistent pulmonary hypertension (**Fig. 1**).

Extremely preterm infants often experience intermittent hypoxemic episodes; however, whether these events are a potentiating factor for pulmonary hypertension development is unknown. Episodes result from many factors, including upregulation of neurotransmitters that inhibit respiratory drive and insensitivity to respiratory stimulants. A prospective study examining the oxygen saturation patterns of extremely low–birth-weight infants during the first 8 postnatal weeks noted an increase in the number of hypoxemic episodes with postnatal age peaking at around 1 month after birth.[18] As previously mentioned, a large prospective cohort study diagnosed more extremely preterm infants with pulmonary hypertension on echocardiograms occurring beyond the first 4 postnatal weeks.[4] As a corollary in older children, intermittent airway obstruction and hypoxemia can occur in children with hypertrophied tonsils and adenoids. Higher pulmonary artery pressures have been observed in prospective

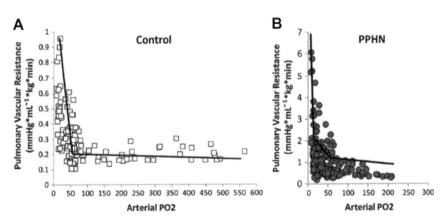

Fig. 1. Pulmonary vascular resistance (PVR) in lambs following exposure to 10% to 50% oxygen. The mean change point for PVR is ~60 mm Hg in control lambs (Panel A) and at ~52 mm Hg in PPHN lambs (Panel B). PPHN, persistent pulmonary hypertension. (*From* Lakshminrusimha S, Swartz DD, Gugino SF, et al. Oxygen concentration and pulmonary hemodynamics in newborn lambs with pulmonary hypertension. Pediatr Res 2009;66:539-44; with permission.)

studies of children with obstructive sleep apnea compared with age- and sex-matched controls.[19]

A critical question remains: what oxygen saturations provide a sufficient acute and/or chronic hypoxemic exposure for development of pulmonary hypertension in extremely preterm infants? When born extremely preterm, infants are between the canalicular and saccular stages of embryologic lung development during which pulmonary vascular resistance decreases. Conversely, when a fetus approaches term gestation, pulmonary vascular resistance becomes increasingly sensitive to hypoxia.[20] Based on a systematic review of prospective cohort studies in extremely preterm infants, this postnatal age corresponds to the time at which many extremely preterm infants develop pulmonary hypertension.[8] In 3 of the 5 trials from the NeO-ProM trials, the median oxygen saturation achieved in the lower target group was less than 90% SpO_2.[21] As perturbations in vascular growth factors contribute to BPD pathogenesis,[22] maintaining oxygen saturations less than an SpO2 of 90%, an inflection point of increased pulmonary vascular resistance may therefore increase infants' risk for developing pulmonary hypertension.

OXYGEN SATURATION TARGETING AND PULMONARY HYPERTENSION: CLUES FROM NeOProM
Oxygen Therapy and the Risk for Late Mortality

In the NeOProM trials, infants in the lower oxygen saturation targets (85%–89%) had an increased risk for death compared with infants in the higher oxygen saturation targets (91%–95%).[23] Furthermore, there is some evidence suggesting an increased risk for late as opposed to early death but limited evidence suggesting that pulmonary causes were the most contributory cause of death. In both the SUPPORT and BOOST trials, estimates for death before discharge show progressive divergence between groups long after birth suggesting that infants in the low saturation group are at increased risk for late death. The risk for pulmonary hypertension was not specifically reported in these trials. The cause of death did not differ between groups including BPD in the SUPPORT trial.[24] In the BOOST trials chronic lung disease contributed to 11% of deaths in the lower saturation target group and 6% of deaths in the higher saturation group.[25,26] A meta-analysis of NeOProM did not demonstrate differences in the rate of BPD between the lower and higher oxygen saturation target groups.[27]

Infants with BPD who also develop pulmonary hypertension are at increased risk for mortality. Meta-analyses of cohort studies report an increased risk for death of around 5-fold.[8,9] A recent retrospective chart review of extremely preterm infants (N = 61) with diagnosed pulmonary hypertension indicates that the severity of pulmonary hypertension is also associated with risk for mortality.[28] A similar retrospective review of extremely preterm infants (N = 42) found that this risk for death remains significant for months after diagnosis.[29] Although the timing of BPD-associated pulmonary hypertension diagnosis varies among extremely preterm infants, most prospective studies report diagnosis as early as 4 to 12 weeks PMA (**Fig. 2**).[8] Many other causes of mortality in extremely preterm infants, including necrotizing enterocolitis, intraventricular hemorrhage, and pulmonary hemorrhage lead to death within the first 28 days of life. Conversely, BPD is one of the most significant contributors to late mortality in extremely preterm infants.[30] It is therefore plausible that exposure to lower oxygen saturation targets, if mechanistically important to the development of BPD-associated pulmonary hypertension, may have contributed to the increased risk for mortality observed in the NeOProM studies.

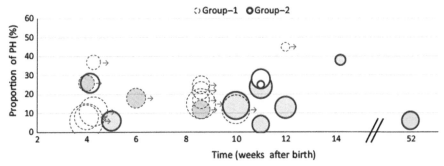

Fig. 2. Timing of pulmonary hypertension (PH) diagnosis in extremely preterm infants. Group 1 indicates studies in which time of diagnosis was not well defined, with arrows signifying the time point of first PH assessment. Group 2 indicates studies that defined when PH assessments were conducted. Prospective studies are shaded. (*From* Arjaans S, Zwart EAH, Ploegstra MJ, et al. Identification of gaps in the current knowledge on pulmonary hypertension in extremely preterm infants: A systematic review and meta-analysis. Paediatr Perinat Epidemiol 2018;32:258-67; with permission.)

Additional analyses from the NeOProM trials detailing causes of death by postnatal age may further support this hypothesis.

Risk for Pulmonary Hypertension–Associated Death in Growth-Restricted Infants

Consideration of BPD-associated pulmonary hypertension in growth-restricted infants may be important, given the possibility of increased risk for death in growth-restricted infants and the timing of infant death. As growth-restricted infants may be exposed to prolonged hypoxia in utero, elevated pulmonary vascular resistance may persist after birth.[31] Several studies have demonstrated an increased risk for pulmonary hypertension in extremely preterm infants who are born small for gestational age (SGA).[4,32–34] However, evidence is conflicting as to whether SGA infants with BPD-associated pulmonary hypertension are also at increased risk for death. A retrospective study of extremely low–birth-weight infants who developed BPD-associated pulmonary hypertension (N = 36) did not find a difference in mortality in SGA infants.[32] Conversely, a retrospective cohort study in infants with moderate to severe BPD (N = 138) observed an increased number of deaths before discharge in infants with BPD-associated PH who were also SGA, with 23% of these deaths occurring after 36 weeks PMA.[33]

Observational Evidence Following NeOProM

Although the NeOProM trials evaluated the influence of 2 oxygen saturation targets on mortality and important morbidities of prematurity, none of the trials specifically evaluated pulmonary hypertension as an outcome.[27] However, changes in clinical practice (eg, increasing oxygen saturation targets) following the NeOProM trials may provide observational evidence. A retrospective chart review of infants born at less than 29 weeks' gestation compared rates of BPD-associated pulmonary hypertension between epochs in which oxygen saturation targets were increased from 88% to 92% to 90% to 95%. At the included centers, infants achieved oxygen saturation targets between 50% and 80% of the time. The rate of BPD-associated pulmonary hypertension decreased by 50% between the 2 time periods.[35] Additional studies evaluating the influence of oxygen saturation targets on the development of BPD-associated pulmonary hypertension are needed.

OXYGEN THERAPY IN EXTREMELY PRETERM INFANTS WITH PULMONARY HYPERTENSION

Randomized controlled trials have not evaluated oxygen saturation targeting in extremely preterm infants diagnosed with pulmonary hypertension. In term infants with persistent pulmonary hypertension, maintaining saturations between 90% and 97% may be optimal given measurements of pulmonary vascular resistance in animal models.[17] A study evaluating clinical practices in infants diagnosed with BPD-associated pulmonary hypertension indicated that 65% of clinicians send infants home on oxygen therapy and that many clinicians tolerate saturation targets of 90% to 92%.[36] The American Heart Association and American Thoracic Society published guidelines in 2015 recommending oxygen saturations of 92% to 95% in infants with BPD-associated pulmonary hypertension to balance the risks of hypoxemia-induced increases in pulmonary vascular resistance at lower saturations with hyperoxic lung inflammation at higher saturations.[37] However, this recommendation was given a Class IIa Level of Evidence C rating reflecting a consensus or expert opinion. Other potential therapeutic strategies (inhaled nitric oxide, vasodilators such as sildenafil or endothelin receptor antagonists, or prostacyclin derivatives) also need to be evaluated systematically.

LONG-TERM EFFECTS OF PULMONARY HYPERTENSION AND BRONCHOPULMONARY DYSPLASIA

Alterations in pulmonary vascular physiology persist beyond the neonatal period in extremely preterm infants diagnosed with pulmonary hypertension. Sensitivity to hypoxia may continue until discharge and may still be present at 5 years of age[38] and into adolescence.[39] A recent study by Goss and colleagues[40] demonstrated pulmonary vascular disease by right heart catheterization even as late as young adult life in individuals who were very low–birth-weight infants (average gestational age 28 weeks) at birth, with 27% (3/11) having borderline pulmonary hypertension and 18% (2/11) meeting criteria for overt pulmonary hypertension. Pulmonary vascular resistance and elastance were higher both at rest and during exercise, indicating stiffer pulmonary vasculature. When compared with control subjects, preterm subjects were less able to augment cardiac index or right ventricular stroke work during exercise.[40] Adult survivors of BPD also have persistent structural and functional lung impairment.[41] These data suggest that BPD and abnormal pulmonary vasculature following preterm birth may prove to be the sword of Damocles that may result in early onset of chronic obstructive pulmonary disease and symptomatic pulmonary hypertension later in adult life.

SUMMARY

Hypoxemia demonstrably induces pulmonary hypertension in animal models and within multiple human contexts. Optimal oxygen target saturations that may prevent the development of pulmonary hypertension in extremely preterm infants are unknown. Maintaining oxygen saturations below 90% increased the risk of mortality in the NeOProM trials, which, although not specifically evaluated, may have been partially due to an increased risk for pulmonary hypertension known to significantly increase the risk for death. After pulmonary hypertension is diagnosed, experts suggest targeting oxygen saturation targets of 92% to 95%. As pulmonary hypertension increases the risk for mortality, randomized controlled trials comparing different oxygen targets as well as potential therapeutic strategies in extremely preterm infants with established pulmonary hypertension would provide the needed clinical guidance.

Best Practices

What is the current practice for pulmonary hypertension in preterm infants?

Best Practice/Guideline/Care Path Objective
- Screen infants with bronchopulmonary dysplasia for pulmonary hypertension
- In infants with established pulmonary hypertension:
  - Maintain oxygen saturations between 92% and 95%
  - Nitric oxide and/or sildenafil may be beneficial

What changes in current practice are likely to improve outcomes?

- As acute and chronic hypoxemia may increase pulmonary vascular resistance, low oxygen saturations should be avoided.

- Initial echocardiograms may be normal in infants developing BPD-associated pulmonary hypertension (PH), so serial echocardiography may be required.

- Cardiac catheterization may be required in infants with severe cardiorespiratory disease, persistent disease despite optimal management, and infants with recurrent pulmonary edema.

Major recommendations

- Infants with established BPD should be screened for PH with echocardiography (Class I; Level of Evidence B)

- Infants with severe cardiorespiratory disease should receive cardiac catheterization to identify other structural and functional contributors to disease including pulmonary vein stenosis and anatomic shunts (Class I; Level of Evidence B)

- Limit hypoxemic events and maintain oxygen saturations between 92% and 95% (Class IIa; Level of Evidence C)

- Inhaled nitric oxide should be considered as an adjunctive therapy in infants with persistent disease (Class IIa; Level of Evidence C)

Summary statement

As pulmonary hypertension is commonly associated with bronchopulmonary dysplasia and significantly increases the risk for mortality, screening and prompt treatment remain critical to improve outcomes.

Bibliographic Source(s): Abman SH, Hansmann G, Archer SL, et al. Pediatric Pulmonary Hypertension: Guidelines From the American Heart Association and American Thoracic Society. Circulation 2015;132:2037-99.

REFERENCES

1. Ambalavanan N, Aschner JL. Management of hypoxemic respiratory failure and pulmonary hypertension in preterm infants. J Perinatol 2016;36(Suppl 2):S20–7.
2. Halliday H, Hirschfeld S, Riggs T, et al. Respiratory distress syndrome: echocardiographic assessment of cardiovascular function and pulmonary vascular resistance. Pediatrics 1977;60:444–9.
3. Kumar VH, Hutchison AA, Lakshminrusimha S, et al. Characteristics of pulmonary hypertension in preterm neonates. J Perinatol 2007;27:214–9.
4. Bhat R, Salas AA, Foster C, et al. Prospective analysis of pulmonary hypertension in extremely low birth weight infants. Pediatrics 2012;129:e682–9.
5. De Paepe ME, Greco D, Mao Q. Angiogenesis-related gene expression profiling in ventilated preterm human lungs. Exp Lung Res 2010;36:399–410.
6. Trittmann JK, Gastier-Foster JM, Zmuda EJ, et al. A single nucleotide polymorphism in the dimethylarginine dimethylaminohydrolase gene is associated with

lower risk of pulmonary hypertension in bronchopulmonary dysplasia. Acta Paediatr 2016;105:e170–5.

7. Walsh-Sukys MC, Tyson JE, Wright LL, et al. Persistent pulmonary hypertension of the newborn in the era before nitric oxide: practice variation and outcomes. Pediatrics 2000;105:14–20.

8. Arjaans S, Zwart EAH, Ploegstra MJ, et al. Identification of gaps in the current knowledge on pulmonary hypertension in extremely preterm infants: a systematic review and meta-analysis. Paediatr Perinat Epidemiol 2018;32:258–67.

9. Al-Ghanem G, Shah P, Thomas S, et al. Bronchopulmonary dysplasia and pulmonary hypertension: a meta-analysis. J Perinatol 2017;37:414–9.

10. Mirza H, Ziegler J, Ford S, et al. Pulmonary hypertension in preterm infants: prevalence and association with bronchopulmonary dysplasia. J Pediatr 2014;165:909–14.e1.

11. Mourani PM, Sontag MK, Younoszai A, et al. Clinical utility of echocardiography for the diagnosis and management of pulmonary vascular disease in young children with chronic lung disease. Pediatrics 2008;121:317–25.

12. Castillo A, Sola A, Baquero H, et al. Pulse oxygen saturation levels and arterial oxygen tension values in newborns receiving oxygen therapy in the neonatal intensive care unit: is 85% to 93% an acceptable range? Pediatrics 2008;121:882–9.

13. Arias-Stella J, Saldana M. The terminal portion of the pulmonary arterial tree in people native to high altitudes. Circulation 1963;28:915–25.

14. Weitzenblum E, Chaouat A. Hypoxic pulmonary hypertension in man: what minimum daily duration of hypoxaemia is required? Eur Respir J 2001;18:251–3.

15. Meyrick B, Reid L. The effect of continued hypoxia on rat pulmonary arterial circulation. An ultrastructural study. Lab Invest 1978;38:188–200.

16. Hislop A, Reid L. New findings in pulmonary arteries of rats with hypoxia-induced pulmonary hypertension. Br J Exp Pathol 1976;57:542–54.

17. Lakshminrusimha S, Swartz DD, Gugino SF, et al. Oxygen concentration and pulmonary hemodynamics in newborn lambs with pulmonary hypertension. Pediatr Res 2009;66:539–44.

18. Abu Jawdeh EG, Martin RJ, Dick TE, et al. The effect of red blood cell transfusion on intermittent hypoxemia in ELBW infants. J Perinatol 2014;34:921–5.

19. Yilmaz MD, Onrat E, Altuntas A, et al. The effects of tonsillectomy and adenoidectomy on pulmonary arterial pressure in children. Am J Otolaryngol 2005;26:18–21.

20. Rasanen J, Wood DC, Weiner S, et al. Role of the pulmonary circulation in the distribution of human fetal cardiac output during the second half of pregnancy. Circulation 1996;94:1068–73.

21. Lakshminrusimha S, Manja V, Mathew B, et al. Oxygen targeting in preterm infants: a physiological interpretation. J Perinatol 2015;35:8–15.

22. Alvira CM, Morty RE. Can we understand the pathobiology of bronchopulmonary dysplasia? J Pediatr 2017;190:27–37.

23. Al-Rubaie ZTA, Askie LM, Hudson HM, et al. Assessment of NICE and USPSTF guidelines for identifying women at high risk of pre-eclampsia for tailoring aspirin prophylaxis in pregnancy: an individual participant data meta-analysis. Eur J Obstet Gynecol Reprod Biol 2018;229:159–66.

24. SUPPORT Study Group of the Eunice Kennedy Shriver NICHD Neonatal Research Network, Carlo WA, Finer NN, Walsh MC, et al. Target ranges of oxygen saturation in extremely preterm infants. N Engl J Med 2010;362:1959–69.

25. Australia B-I, United Kingdom Collaborative G, Tarnow-Mordi W, et al. Outcomes of two trials of oxygen-saturation targets in preterm infants. N Engl J Med 2016; 374:749–60.
26. Group BIUKC, Group BIAC, Group BINZC, et al. Oxygen saturation and outcomes in preterm infants. N Engl J Med 2013;368:2094–104.
27. Manja V, Lakshminrusimha S, Cook DJ. Oxygen saturation target range for extremely preterm infants: a systematic review and meta-analysis. JAMA Pediatr 2015;169:332–40.
28. Altit G, Bhombal S, Hopper RK, et al. Death or resolution: the "natural history" of pulmonary hypertension in bronchopulmonary dysplasia. J Perinatol 2019;39(3): 415–25.
29. Khemani E, McElhinney DB, Rhein L, et al. Pulmonary artery hypertension in formerly premature infants with bronchopulmonary dysplasia: clinical features and outcomes in the surfactant era. Pediatrics 2007;120:1260–9.
30. Park JH, Chang YS, Sung S, et al. Trends in overall mortality, and timing and cause of death among extremely preterm infants near the limit of viability. PLoS One 2017;12:e0170220.
31. Thibeault DW, Hall FK, Sheehan MB, et al. Postasphyxial lung disease in newborn infants with severe perinatal acidosis. Am J Obstet Gynecol 1984;150:393–9.
32. Cuna A, Kandasamy J, Sims B. B-type natriuretic peptide and mortality in extremely low birth weight infants with pulmonary hypertension: a retrospective cohort analysis. BMC Pediatr 2014;14:68.
33. Check J, Gotteiner N, Liu X, et al. Fetal growth restriction and pulmonary hypertension in premature infants with bronchopulmonary dysplasia. J Perinatol 2013; 33:553–7.
34. Danhaive O, Margossian R, Geva T, et al. Pulmonary hypertension and right ventricular dysfunction in growth-restricted, extremely low birth weight neonates. J Perinatol 2005;25:495–9.
35. Laliberte C, Hanna Y, Ben Fadel N, et al. Target oxygen saturation and development of pulmonary hypertension and increased pulmonary vascular resistance in preterm infants. Pediatr Pulmonol 2019;54:73–81.
36. Altit G, Lee HC, Hintz S, et al. Practices surrounding pulmonary hypertension and bronchopulmonary dysplasia amongst neonatologists caring for premature infants. J Perinatol 2018;38:361–7.
37. Abman SH, Hansmann G, Archer SL, et al. Pediatric pulmonary hypertension: guidelines from the American Heart Association and American Thoracic Society. Circulation 2015;132:2037–99.
38. Poon CY, Edwards MO, Kotecha S. Long term cardiovascular consequences of chronic lung disease of prematurity. Paediatr Respir Rev 2013;14:242–9.
39. Mourani PM, Ivy DD, Gao D, et al. Pulmonary vascular effects of inhaled nitric oxide and oxygen tension in bronchopulmonary dysplasia. Am J Respir Crit Care Med 2004;170:1006–13.
40. Goss KN, Beshish AG, Barton GP, et al. Early pulmonary vascular disease in young adults born preterm. Am J Respir Crit Care Med 2018;198(12).
41. Caskey S, Gough A, Rowan S, et al. Structural and functional lung impairment in adult survivors of bronchopulmonary dysplasia. Ann Am Thorac Soc 2016;13: 1262–70.

Current Recommendations and Practice of Oxygen Therapy in Preterm Infants

William Tarnow-Mordi, BA, MB BChir, MRCP (UK), DCH*,
Adrienne Kirby, MSc

KEYWORDS

- Oxygen • Oxygenation • Oximetry • Infant mortality • Necrotizing enterocolitis
- Retinopathy of prematurity • Extremely premature infant

KEY POINTS

- Because low-oxygen saturation targets increased mortality in extremely preterm infants, all guidelines since 2011, except one, have recommended targeting oxygen saturation ranges of 91% to 95% or 90% to 95%, or avoiding 85% to 89%.
- The quality of the evidence that the low target increased mortality has been rated as "high," "moderate," or "low" despite the low heterogeneity between randomized trials of oxygen saturation targeting, suggesting key differences in interpreting the GRADE guidelines.
- International surveys in 2015 and 2016 showed that oxygen saturation target ranges had increased to levels that are more consistent with the evidence.
- Randomized controlled trials on oxygen saturation targeting have excluded moderately and late preterm infants. This is a major evidence gap.
- Systematic reviews, guidelines, and consensus statements without biostatisticians or epidemiologists as coauthors should be considered potentially problematic.

INTRODUCTION

Authors of systematic reviews, editorial commentaries, opinions, consensus statements, and guidelines render a valuable service in summarizing the best available evidence for clinical practice. Similarly, those who undertake periodic questionnaire surveys reveal whether this appraisal of the evidence subsequently impacts clinical practice. After 2 systematic reviews, which were published in 2017 and 2018,[1,2] had

Disclosure Statement: W. Tarnow-Mordi and A. Kirby were Chief Investigators of the BOOST II Study, funded by the Australian National Health and Medical Research Council and coinvestigators of the NeOProM Collaboration.
NHMRC Clinical Trials Centre, University of Sydney, Sydney, New South Wales, Australia
* Corresponding author.
E-mail addresses: williamtm@med.usyd.edu.au; wotarnowmordi@gmail.com

assessed the 5 Neonatal Oxygen Prospective Meta-analysis (NeOProM) trials of low- (85%–89%) versus high- (91%–95%) oxygen saturation target ranges in infants of less than 28 weeks' gestation,[3–7] the authors evaluated published (i) recommendations for oxygen-saturation target ranges in these infants during oxygen therapy after admission to the neonatal unit and (ii) surveys of practice.

The GRADE Working Group Guidelines

Several systematic reviews, commentaries, and consensus statements have cited the GRADE guidelines[8–10] in assessing (a) the quality of evidence and (b) the strength of recommendations made. The 4 grades of evidence in the GRADE guidelines are high quality (indicating that further research is very unlikely to change the confidence in the estimate of effect), moderate quality (further research is likely to have an important impact on the confidence in the estimate of effect and may change the estimate), low quality (further research is very likely to have an important impact on the confidence in the estimate of effect and is likely to change the estimate), and very low quality (very uncertain about the estimate). Evidence from observational studies is initially rated as of low quality, but ratings can be modified upward, while evidence from randomized studies is initially rated as of high quality, but ratings can be modified downward. After assessing the quality of evidence, GRADE gives criteria to rate recommendations for practice as "strong" or "weak."[11]

The GRADE process begins with a Health Care Question (Patient Intervention, Comparator, Outcome), progresses through systematic reviews of all evidence addressing that question, rates the quality of evidence of each outcome across studies and overall, and then rates the strength of the resulting recommendations, as summarized in **Fig. 1**.

OXYGEN SATURATION TARGETS IN INFANTS LESS THAN 28 WEEKS' GESTATION
Methods

Search strategy

The authors searched PubMed for systematic reviews, editorial commentaries, opinions, consensus statements, and guidelines on oxygen therapy in infants less than 28 weeks' gestation, excluding (i) reports of individual randomized controlled trials (RCTs) of low- versus high-oxygen saturation targets, (ii) guidelines focusing on a single measure of outcome, for example, retinopathy of prematurity (ROP), bronchopulmonary dysplasia (BPD), and (iii) systematic reviews or commentaries on oxygen targeting during resuscitation or delivery room care. Further relevant articles were obtained from the reference lists of publications identified as above. The search was limited to the period since the publication in 2010 of SUPPORT,[3] the first of the NeOProM trials.[12] The search terms were "((clinical practice guidelines) AND preterm AND oxygen) NOT resuscitation," which yielded 18 hits and "systematic review AND preterm AND oxygen NOT resuscitation," which yielded 90 hits. Guidelines, systematic reviews, narrative reviews, commentaries, opinions, and consensus statements were selected from among these 108 hits. This search strategy yielded 23 publications **(Table 1)**.[1,2,13–33] The authors also searched CINAHL using the terms ("Infant, Premature") AND ("Practice Guidelines"), which yielded 28 hits, none of which were relevant.

These strategies also yielded 2 surveys of clinical practice, one conducted between November 2015 and February 2016 in 193 European neonatal intensive care units (NICUs),[34] and another among representatives of 329/390 NICUs of the International Network for Evaluating Outcomes in Neonates (iNeo), conducted in 2015.[35]

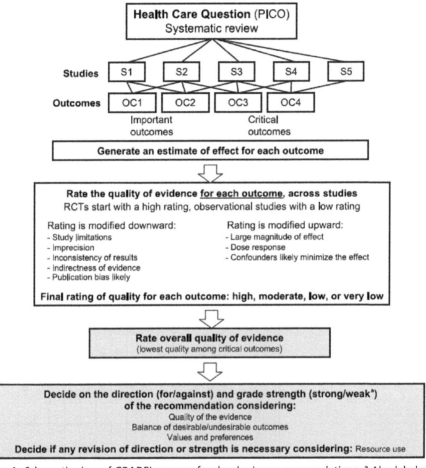

Fig. 1. Schematic view of GRADE's process for developing recommendations. [a] Also labeled "conditional" or "discretionary". PICO, patient, intervention, comparator, outcome. (*From* Guyatt G, Oxman AD, Akl EA, et al. GRADE guidelines: 1. Introduction-GRADE evidence profiles and summary of findings tables. J Clin Epidemiol 2011;64:383–94; with permission.)

Results

Recommendations for practice

The authors found 2 consensus guidelines,[19,29] a clinical report from the Committee on Fetus and Newborn of the American Academy of Pediatrics (AAP),[26] 5 systematic reviews,[1,2,20,22,28] and 13 commentaries or opinions (see **Table 1**).

European Consensus guidelines and American Academy of Pediatrics Clinical Report

In 2016, the European Consensus Guidelines on Management of Respiratory Distress Syndrome,[29] in an update of its earlier consensus statement,[19] suggested an oxygen saturation target of 90% to 94% for all preterm infants less than 28 weeks' gestation. Using the GRADE guidelines,[8] the European Consensus group assessed the overall quality of evidence for this recommendation overall, rather than for specific outcomes, as "moderate" and the strength of this recommendation as "weak."

In 2016, the AAP Committee on Fetus and Newborn[26] concluded that an oxygen saturation target range greater than 89% may be safer, at least for some infants.

Table 1
Recommendations for oxygen saturation target ranges and alarm limits

First Author, Year	Type of Publication	Recommended Target Range	Quality of Evidence (Strength of Recommendation)
Saugstad et al,[13] 2011	Commentary	>89%	-
Bashambu et al,[14] 2012	Narrative review	>89%	-
Askie,[15] 2013	Opinion	>90%	-
Polin & Bateman[16] 2013	Commentary	90%–95%	-
Bancalari & Claure,[17] 2013	Commentary	90%–95%	-
Stenson,[18] 2013	Opinion	90–95	-
Sweet et al,[19] 2013	Consensus statement	90%–95%	Moderate
Saugstad & Aune,[20] 2014	**Systematic review**	**90%–95%**	-
Schmidt et al,[21] 2014	Commentary	85%–88% to 93%–94%[a] 89%–90% to 95%[b]	-
Manja et al,[22] 2015	**Systematic review**	-	**Low[c]**
Synnes & Miller,[23] 2015	Commentary	85%–95%	-
Isaacs[24] 2016	Commentary	91%–95%	-
Stenson[25] 2016	Commentary	90%–95%	-
Cummings et al,[26] 2016	Committee clinical report	90% to 95%[d,e]	-

Deschmann & Norman,[27] 2017	Commentary	91%–95%	-
Manja,[28] 2017	**Systematic review**	**91%–95%[e]**	**Moderate[c]**
Sweet,[29] 2017	Consensus statement	90%–94%[e]	Moderate (weak)
Askie,[1] 2017	**Systematic review**	-	**High[c]**
Kayton,[32] 2018	Commentary	91%–95%	-
Askie et al,[2] 2018	Systematic review	-	-
Bizzarro,[30] 2018	Commentary	91%–95%	-
Einhorn,[33] 2018	Commentary	91%–95%	-
Stenson & Saugstad,[31] 2018	Commentary	91–95[e]	-

Bold indicates systematic review; italics indicates an outlier commentary which recommends 85-95% in contrast to other commentaries which recommend ranges above 89%.

[a] e.g. alarm limits in hospitals with low rates of mortality and necrotizing enterocolitis but high rates of severe ROP.
[b] e.g. alarm limits in hospitals with low rates of severe ROP, but high rates of mortality and necrotizing enterocolitis.
[c] For effect on mortality.
[d] 90 to 95% may be safer than 85% to 89% in some infants.
[e] Lower alarm limit will generally need to extend somewhat below the lower target.

Although the disproportionately high rate of mortality in small-for-gestational-age infants in the low-target group was discussed, the committee did not define those infants in whom it considered a higher saturation target safer. The AAP Committee on Fetus and Newborn did not apply the GRADE guidelines.

Systematic reviews

In 2014, Saugstad and Aune[20] published a systematic review and meta-analysis on infants less than 28 weeks' gestation reported in the 5 NeOProM trials. They reported no difference in death or disability up to 24 months corrected gestational age in 2463 infants in SUPPORT[3] and COT,[5] the 2 trials that had reported this outcome. However, all 5 trials reported an increased relative risk (RR) for mortality at discharge or follow-up (4884 infants; RR 1.41; 95% confidence interval [CI] 1.14–1.74) and for necrotizing enterocolitis (NEC) (4929 infants; RR 1.25, 95% CI 1.05–1.49). Results were inconclusive for ROP, BPD, brain injury, and patent ductus arteriosus. They recommended adoption of an oxygen saturation target range of 90% to 95% until 36 weeks' gestation but did not use the GRADE guidelines to assess the quality of evidence or strength of this recommendation.

In 2015, Manja and colleagues[22] published a systematic review in 4929 infants reported in the 5 NeOProM trials, which was the first to use the GRADE guidelines[8] to assess the quality of evidence for each outcome. It reported (i) no effect for death or disability up to 24 months corrected gestational age in 3 trials (2716 infants; RR 1.02, 95% CI 0.94–1.14: quality of evidence downgraded to moderate[8]); (ii) increased hospital mortality in the low-target group across 4 trials (3757 infants; RR 1.18, 95% CI 1.03–1.36: quality of evidence downgraded to low[8] because, among other reasons, the separation in oxygen saturation achieved between low- and high-target groups was less than planned); (iii) that the low target increased NEC in 5 trials (4929 infants; RR 1.24%, 95% 1.05–1.47; quality of evidence downgraded to moderate); (iv) no effect for severe ROP in 5 trials (4066 infants; RR 0.72, 95% CI 0.5–1.04; quality of evidence downgraded to low[8] because of unexplained heterogeneity); and (v) no effect for BPD, neurodevelopmental outcomes at 18 to 24 months, and hearing loss (quality of evidence downgraded to moderate[8]).

In 2017, Manja and colleagues[28] published a systematic review of RCTs evaluating the effect of lower (85%–89%) versus higher (91%–95%) pulse oxygen saturation (Spo_2) target on mortality and neurodevelopmental impairment at 18 to 24 months.[28] They concluded that the risks associated with restricting the upper Spo_2 target limit to 89% outweighed the benefits. The quality of evidence was moderate. They speculated that a wider target range (lower alarm limit, 89%, and upper alarm limit, 96%) might increase time spent within the 91% to 95% range.

In 2017, Askie and colleagues[1] published a Cochrane Review of the effects of targeting lower versus higher arterial oxygen saturations on death or disability in preterm infants, based on the 5 NeOProM trials, in a total of 4965 infants less than 28 weeks' gestation. They applied the GRADE guidelines to assess the quality of evidence for estimates of the effect of the low-target range on individual outcomes. Their assessments of the quality of evidence for these outcomes have been summarized alongside the assessments of Manja and colleagues[22] in **Table 2**.

In 2018, Askie and colleagues[2] published the results of the previously planned[12] prospective individual patient data meta-analysis of the effects of targeting 85% to 89% versus 91% to 95% oxygen saturation in all 4965 infants less than 28 weeks' gestation in the 5 NeOProM Collaboration trials. This publication[2] (which did not apply the GRADE guidelines[12]) and the Cochrane Review by Askie and colleagues[1] suggest that for every 1000 infants, targeting low- versus high-oxygen saturation made no difference in death or major disability up to 18 to 24 months, nor in major disability,

Table 2
Observed effects of the low-target range 85% to 89% on individual outcomes in 2 systematic reviews of 5 trials, with quality of evidence assessed by GRADE

Outcome	Observed Effect of 85%–89% Target on This Outcome in Manja et al,[22] 2015	Quality of Evidence as Assessed in Manja et al,[22] 2015	Observed Effect of 85%–89% Target on This Outcome in Askie et al,[1] 2017	Quality of Evidence as Assessed in Askie et al,[1] 2017
Death or disability at 24 mo	No effect	Moderate	No effect	High
Hospital death	Increased	Low	Increased	High
Disability at 18–24 mo	No effect	Moderate	No effect	High
NEC	Increased	Moderate	Increased	High
Treated ROP	No effect	Low	No effect	Moderate
Hearing loss	No effect	Moderate	No effect	Not assessed
Blindness	No effect	Moderate	No effect	Not assessed

including blindness, but led to 28 more deaths, 22 more cases of NEC, and 42 fewer infants being treated for ROP.[1,2,36]

Table 3 presents the authors' reasons for uprating the Quality of Evidence that the low target increases mortality in the NeOProM trials in 2 systematic reviews using GRADE from "low"[22] to "high."[1]

SURVEYS OF CLINICAL PRACTICE IN OXYGEN TARGETING AMONG INFANTS LESS THAN 28 WEEKS' GESTATION

In a Web-based survey among representatives of 390 NICUs of the International Network for Evaluating Outcomes in Neonates (iNeo) conducted in 2015, responses were received from 329 (84%).[35] Of these, 60% had recently made changes to their upper and lower SpO_2 target limits, with the median value of the target range set higher than previously by 2% to 3% in 8 of 10 networks.

In a similar survey of 193 European NICUs conducted in 2015 and 2016,[34] there was considerable variation in practice. The most frequently targeted oxygen-saturation ranges were 90% to 95% (28%), 88% to 95% (12%), 90% to 94% (5%), and 91% to 95% (5%), reflecting the most commonly recommended target ranges shown in **Table 1**. A total of 156 NICUs (81%) had recently changed their oxygen saturation target limits. The median values for the oxygen-saturation ranges in clinical practice had increased by between 3% and 5% within the last 10 years.

Neither survey determined current practice in setting alarm limits nor in oxygen saturation targeting for preterm infants of 30 to 36 weeks' gestation.

Discussion

All 5 systematic reviews of trials of oxygen saturation targeting for infants of less than 28 weeks' gestation that were identified since 2010 concluded that the low target 85% to 89% increased mortality.[1,2,20,22,28] **Table 1** shows notable uniformity in recommendations for practice. Of 16 guidelines, commentaries, or opinions published since SUPPORT in 2010 (see **Table 1**), 15 recommended targeting a range greater than

Table 3
Contrasting interpretations of the quality of evidence that the low target increased mortality in randomized controlled trials of oxygen saturation targets in infants less than 28 wk using GRADE[8]

Initial Reason for Downgrading Quality of Evidence[22]	Reinterpretation Using the GRADE Guidelines	Our Interpretation of the Effect on Quality of Evidence
1. Separation of achieved Spo_2 values was less than planned	Despite less than expected separation, mortality effects were still observed. This confounding is likely to have reduced the effect (see **Fig. 1**[8])	Rating should be modified upward
2. The oximeter algorithm was revised during enrollment to 3 trials[5,7]	The revised algorithm improved separation in oxygen saturation[36] and thus study power. The original algorithm reduced separation (see **Fig. 1**[8]), thus underestimating the average estimate of effect[36]	Rating should be modified upward
3. Mortality in infants on the revised algorithm was not a prespecified outcome; yet 2 BOOST II trials[7,37] were stopped early because of an increase in this outcome	The BOOST II protocols specified a difference in a major endpoint of >3 standard errors or >3 standard deviations (equivalent to $P<.0027$) to justify early stopping. After SUPPORT showed excess mortality,[3] the BOOST II trials[7,37] were stopped early because of a highly significant increase in pooled mortality in infants on revised oximeters (RR 1.65; $P = .0003$)[38]	Rating should be modified upward
4. Only 4[3,6,37] of 5 trials reported hospital death	The estimates of effect on hospital death in these 4 trials demonstrate low to moderate heterogeneity[39] (χ^2 4.76, $P = .19$; $I^2 = 37\%$)	No effect on rating

Other issues

5. Effects on mortality using revised vs original oximeters; among infants on revised oximeters, low-target infants had consistently higher mortality than high-target infants, with (a) statistically significant interactions in 3 meta-analyses of mortality in low- vs high-target infants stratified by use of original vs revised oximeters ($P = .006$[38]; $P = .03$[1,20]; $P = .04$[22]) (but interactions were unreported in 2 meta-analyses[20,22]); (b) Infants using revised oximeters spent more time in their assigned target ranges than those on original oximeters[36]	The mortality risk for low- vs high-target infants was greater in those using revised vs original oximeters.[8] This, and the finding that targeting was more accurate in infants using revised oximeters,[36] is likely to have caused the average effect of the low target on mortality in infants on original oximeters to have been underestimated, as in 1 above (see **Fig. 1**[8])	Rating should be modified upward

(continued on next page)

| | | Our Interpretation |
Initial Reason for Downgrading Quality of Evidence[22]	Reinterpretation Using the GRADE Guidelines	of the Effect on Quality of Evidence
6. What was the potential for biased assessment of mortality?	None. Death was assessed without interobserver variation or bias	Shows high quality
7. Was there loss to follow-up in ascertainment of mortality?	No. 100% ascertainment of death at 36 wk and before hospital discharge	Shows high quality
8. Was the magnitude of the effect on mortality large?	Yes. The low target shows a 38% increase in RR of death in infants on revised oximeters (RR 1.38, 95% CI 1.13–1.68; $P = .014$)[1] (see **Fig. 1**[8])	Rating should be modified upward

Table 3 *(continued)*

90% or avoiding the low-target range of 85% to 89%. The exception was an editorial commentary,[23] which suggested that targeting an oxygen-saturation range between 85% and 95% remained acceptable. Two international surveys[34,35] in approximately 500 neonatal units reported considerable variation in clinical practice, but documented recent increases of 2% to 5% in the median values for target oxygen-saturation ranges.

CONTRASTING INTERPRETATIONS OF CURRENT RANDOMIZED EVIDENCE

The recommendation[23] that an oxygen-saturation target range of 85% to 89% remained acceptable[23] reflects a judgment in the systematic review of Manja and colleagues[22] that the GRADE quality of evidence that the low target increased mortality was low. This conclusion merits reconsideration. Reviewers may legitimately disagree when interpreting quality of evidence using GRADE, which provides a transparent framework guiding the assessment process (see **Fig. 1**).[8,9] **Table 2** shows judgments from 2 systematic reviews[1,22] about the quality of evidence for the effect of the low target on various outcomes. **Table 3** outlines the present authors' reasons for reinterpreting the quality of evidence for the effect of the low target on mortality as "high" rather than "low," using GRADE. For example, a treatment effect for mortality was observed *despite* the confounding effect of achieving less separation between study arms in actual oxygen saturation than planned. This result supports an upward modification of the rating for quality (see **Fig. 1**).

Neither the European Consensus Guidelines nor the AAP Guidance has been updated since these most recent data were published.[1,2] Future recommendations may benefit from inviting coauthorship by colleagues with advanced biostatistic and epidemiologic expertise. Indeed, attempting to synthesise and interpret complex trial data without such expertise might be compared with attempting brain surgery without a neurosurgeon.

Future international clinical surveys[32–35] and other evidence[36,40] are warranted, to assess the impact on practice of the final results of the NeOProM trials.[1,2] Future practice may also be influenced by increasing attention to 5 questions:

i. Did the pulse oximeters which were used in the NeOProM trials estimate hypoxemia with progressively wider limits of accuracy as true oxygen-saturation values (Sao_2) decreased from 93% to 80%, as reported in 2012 by Rosychuk et al (**Fig. 2**)?[41] Did the pulse oximeters expose substantially more infants in the lower-target group to values of oxygen tension less than 50 mm Hg (6.7 kPa).[42] The study authors[41] wrote, *"The large sample size of each of these (NeOProM) trials and the planned meta-analysis should address the question of whether infants assigned to the lower range are at higher risk of low Pao₂-induced pulmonary vaso-constriction, patent ductus arteriosus, abnormal neuro-developmental outcome, and potentially death. Our data may provide partial explanations if differences in short- or long-term outcomes are observed."*[41]

ii. Could targeting an untested intermediate oxygen-saturation range, such as 87 to 93%, increase mortality versus a higher range because current oximeters inadvertently permit increasingly disproportionate exposure to hypoxemia as true oxygen saturation decreases below 93%? (see **Fig. 2**).[40,41] At present, the most rigorously evaluated evidence for policy is that targeting oxygen saturations of 91 to 95% is safer overall than targeting oxygen saturations of 85% to 89%.[1,2,40] The most reliable evidence for an intermediate range will come from an adequately powered RCT of two pre-specified target ranges, defined by pre-specified alarm settings.

iii. Will future practice reflect recent analyses showing that infants with revised oximeters in the Australian and UK Benefits of Oxygen Saturation Targeting-II (BOOST II) trials spent longer in their planned pulse oximeter saturation target ranges than infants with the original oximeters (P<0.001)?[36] There was no difference in separation of median oxygen saturation between infants with original vs revised oximeters,[43] but the increased targeting accuracy in the low-target range

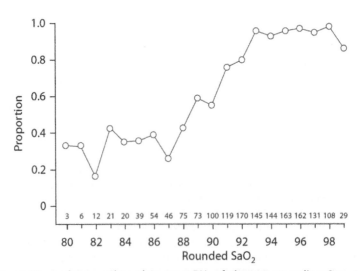

Fig. 2. Proportions of Spo₂ values that are ±3% of the corresponding Sao₂ value are plotted. The numbers above the x-axis on the graph denote the number of measurements at each value of Sao₂, i.e. a total of 1,620 measurements. There is a highly significant difference in the proportions of measurements in which Spo₂ is within ± 3% of the corresponding Sao₂ value for values of Sao₂ of ≤92% versus values of Sao₂ >92% (Chi squared >63, p<0.0001). Further analyses adjusted for clustering by infant will be valuable. (*From* Rosychuk RJ, Hudson-Mason A, Eklund D, Lacaze-Masmonteil T. Discrepancies between arterial oxygen saturation and functional oxygen saturation measured with pulse oximetry in very preterm infants. Neonatology 2012;101:14–9; with permission.)

Table 4
Sample sizes to show 10% or 20% reductions in relative risk of mortality or disability

Event Rate in Control Group (C), %	Event Rate in Treatment Group (T), %	Risk Difference (C − T = Δ), %	Relative Risk or Risk Ratio (RR = T/C)	Relative Risk Reduction (1 − RR)	Number Needed to Benefit or Harm (100/Δ)	Total Sample to Show Effect in a 2-Arm Comparison with 90% Power, 2P = .05 and Nonadherence to Protocol Due to:		
						0% Crossover in Each Group (Perfect Adherence to Protocol)	5% Crossover in Each Group (Total 10% Crossover)	10% Crossover in Each Group (Total 20% Crossover)
20	16	4	0.8	0.2	25	3868	4776	6044
20	18	2	0.9	0.1	50	16,166	19,960	25,260
10	8	2	0.8	0.2	50	8598	10,616	13,436
10	9	1	0.9	0.1	100	36,136	44,164	56,464

Data from Sealed envelope. Trial sample size calculator. Available at: https://www.sealedenvelope.com/power/. Accessed 24 Jan 2018.

with revised oximeters[36] may explain the larger mortality difference between low- and high-target infants with revised oximeters. It also suggests that average treatment effects in the BOOST II trials are underestimates, as they include data from infants on the original oximeters.[36]

iv. Should future clinical policy be based on observational studies? No. David Sackett, an early advocate of Evidence-Based Medicine, stated *"If you're scanning an article about therapy and it is not a randomized trial, why on earth are you wasting your time?"*[44] Two major threats to the validity of therapeutic comparisons are random error and systematic bias. Randomization is the most reliable way to protect therapeutic comparisons from systematic bias, because it tends to balance all confounding variables, including those which are currently unknown, evenly between intervention and control groups.[45] Large observational analyses can minimize random error, but cannot overcome errors arising from systematic bias. Hence the most reliable evidence for future policy will come from large randomized trials, preferably those which incorporate automated targeting of oxygen saturation with predefined settings for alarm limits around each target.

v. What do parents and former patients think of the trade-offs between lower mortality and NEC vs lower survival and less ROP, or future trade-offs? Increasingly, using digital technology to seek input from parents and patients will allow their voices to be heard in discussions about trade-offs between competing outcomes in oxygen trials. Such methods could allow parents, former patients, professionals, policymakers and other stakeholders to help prioritize core questions for large international trials. Such trials could evaluate the effects of different oxygen targeting policies on survival as primary outcome, and on disability in survivors as a key secondary outcome.[46–48]

LACK OF EVIDENCE FROM TRIALS IN MODERATELY PRETERM OR LATE PRETERM INFANTS

No trials or systematic reviews have evaluated the effects of different oxygen saturation targets or saturation alarm limits on short- or long-term outcomes in preterm infants of 28 to 36 weeks' gestation, who may outnumber extremely preterm infants of less than 28 weeks' gestation by 10-fold or 20-fold.[49] This represents a major evidence gap.

OBTAINING EVIDENCE FOR FUTURE RECOMMENDATIONS ON OXYGEN TARGETS IN PRETERM INFANTS

In 1998, Peto and Baigent wrote,[50] *"...medical research needs to find practicable ways of greatly increasing the size of randomized studies; otherwise moderate but worthwhile benefits will continue to be missed ..."* As event rates fall, if mortality and disability are to improve further, large, well-designed perinatal trials with increasingly large sample sizes will be needed.[51] **Table 4** illustrates the sample sizes needed to detect moderate, worthwhile reductions of 10% and 20% in key outcomes, such as mortality or disability, with adequate power and realistic rates of nonadherence to protocol.[52] These sample sizes might mean about 1 additional survivor without major disability for every 50 to 100 patients treated, which many would consider worthwhile for a widely available, affordable treatment like oxygen. All this underlines the need for increasing international collaboration, a major goal of the newly conceived ALPHA Collaboration for *A*dvancing *L*arge, collectively *P*rioritized perinatal trials of *H*ealth outcomes *A*ssessment.[46–48]

Best Practices

What is the current practice for oxygen saturation targeting in infants of less than 28 weeks' gestation?

Surveys conducted in 2015 and 2016 in more than 500 NICUs showed wide variation in practice, with between 60% and 81% of NICUs having increased their median oxygen saturation target ranges by 2% to 5%.[34,35] The most up-to-date guidance for practice, published since the NeOProM Collaboration results in 2017 and 2018,[1,2] recommends a target range of 91 to 95.[30,31]

What changes in current practice are likely to improve outcomes?

Targeting an oxygen saturation of 91% to 95% will reduce mortality and NEC and increase retinopathy without increasing blindness or disability, compared with targeting an oxygen saturation of 85% to 89%.[1,2,7] Targeting an intermediate oxygen-saturation range, such as 87% to 93%, is an untested practice that may increase mortality compared with targeting 91% to 95%, because current oximeters permit increasingly disproportionate exposure to hypoxemia as oxygen saturation decreases to less than 93%.[7,41]

Is there a Clinical Algorithm? No.

New trials are needed in infants of 28 weeks and 0 days to 35 weeks and 6 days gestation to determine which targets minimize mortality and NEC and ROP. However, the incidence of ROP is likely to be proportionately much lower than the incidence of the first 2 outcomes in these infants.

Major Recommendations:

Adopt a target range of 91% to 95% for oxygen saturation in infants less than 28 weeks' gestation.

Rating for the Strength of the Evidence: High.[1]

Bibliographic Source(s): Refs.[1,2,36,41]

ACKNOWLEDGMENT

We acknowledge valuable comments by Dr Balpreet Singh, IWK Hospital, Halifax.

REFERENCES

1. Askie LM, Darlow BA, Davis PG, et al. Effects of targeting lower versus higher arterial oxygen saturations on death or disability in preterm infants. Cochrane Database Syst Rev 2017;(4):CD011190.
2. Askie LM, Darlow BA, Finer N, et al. Association between oxygen saturation targeting and death or disability in extremely preterm infants in the neonatal oxygenation prospective meta-analysis collaboration. JAMA 2018;319:2190–201.
3. Carlo WA, Finer NN, Walsh MC, et al. Target ranges of oxygen saturation in extremely preterm infants. N Engl J Med 2010;362:1959–69.
4. Vaucher YE, Peralta-Carcelen M, Finer NN, et al. Neurodevelopmental outcomes in the early CPAP and pulse oximetry trial. N Engl J Med 2012;367: 2495–504.
5. Schmidt B, Whyte RK, Asztalos EV, et al. Effects of targeting higher vs lower arterial oxygen saturations on death or disability in extremely preterm infants: a randomized clinical trial. JAMA 2013;309:2111–20.
6. Darlow BA, Marschner SL, Donoghoe M, et al. Randomized controlled trial of oxygen saturation targets in very preterm infants: two year outcomes. J Pediatr 2014;165:30–5.e2.

7. Tarnow-Mordi W, Stenson B, Kirby A, et al, BOOST II Australia and BOOST II UK Collaborative Study Groups. Outcomes of two trials of oxygen-saturation targets in preterm infants. N Engl J Med 2016;374:749–60.

8. Guyatt G, Oxman AD, Akl EA, et al. GRADE guidelines: 1. Introduction-GRADE evidence profiles and summary of findings tables. J Clin Epidemiol 2011;64: 383–94.

9. Balshem H, Helfand M, Schunemann HJ, et al. GRADE guidelines: 3. Rating the quality of evidence. J Clin Epidemiol 2011;64:401–6.

10. Guyatt GH, Oxman AD, Kunz R, et al. What is "quality of evidence" and why is it important to clinicians? BMJ 2008;336:995–8.

11. Guyatt GH, Oxman AD, Kunz R, et al. Going from evidence to recommendations. BMJ 2008;336:1049–51.

12. Askie LM, Brocklehurst P, Darlow BA, et al. NeOProM: neonatal oxygenation prospective meta-analysis collaboration study protocol. BMC Pediatr 2011;11:6.

13. Saugstad OD, Speer CP, Halliday HL. Oxygen saturation in immature babies: revisited with updated recommendations. Neonatology 2011;100:217–8.

14. Bashambu MT, Bhola M, Walsh M. Evidence for oxygen use in preterm infants. Acta Paediatr 2012;101:29–33.

15. Askie LM. Optimal oxygen saturations in preterm infants: a moving target. Curr Opin Pediatr 2013;25:188–92.

16. Polin RA, Bateman D. Oxygen-saturation targets in preterm infants. N Engl J Med 2013;368:2141–2.

17. Bancalari E, Claure N. Oxygenation targets and outcomes in premature infants. JAMA 2013;309:2161–2.

18. Stenson BJ. Oxygen targets for preterm infants. Neonatology 2013;103:341–5.

19. Sweet DG, Carnielli V, Greisen G, et al. European consensus guidelines on the management of neonatal respiratory distress syndrome in preterm infants–2013 update. Neonatology 2013;103:353–68.

20. Saugstad OD, Aune D. Optimal oxygenation of extremely low birth weight infants: a meta-analysis and systematic review of the oxygen saturation target studies. Neonatology 2014;105:55–63.

21. Schmidt B, Whyte RK, Roberts RS. Trade-off between lower or higher oxygen saturations for extremely preterm infants: the first benefits of oxygen saturation targeting (BOOST) II trial reports its primary outcome. J Pediatr 2014;165:6–8.

22. Manja V, Lakshminrusimha S, Cook DJ. Oxygen saturation target range for extremely preterm infants: a systematic review and meta-analysis. JAMA Pediatr 2015;169:332–40.

23. Synnes A, Miller SP. Oxygen therapy for preterm neonates: the elusive optimal target. JAMA Pediatr 2015;169:311–3.

24. Isaacs D. Optimal oxygen saturation target for preterm infants. J Paediatr Child Health 2016;52:783.

25. Stenson BJ. Oxygen saturation targets for extremely preterm infants after the NeOProM trials. Neonatology 2016;109:352–8.

26. Cummings JJ, Polin RA, Committee On F, et al. Oxygen targeting in extremely low birth weight infants. Pediatrics 2016;138 [pii:e20161576].

27. Deschmann E, Norman M. Oxygen-saturation targets in extremely preterm infants. Acta Paediatr 2017;106:1014.

28. Manja V, Saugstad OD, Lakshminrusimha S. Oxygen saturation targets in preterm infants and outcomes at 18-24 months: a systematic review. Pediatrics 2017;139 [pii:e20161609].

29. Sweet DG, Carnielli V, Greisen G, et al. European consensus guidelines on the management of respiratory distress syndrome—2016 update. Neonatology 2017;111:107–25.

30. Bizzarro MJ. Optimizing oxygen saturation targets in extremely preterm infants. JAMA 2018;319:2173–4.

31. Stenson B, Saugstad OD. Oxygen treatment for immature infants beyond the delivery room: lessons from randomized studies. J Pediatr 2018;200:12–8.

32. Kayton A, Timoney P, Vargo L, et al. A review of oxygen Physiology and Appropriate management of oxygen levels in premature neonates. Adv Neonatal Care 2018;18:98–104.

33. Einhorn, J. Oxygen Saturation Limits for Premature Babies: The Final Word for Now. NEJM Journal Watch. 25 June 2018. Available at: https://www.jwatch.org/na46890/2018/06/25/oxygen-saturation-limits-premature-babies-final-word-now. Accessed May 27, 2019.

34. Huizing MJ, Villamor-Martinez E, Vento M, et al. Pulse oximeter saturation target limits for preterm infants: a survey among European neonatal intensive care units. Eur J Pediatr 2017;176:51–6.

35. Darlow BA, Vento M, Beltempo M, et al. Variations in oxygen saturation targeting, and retinopathy of prematurity screening and treatment criteria in neonatal intensive care units: an international survey. Neonatology 2018;114:323–31.

36. Stenson BJ, Donoghoe M, Brocklehurst P, et al. Pulse oximeter saturation targeting and oximeter changes in the benefits of oxygen saturation targeting (BOOST)-II Australia and BOOST-II UK oxygen trials. J Pediatr 2019;204:301–4.e2.

37. Stenson BJ, Tarnow-Mordi WO, Darlow BA, et al, for the Boost II United Kingdom, Australian and New Zealand Collaborative Groups. Oxygen saturation and outcomes in preterm infants. N Engl J Med 2013;368:2094–104.

38. Stenson B, Brocklehurst P, Tarnow-Mordi W. Increased 36-week survival with high oxygen saturation target in extremely preterm infants. N Engl J Med 2011;364:1680–2.

39. Ryan R, Hill S. How to GRADE the quality of the evidence. Cochrane Consumers and Communication Group; 2016. Available at: http://cccrg.cochrane.org/author-resources. Accessed June 14, 2019.

40. Tarnow Mordi W, Stenson B, for BOOST II Australia and BOOST II UK Collaborative Groups. Outcomes of two trials of oxygen saturation targets in preterm infants. N Engl J Med 2016;374:749–60.

41. Rosychuk RJ, Hudson-Mason A, Eklund D, et al. Discrepancies between arterial oxygen saturation and functional oxygen saturation measured with pulse oximetry in very preterm infants. Neonatology 2012;101:14–9.

42. Quine D, Stenson BJ. Arterial oxygen tension (Pao_2) values in infants <29 weeks of gestation at currently targeted saturations. Arch Dis Child Fetal Neonatal Ed 2009;94:F51–3.

43. Whyte RK, Nelson H, Roberts RS, et al. Benefits of oxygen saturation targeting trials: oximeter calibration software revision and infant saturations. J Pediatr 2017;182:382–4.

44. Vines G. Quotation attributed to David Sackett. In: Is there a database in the house? New Scientist 1995. Available at: https://www.newscientist.com/article/mg14519612-300-is-there-a-database-in-the-house/. Accessed May 27, 2019.

45. Byar DP, Simon RM, Friedewald WT, et al. Randomized clinical trials. Perspectives on some recent ideas. N Engl J Med 1976;295:74–80.

46. Tarnow-Mordi W, Cruz M, Morris JM, et al. RCT evidence should drive clinical practice: a day without randomisation is a day without progress. BJOG 2017; 124:613.

47. Fogarty M, Osborn DA, Askie L, et al. Delayed vs early umbilical cord clamping for preterm infants: a systematic review and meta-analysis. Am J Obstet Gynecol 2018;218:1–18.

48. NHMRC Clinical Trials Centre, University of Sydney. Saving millions more lives through megatrials; Introducing the ALPHA Collaboration. Available at: https://www.youtube.com/watch?v=oy3J6iZzOfE. Accessed July 5, 2018.

49. Blencowe H, Cousens S, Oestergaard MZ, et al. National, regional, and worldwide estimates of preterm birth rates in the year 2010 with time trends since 1990 for selected countries: a systematic analysis and implications. Lancet 2012;379:2162–72.

50. Peto R, Baigent C. Trials: the next 50 years. Large scale randomised evidence of moderate benefits. BMJ 1998;317:1170–1.

51. Tarnow-Mordi W, Cruz M, Morris J. Design and conduct of a large obstetric or neonatal randomized controlled trial. Semin Fetal Neonatal Med 2015;20: 389–402.

52. Sealed envelope. Trial sample size calculator. Available at: https://www.sealedenvelope.com/power/. Accessed January 24, 2018.

Moving?

Make sure your subscription moves with you!

To notify us of your new address, find your **Clinics Account Number** (located on your mailing label above your name), and contact customer service at:

Email: **journalscustomerservice-usa@elsevier.com**

800-654-2452 (subscribers in the U.S. & Canada)
314-447-8871 (subscribers outside of the U.S. & Canada)

Fax number: **314-447-8029**

Elsevier Health Sciences Division
Subscription Customer Service
3251 Riverport Lane
Maryland Heights, MO 63043

*To ensure uninterrupted delivery of your subscription, please notify us at least 4 weeks in advance of move.

Printed and bound by CPI Group (UK) Ltd, Croydon, CR0 4YY

18/10/2024

01776288-0001